Unlearning

Unlearning

Rethinking Poetics, Pandemics, and the Politics of Knowledge

Charles L. Briggs

Utah State University Press
Logan

© 2021 by University Press of Colorado

Published by Utah State University Press
An imprint of University Press of Colorado
245 Century Circle, Suite 202
Louisville, Colorado 80027

All rights reserved

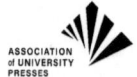 The University Press of Colorado is a proud member of the Association of University Presses..

The University Press of Colorado is a cooperative publishing enterprise supported, in part, by Adams State University, Colorado State University, Fort Lewis College, Metropolitan State University of Denver, Regis University, University of Colorado, University of Northern Colorado, University of Wyoming, Utah State University, and Western Colorado University.

ISBN: 978-1-64642-101-5 (paperback)
ISBN: 978-1-64642-102-2 (ebook)
https://doi.org/10.7330/9781646421022

Library of Congress Cataloging-in-Publication Data

Names: Briggs, Charles L., 1953– author.
Title: Unlearning : rethinking poetics, pandemics, and the politics of knowledge / Charles L. Briggs.
Description: Logan : Utah State University Press, [2021] | Includes bibliographical references and index.
Identifiers: LCCN 2021001139 (print) | LCCN 2021001140 (ebook) | ISBN 9781646421015 (paperback) | ISBN 9781646421022 (ebook)
Subjects: LCSH: Folklorists. | Folklore—Study and teaching. | Mass media and folklore. | Applied folklore—Study and teaching. | Communication in folklore.
Classification: LCC GR49 .B75 2021 (print) | LCC GR49 (ebook) | DDC 398.092—dc23
LC record available at https://lccn.loc.gov/2021001139
LC ebook record available at https://lccn.loc.gov/2021001140

The University Press of Colorado gratefully acknowledges the support of the University of California, Berkeley, toward the publication of this book.

All photographs are by the author, unless otherwise noted.

Cover photograph by Clara Mantini-Briggs

for Feliciana, always

Contents

List of Figures   ix
Introduction   3

PART I: UNLEARNING RACIALIZED DISCIPLINARY GENEALOGIES

1. Disciplining Folkloristics   53
2. Contested Mobilities: On the Politics and Ethnopoetics of Circulation   66
3. What We Should Have Learned from Américo Paredes: The Politics of Communicability and the Making of Folkloristics   78
4. The Coloniality of Folkloristics: Toward a Multi-Genealogical Practice
   with Sadhana Naithani   100

PART II: RETHINKING PSYCHOANALYSIS, POETICS, AND PERFORMANCE

5. Reconnecting Psychoanalysis with Poetics and Performance   135
6. Dear Dr. Freud   161

PART III: A NEW POETICS OF HEALTH, MULTISPECIES RELATIONS, AND ENVIRONMENTS

7. Toward a New Folkloristics of Health   193
8. Moving beyond "the Media": From Traditionalization to Mediatization   213
9. Germ Wordfare: The Poetic Production of Medical Panics   235

10. From Progressive Extractivism to Phyto-Socialism: Trees, Bodies, and Discrepant Phytocommunicabilities in a Mysterious Epidemic   264

Epilogue   287
Acknowledgments   293
References   297
Index   323

Figures

0.1.	Dump rake	7
0.2.	John Donald and Harriet Robb	15
0.3.	Córdova, New Mexico	16
0.4.	Map of Córdova and its surroundings	16
0.5.	George López—wood-carver of Córdova	17
0.6.	*Our Lady of Light* by José Dolores López	18
0.7.	Silvianita López shows a carving to customers	19
0.8.	George López's first image of St. Isidore, 1949	23
0.9.	Map of Delta Amacuro State, Venezuela	30
0.10.	Hana Hubasuhuru	31
0.11.	The author and son Gabriel operating their motorized dugout canoe	32
0.12.	Teodoro Moraleda playing a bone flute	33
0.13.	Librado Moraleda	34
0.14.	Conrado Moraleda	34
0.15.	A *wisidatu* healer performing in the *nahanamu* festival	35
0.16.	Clara Mantini-Briggs with healer Paulino Zapata	38
0.17.	Tirso Gómez	41
0.18.	Norbelys Gómez	41
6.1.	Muaina	165
6.2.	Florencia Macotera and Indalesio Pizarro	166
6.3.	Mamerto Pizarro at the Indigenous University of Venezuela	167
6.4.	Singing laments for Elbia Torres Rivas, Barranquita	168
6.5.	The contractors' sawmill at Muaina	170
6.6.	Enrique Moraleda	176
6.7.	Florencia Macotera telling the story of Dalvi's death	177
6.8.	The Uyapar Hospital in Puerto Ordaz	179
6.9.	Elbia Torres Rivas with her mother, Anita Rivas	183
6.10.	*El Nacional* photograph of team with pictures of Elbia Torres Rivas and her family	185
9.1.	CBS anchor Katie Couric, April 24, 2009	242
9.2.	ICE Agents scrutinize crossers at US-Mexico border	243
9.3.	Acting director Richard Besser at CDC news conference	244
9.4.	Dr. William Schaffner performs a sound bite	245
9.5.	Dr. Jon LaPook with anchor Katie Couric	246
9.6.	Mexican crowd and face masks	248

9.7.	Pigs appearing in the CBS broadcast	249
9.8.	Shot of high-security laboratory in opening scenes of *Outbreak*	252
9.9.	Jon Stewart's *The Daily Show*, April 27, 2009	256
10.1.	A Delta house	270
10.2.	Houses built by the contractor in Muaina, unfinished but already decaying	271
10.3.	A dugout canoe under construction	274
10.4.	Mukoboina	280
10.5.	Odilia Torres and Yunelis	280
10.6.	The grandmother's house	281

Unlearning

Introduction

This book brings together efforts to open up new ways of thinking, reading, writing, and practice. Focusing on core assumptions and theoretical approaches in folkloristics, linguistic anthropology, medical anthropology, and psychoanalysis, I try to build a deeper and broader dialogue by linking classic perspectives on poetics and performance with challenges presented by colonialism and the politics of knowledge in exploring new points of departure for researching cultural forms, health, media, mourning, and the more-than-human.

This work extends the relationship between two of the things I hold dearest as a scholar: theory and ethnographic engagement with the worlds around and within us. This dual orientation is characteristic of much work in anthropology, folkloristics, and other fields. A difference lies in my sources of theoretical inspiration. Some are academic. Starting long before I first conducted ethnographic research at nineteen years of age and continuing through the present, however, many of the people who have affected my thinking the most are not scholars, never published, and, in some cases, never had access to formal schooling. Mentors in New Mexico and the Delta Amacuro rainforest of eastern Venezuela were some of the most profound, abstract, subtle, and creative thinkers I have known. In conversations that ranged from two hours to two decades, they criticized my core assumptions about knowledge and the world and opened doors to ways of thinking, feeling, writing, and being that, without them, I would never have imagined. Here again, I don't think that I am alone: I would assert that folkloristics, anthropology, ethnomusicology, and other fields gain their analytic power, in part, by appropriating theoretical insights developed by people outside the academy. The problem is that scholars often then take the credit for their insights and eliminate the challenges to scholarly authority that often come with their ideas. My practice has long been to acknowledge synergies between insights coming from academic domains and farmers, healers, forest dwellers, and wood-carvers.

Introductions are charged with announcing the principal concerns advanced by the author and placing them in broader contexts; that is exactly what I do here. In academic books—and this is surely one—this work of contextualization emerges through business-as-usual scholarly rhetorics, distanced orchestrations of authors and frameworks. Introductions are metatexts or, in Jacques Derrida's ([1967] 1976) terms, subtexts that tell origin stories about how a particular book came into being, thereby seducing readers into interpreting it in particular ways. Telling an origin story whose characters are all prominent academics would imbue this book with a fatal contradiction from the start. If the succeeding chapters are to challenge practices enabling researchers to appropriate analytics produced outside scholarly domains and claim them as their own, an introduction that presents a dialogue only with other academics would be metacommunicative, in Gregory Bateson's (1972) sense: it would signal that I really don't mean it, that only academic interlocutors really count. The task that I have set for myself in this book centers, as the title suggests, on *unlearning*; starting with a purely academic genealogy would limit the scope and traction of the unlearning process in advance.

I have no magic wand that would transform the parameters of the introduction genre. Nor do I wish to do so. I want to tell you an origin story, a tale that purports to recount not just how this book came into being but my own circuitous route to becoming a strange mix of scholar and practitioner. It is not a story of *self*-fashioning, but rather one of the people, nonhumans, ideas, and experiences that shaped me. Some of the characters I introduce are scholars who are probably known to you, personally or at least through their writings. Others you may know through cultural productions, such as wood carvings that grace major museums. Others are people you've never met, because their extraordinary contributions to global knowledge have been stopped in their tracks by boundaries of language, education, mobility, race, and class. Nonhumans include aspen and palm trees, vampire bats, bacteria, viruses, and nonhuman entities that fall so far outside of dominant ontologies that they get lumped into the category of "spirits."

My story doesn't start when I got a PhD or even when I entered college but rather in my childhood. I place some of my most important mentors in dialogue, taking the sorts of horizontally organized, creative exchanges of knowledge that I think lie at the heart of transformative scholarly endeavors out of the realm of the unsaid. Here I need to make a confession. I wanted to finish this project three years earlier. Everything was in place, except this introduction. Frankly, I've shielded my self with academic styles of writing for so long that the task of "writing an introduction" put me on autopilot, into construct-an-academic-genealogy mode. And then came the resistance—I could not force myself to start writing it. Well, if you think a lot about psychoanalysis, sometimes you just cannot help looking inside, even though you know that self-analysis is tricky. Fortunately, I remembered my experience in writing the essay that appears as chapter 6. There a failed attempt to place Sigmund Freud's classic essay "Mourning and Melancholia" in dialogue with the laments and narratives of Delta Amacuro women who lost children in a rabies epidemic prompted me to experiment. I thus developed a new rule of thumb; when something inside you says no, when there is fundamental resistance to a writing project: Stop! Think! Resist the sense that it is your own personal failing. Ask yourself if the generic structures of academic writing are getting in the way. If so, experiment! Create a new way of writing and see how it feels, if words not only begin to flow but break apart the conceptual, rhetorical, and emotional constraints getting in the way. And, once you have finished, think about whether your breakthrough might be of value to your readers. (I do just this at the end of this introduction.)

So, I want to try something different, even if I'm feeling a bit vulnerable as I begin. Many of the points of origin I recount here are not authorized by academic genealogies. Rather than projecting singular, bounded points of origin and linear progressions of ideas and perspectives, each gets multiplied as I recount synergies and long-term effects of what these individuals taught me. The times I have confronted the most profound philosophical challenges have often come when friends demanded that I join them in helping people keep their family members and neighbors from dying in epidemics or enlisted my help in confronting governments and corporations that steal the land and destroy the environments in which they live. These engagements forced me to identify the commonsense frameworks and practices that produced and normalized these profound inequalities and ally with others in imagining alternative futures. This introduction consists, in short, of a memoir, admittedly one that is as idiosyncratic as the life and mind upon which it reflects. Participating in current efforts to stop perplexing pandemics and confront pervasive and entrenched forms of racism and racialized violence, I find that my *un*learning curve grows steeper every day. This introduction retraces some of my steps in unlearning assumptions that I thought self-evident and rethinking the politics of knowledge making. It ends in a set of proposals for using these sorts of quirky, often disconcerting encounters in developing theoretically innovative intellectual practices.

ON FRUIT TREES, BEES, AND ALFALFA: MULTISPECIES ONTOLOGIES AND RELATIONS

Stories, memory, and landscape haunted my childhood. I spent a lot of time with elderly people, and I liked talking with them. My maternal grandparents, John Donald and Harriet Robb, lived on one end of a small street, and my paternal grandparents, Leslie and Edith Briggs, on the other, two blocks apart. During periods when my parents were separated, my father Bill Briggs, my older brother Chris, and I with lived with my paternal grandparents. John Robb was a composer, conductor, and professor of music at the University of New Mexico. He was also an avid collector of folk music, and I'll say more about that shortly. Leslie Briggs worked for years as a county extension agent, teaching ranchers and farmers in southeastern New Mexico how to grow fatter cattle and more abundant crops. His job was to transform complex "traditional" relations between humans, plants, animals, machinery, and environments, displacing "outmoded" multispecies ontologies in favor of modern, scientific, profitable ones. A century later, the sustainable agriculture movement is trying to counter the perspectives and practices he promoted. Born a city slicker, one of the ways he built street cred with rural residents was by using proverbs often and skillfully. I remember times that his proverbs stopped my childhood pretensions in their tracks. He and my father were both remarkable storytellers and my father was a good ballad singer—memories and histories constantly inflected their words in unexpected ways.

Most of the time I lived with my parents in the Los Candelarias section of the North Valley of Albuquerque, a mile east of the Rio Grande. Much of the land around our home was still agricultural, and many houses were built of sun-dried adobe mud bricks and occupied by the Chicano families who had built them. I attended the local high school, Valley High; the students were predominantly Chicano/a and Native American. Many of my friends' grandparents were Spanish speakers, and their parents were symmetrical bilinguals, as comfortable in English as in Spanish. They had been told, however, that their children would "speak with an accent" if they taught them Spanish, so most of my peers spoke only Chicano English, which certainly did not vaccinate them against racism.

The neighborhood was in the middle of a slow process of urbanization, resulting in spaces—from a half acre to over a square mile—that reinserted fragments of the North Valley's agricultural past into the increasingly middle-class, white, gentrified present. In the 1950s and 1960s, middle-class families leaving already urbanized parts of the city bought a few acres from working-class Chicano/a families. The new owners nostalgically viewed the semi-rural landscape they were displacing in romantic terms, somehow overlooking their own role in disrupting its historical cartography. My family formed part of this racialized political economy, and my experiences with neighbors and classmates often made me aware of my own positionality.

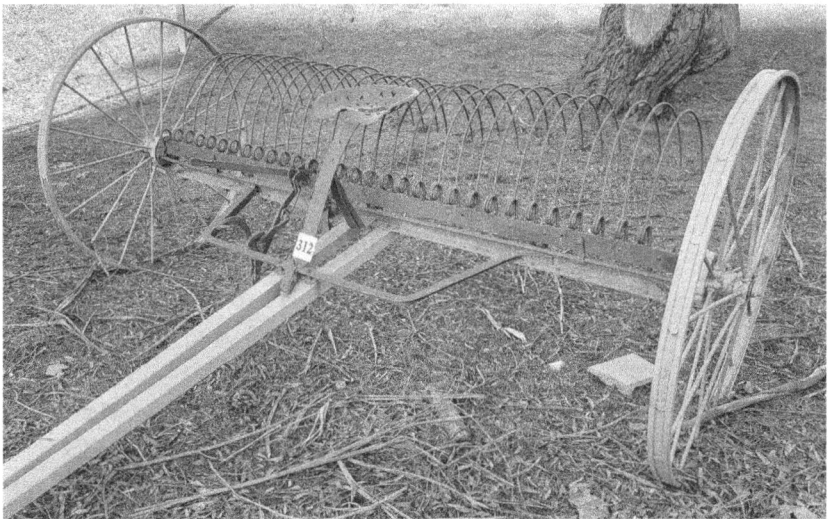

Figure 0.1. Dump rake (photograph by Sharon Turner; courtesy of the Monterey County Agricultural and Rural Life Museum)

That's how I met Señor Olguín, my first mentor in the neighborhood. I saw him when he came down the dirt road beside our house atop an alfalfa dump rake, a rusted contraption with metal wheels and large arching loops bouncing behind a horse that seemed just as ancient as its owner (see figure 0.1). In my child eye's view, he was very old, probably in his seventies, tall and thin, with an erect posture, dark black hair, an angular nose, and eyes that seemed to suggest both warmth and an otherworldly vision. He was, as all the other times I saw him, wearing jean overalls. Struggling to maintain an economic foothold in this increasingly alien landscape, he contracted with several neighbors to keep the fields around their adobe houses—now refitted to suit middle-class white tastes—green and pastoral by planting alfalfa. My family situation left me with too much unsupervised time, and I impulsively ran after him as he approached an adjacent field. I caught up when he got down to open the gate, and my wide-open eyes danced between horse and rake. *Buenos días*, he greeted me. Señor Olguín knew very little English. Elementary-school classes in a juridically bilingual state had provided me with a foundation in Spanish (although certainly not much agricultural terminology), and we began a conversation that lasted half a decade.

When Señor Olguín invited me to join him in the field, I probably figured that I could perch alongside him, maybe even take the reins. But the device had only one seat, and hindsight suggests that the last thing he wanted was to have a young gringo fall off and get mangled by the rake. So I could only lean up again the wooden fence and watch as he dropped the long curves of the rake until they scooped up the alfalfa he had cut a few days earlier and allowed to dry. I was enthralled by the ballet unfolding before me: the horse's head, Señor Olguín's body, and the gap between the rake's metal fingers and the soil seemed to move up and down in perfect synchrony, magically drawing the pungent, fresh-cut alfalfa along. Once the rake was full, he would pull a lever that used the turning of the metal wheels to raise the hay and then dump it in a line. As I watched him follow the curved contours of the adjacent fence and irrigation ditch, I could see that the perfect coordination between Señor Olguín's hand and eye, his horse, and the dump rake was leaving straight lines at equal intervals. My amazement grew as I saw that on his return from the end of the field he traced a perfect parallel line and dumped each load of alfalfa hay with precision; soon straight, parallel lines cross-sected the field. Fortunately, the field—just under two acres in total—was small enough that I could watch the entire operation. If he thought that his young visitor would soon grow bored and return home to watch television, Señor Olguín had underestimated my patience, curiosity, and idiosyncrasy. I was there when he finished, my head bursting with questions. Where did he live? Did his horse eat all that alfalfa? How had he cut it? What would happen next? He stopped before opening the gate, probably as much through curiosity about my persistence as resting. I didn't immediately pester him with my questions—living with my grandparents had taught me that you can learn more when knowledge emerges from the rhythms of work, interaction, memory, and a mentor's sense of what is most worthwhile to impart, how and when to tell it.

All of my questions were answered in the ensuing years. I saw him return with his sons to bale the alfalfa and load it onto a pickup. I missed Señor Olguín and his horse when winter came. Early the next spring, when he returned, he stopped next to our house. When I wasn't in school, I ran down the driveway—as fast as my uncoordinated, chubby body could carry me—to walk beside him to the field. I tried to help him shake off the winter's legacy of immobility and turn the rusty metal circular handle to liberate the first stream of water from the *acequia*, one of the ditches bringing water from the Rio Grande. His gaunt face lit up as the brown liquid flowed—first hesitantly and then with steady force—into what seemed a moribund field.

Señor Olguín loved to tell stories, punctuating the work his increasingly frail body performed by leaning against a fence or rake to reveal hidden worlds. He served for decades as the *mayordomo*, or ditch boss, a position that became a friction point for multiracial and cross-class tensions in a changing landscape as he divvied up the hours available for irrigation. His stories of the shifting histories of conflicts between subsistence agriculturalists, small-scale market-oriented producers, middle-class gringos and, increasingly, the land-grabbing demands of developers and urban planners fused with smells (as much of fresh horse manure as of fresh-cut alfalfa), sights, sounds, and textures emerging from his interactions with horse, land, plants, and water. The way I saw the landscape became increasingly layered as the fields were reanimated by the people, animals, buildings, technologies, and activities he brought to life through words.

Not all of my mentors opened floodgates of words like the first spring gush of irrigation water. One of the people from whom I learned the most lived right across the tall ditch bank that separated our house from the paved street on the other side. For years I walked most afternoons along our driveway, did a U-turn around the ditch, and proceeded to the second house on what had become a small, peri-urban, dead-end street to play with the children of a medical student. They were a Mormon family; their kids were two boys who were roughly my age and, magically to me, lacking sisters of my own, two girls. I can only guess that they moved to a more affluent neighborhood after the father graduated or finished his residency, but all I remember is learning that they would be moving. I missed them. One day, bored, I took the same route but continued fifty feet past my friends' old house. My eyes were arrested by a man surrounded by trees and—strikingly—bees. A human body, wearing ordinary clothing, was ensconced amid some ten white wooden boxes and thousands of bees. It was his warm smile that stung me.

I was a couple of decades away from being bitten—again with apologies—by Antonio Gramsci's (1971) notion of resistance, but here lay the property of a couple that refused to sell to the developers who had plopped small, nondescript cinderblock houses on either side of the small orchard. My only point of reference for making sense of this scene was A. A. Milne's *Winnie-the-Pooh*, which my father had read to me often and then used in spinning the myriad imaginative worlds that we inhabited as we walked each evening with our Labrador in the surrounding fields. Señor Olguín's map of the neighborhood contrasted the wild space on my eastern side of the ditch with paved streets on the west side populated with houses, an area that extended nearly to the Rio Grande. Thus, seeing a man surrounded by trees and bees in what I classified as urban space transfixed me. Maybe it was his warm smile or perhaps the loneliness induced by losing my friends, but I stepped off the sidewalk and walked—ever so slowly—toward him, stopping as my approach began to attract the bees' attention. I stood there, watching, my face alternating between reflecting his smile and a look of terror.

Without saying a word, the mysterious man disappeared into the small house nestled into the trees to his left. I lingered, refusing to let his departure squash my curiosity or exacerbate my solitude. And then he returned. As bees buzzed around him, he gently—and wordlessly—placed a full-body covering and white screened hood on me and handed me a pair of gloves. My body was transformed. And then he walked back toward the hives. Suddenly, two human bodies were sharing space with bees, honey, hives, and fruit trees. Like Señor Olguín's, the words he spoke were all in Spanish; they emerged, however, not in long, well-crafted stories but slowly, parsimoniously, tied to bees, hives, and trees. Stepping closer to the hives, he slowly lifted the frames, which were filled with wax and honey, using his eyes and shoulders to suggest to me how I should help extract them. In the coming months, my eyes and body came to accept the rhythms of approaching bees, their sometimes frenetic energies, and their relationship to the honey we extracted, but I never took off the garb, even as I began to fathom why my mentor needed no protection.

Señor Olguín never took me to his house, nor did I meet his wife, but the beekeeper led me through the small grove to his tiny house. His wife, who had probably been watching from the start, showed me rows of jars of honey and honeycomb they would sell. Her homemade bread with honeycomb was one of the most delicious childhood treats I remember. She was less taciturn, telling me stories of children who had left for Colorado and Wyoming, who followed harvests and never returned to a neighborhood whose future did not seem to include them. I was probably about the age of her grandchildren, but I never met them. And she told me about constant pressure from developers to sell their tiny enclave of resistance to urbanization, first with sweet talk and cash offers and then with threats. The beekeeper chimed in, angrily: "No, we'll never sell! Now they're just waiting for us to die!"

I'm embarrassed to say that I never learned their names, or at least I don't remember them if I did. Now I have big words to convey what I learned in that orchard—*materiality*, *embodiment*, and *multispecies relations*. As when I watched the ballet Señor Olguín danced with horse, water, and alfalfa plants, I learned how human lives come to be defined and transformed through intimate relations with other species. I continued to learn this lesson in a Venezuelan rainforest decades later, as I explore in the final chapter of this book.

Not all of my mentors spoke Spanish. I met Old Man Hawkins when I was about ten through my friends, indirectly. We roamed on top of the larger acequias, moving between each other's houses, the small general store on Rio Grande Boulevard, and sites where adventures might lurk. The streets belonged to cars, parents, and the city, but boys ruled the ditch banks. We sometimes accompanied a friend home in the late afternoon to watch his mother milk the goats; she would give us a glass of the warm, thick, frothy liquid. Most trips took us past Old Man Hawkins's small house and orchard, which lay only a few hundred yards south of my home. A new story about him seemed to emerge each time, each one more terrifying than the last. Old Man Hawkins was mean and he was dangerous. He hated children, and he would shoot them if they tried to steal his fruit. He had killed his wife and buried her under the big apple tree; there were probably neighbor children there too. He usually sat in a chair next to his front door, and sure enough, he was cradling a rifle. When we saw him, we would either detour out of range or run breathlessly along the soft, brown, sandy soil on top of the acequia until we had passed his house.

Frankly, I didn't like those stories. Old Man Hawkins looked lonely, and he lived a meager life. My curiosity was getting the better of me. Walking the ditch alone late one summer afternoon, I saw him in his chair, and—impulsively and a bit scared—slid down the deep sand onto his property. As I walked slowly up to him, he didn't raise his gun but rather disappeared with it into his house. I began to think, maybe he does hate children. Maybe I will never find out what he's like. Maybe he would . . . Then he emerged with another simple wooden chair and two delicious peaches, one for each of us. If I had been a fieldworker with a tape recorder, I could have published a rich collection based on the stories he told me during the next several hours. Living practically next door, he gave me new perspectives on the history of my neighborhood, on who had owned the large expanse of agricultural land and how it had been farmed.

Old Man Hawkins also introduced me to his family: the pear, apple, and apricot trees he had planted decades earlier. The study of multispecies relations, including the ways that people fashion themselves and their worlds through intimate, nurturing, and sometimes destructive relations with plants, now forms an important focus in the social sciences and humanities. Looking back, I understand he was teaching me that lesson fifty years ago. Old Man Hawkins did not trace his life through human kinship (he had never married), nor through his work history (he had always been a small-scale farmer), but through decades of intimacy with the trees we were seeing, smelling, touching, and tasting. I learned that plants have social lives, individual biographies, and—at least in his view—personalities. Even trees obtained from the same source and planted simultaneously grew at different rates, not all equally willing to afford the fruit that provided his source of income. I came to see that he was as enmeshed in their lives as they were in his actions, sense of self, time, and place, and economic well-being.

Multispecies relations also explained the presence of the gun, a .22 caliber short. It reappeared suddenly when he was visited by the species that evoked the anger the boys had mistakenly attributed to his relations with other human beings: crows. The erratic descent of dozens of crows was highlighted by the valley's level landscape and the 5,000-foot rise of the Sandia Mountains. A crow invasion could wipe out his source of livelihood. Old Man Hawkins was a good shot: each time a crow perched in one of his trees, it lay, seconds later, in a pile of black feathers and bright red blood. The other side of an act of arboreal care was violence directed at "those damn crows." I finally got it: Old Man Hawkins was socially isolated but not alone, living in a world of intimate relations, of complex and opposing affects, crafted anew each day as he cared for trees, shot crows, and watched changes in the world around him.

Old Man Hawkins talked about growing struggles with age and poverty, feeling isolated from other people. He scrutinized me while saying, "I know the kids tell wild stories about me. They even say I killed my wife—even though I never married." I looked at the ground. In graduate school, I would embrace Richard Bauman's (1977) performance-centered approach, which emphasizes the role of audience members as coauthors of narratives, shaping how they unfold through their bodily, verbal, and nonverbal engagement. I recalled all the times that I had repressed my urge to challenge Old Man Hawkins stories. My silence signaled complicity, helping stories circulate. Subsequently, I became a raconteur of a new repertoire of Old Man Hawkins stories; they mirrored stylistic features of the Scary Old Man Hawkins legends they were designed to crowd out, told with a similarly animated voice, face, and body, just as aesthetically marked and communicatively heightened, just as much designed for display for an audience (Bauman 1977). To use a term I later colluded with Dick Bauman in crafting, my stories were equally designed to be extracted and recontextualized, inserted into conversations with other kids, parents, and neighbors.

Maybe it was less the power of my narratives than the sensory appeal of tree-ripened peaches that convinced several friends to visit Old Man Hawkins. He only had two chairs, so pairs and trios of boys periodically populated the steps in front of his front door. Some neighborhood kids never descended the ditch bank. Maybe they preferred the Scary Old Man Hawkins legends, or maybe their parents were as distrustful of an elderly man living alone in what seemed like a bygone world as fearful of the .22 that retained its prominent role in new Old Man Hawkins stories.

Here we have painful evidence of the power of narratives. Just as years of Scary Old Man Hawkins stories led him to be shunned, new stories—and peaches, apples, and pears—turned Old Man Hawkins into a sort of communal grandfather. Even when kids didn't interrupt the important missions that prompted their passage in front of his house, detours and frightened sprints gave way to waves and friendly greetings: "Hey, Old Man Hawkins, got any peaches?" The fruits of mentorship, as I have come to learn, are not unidirectional: our relationship transformed his world even as his stories opened up mine.

In high school, I grew close to the family of Peter Griego Jr., the best friend I have ever had. I spent time in Peter's room, generally in the company of our group of eight adolescent boys, representing the ethnic mix of our neighborhood: four Chicanos, two Native Americans (Laguna), and two gringos. I also sat around the kitchen table with his parents and grandparents. My appreciation for space, species, environments, and history grew as Peter and I helped his grandfather cultivate the family garden. One of my favorite events was the annual pinto bean harvest on the driveway of the Griegos' home: shelling them, removing sticks and stones, filling the burlap bags as tightly with stories as with beans. From Señor Olguín, Old Man Hawkins, Peter's grandfather, and a Lebanese family that lived next to my paternal grandparents, I learned a fair amount about gardening. Starting around thirteen years of age, I cultivated fruit trees, a strawberry patch, several species of melons, vegetables, and other crops in the valley's rich brown soil and plentiful sunshine.

During my senior year, the world suddenly snatched away the ideas about life and death that the Griegos and I had held. Peter, school president and star student, had graduated the previous spring and started University of New Mexico summer classes. He was killed when his motorcycle was struck from behind. Another Valley High student, driving his dad's pickup, had his head turned to the left, surveying the current occupants of the local hangout, a drive-in hamburger joint. The Griegos lost their only child. Mr. Griego's grief largely unfolded in the form of a burning rage directed against the adolescent, played out in angry monologues and glaring looks delivered silently in courtroom hearings. Mrs. Griego's grief became pain articulated through the poetics of mourning. She performed grieving practices that, I would see decades later, embodied Sigmund Freud's ([1917] 1957) insightful account of the twofold, contradictory aspects of mourning. She sought to hold onto her son, to bring him back to life, a process that Freud refers to as hyper-cathexis. Recruiting me in this process, she asked me to take the role of her son temporarily. For a week, I accompanied the family almost constantly. (I spent time in Peter's room, but didn't sleep there, which she would have liked. That, I felt, would have crossed an unsettling threshold.) Mrs. Griego's parents-in-law were feeble; caring for them forced her to find new ways of getting on with life, part of the work of mourning that Freud called reality-testing. I accompanied the Griegos in a week of masses and rosary services at the nearby Our Lady of Guadalupe Church, my first lesson in how bodies and voices, some no longer physically present, come together through recurrent patterns of words, sounds, gestures, objects, and bodily movements. An appreciation for the poetics of mourning that Peter's mother instilled in me would resonate decades later with what I learned from women in a Venezuelan rainforest.

LEARNING TO LEARN IN CÓRDOVA, NEW MEXICO

Now it's time to bring my maternal grandparents back into the story (see figure 0.2). A giant standing six foot four and weighing well over 200 pounds, John Donald Robb periodically towered over an assembly of grandchildren, declaring: "I'm going to collect folk music. Who wants to come along?" Cousins looked anxiously at one another or their parents, asking silently, "Do I have to go?" My hand shot up, accompanied by an excited "I'll go!" My mother, Nancy Gay, loved these trips, so we would pile into the back seat of my grandparents' Rambler station wagon. I particularly remember the first time my grandfather took me to Córdova, a community of about 400 inhabitants near the famed pilgrimage site of the Santuario de Chimayó (see figure 0.4).[1] Accessible by a short spur off the picturesque "High Road" (State Highway 76) between Santa Fe and Taos, it is bordered on the east by the Sangre de Cristo Mountains. Lying in a small canyon, Córdova was founded between 1725 and 1743; modest harvests of corn, wheat, beans, legumes, and other crops were supplemented by raising goats and sheep (Briggs 1987).

When I first saw Córdova, nearly all of the houses were grouped around the chapel on the hillside. My grandfather visited Córdova many times, principally to see George López (see figure 0.5), known as the leading practitioner of the Córdovan style of wood carving started by his father, José Dolores López (see figure 0.6). Middle-class white artists, writers, art patrons, museum professionals, and tourists came to see George and his wife Silvianita. My grandparents purchased several of their carvings. I made a number of trips with them, but I particularly remember the first, when I was eight or nine. Perhaps it was my own diminutive size, the low height of the doorway in which he was standing, or the stories my grandfather told us during the trip from Albuquerque, but George struck me as a tall and

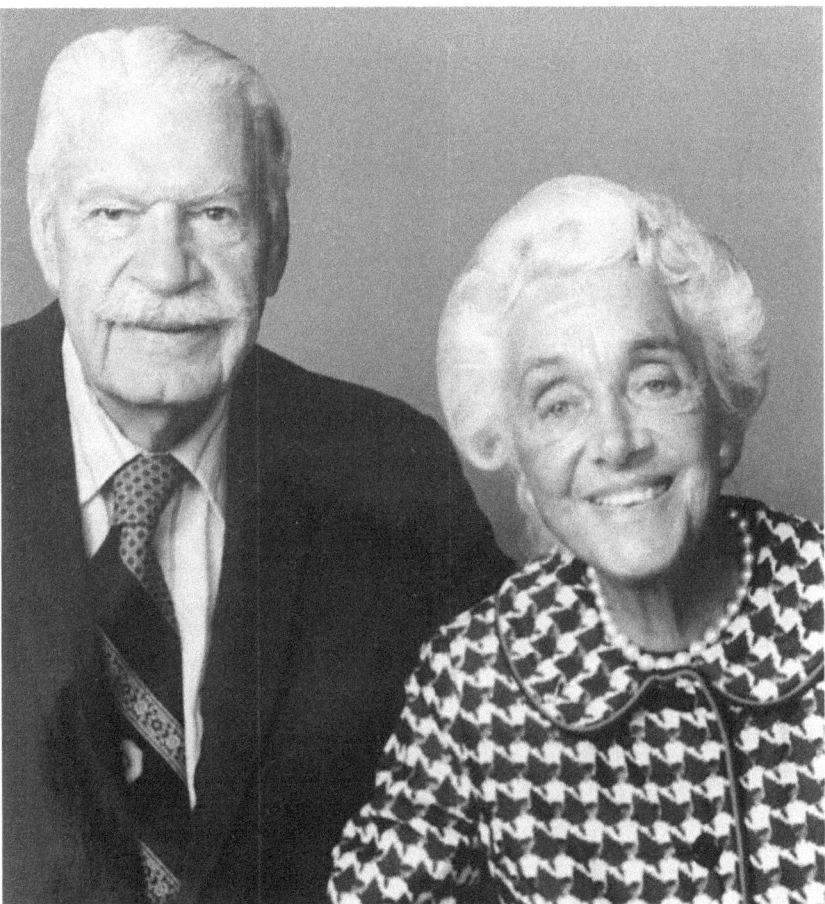

Figure 0.2. John Donald and Harriet Robb (date and photographer unknown)

compelling figure, despite the fact—I realized later—that he was actually fairly short.[2]

My grandfather and George shared an interest in music. Like many Córdovan men, George was a member of a lay religious organization called La Cofradía de Nuestro Padre Jesús Nazareno (The Confraternity of Our Father Jesus the Nazarene), pejoratively called the Penitentes by English speakers, thereby exoticizing their ritual enactments of the Crucifixion during Holy Week. The brothers' Lenten practices included collective singing of *alabados*, hymns whose textual and musical features evoke the passion of Christ and the Virgin Mary's suffering. My first extended encounter with the Lópezes came in 1966 when my grandfather recorded alabados. Their interaction intrigued me. George spoke virtually no English, and my grandfather's

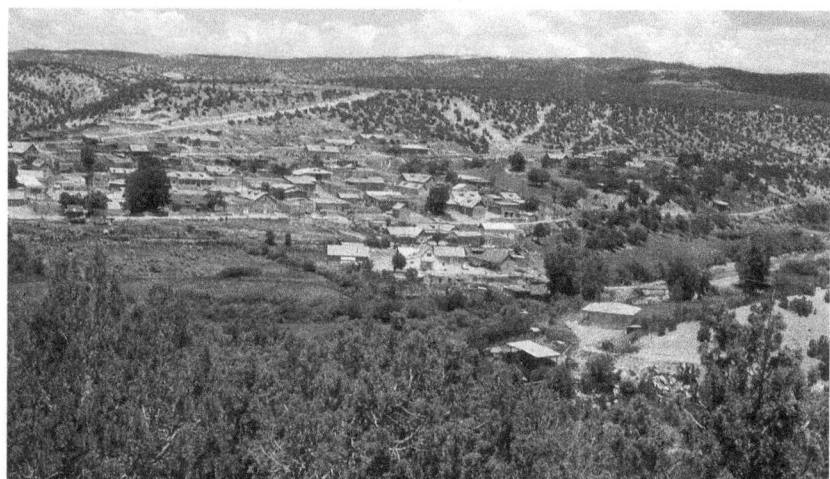

Figure 0.3. Córdova, New Mexico

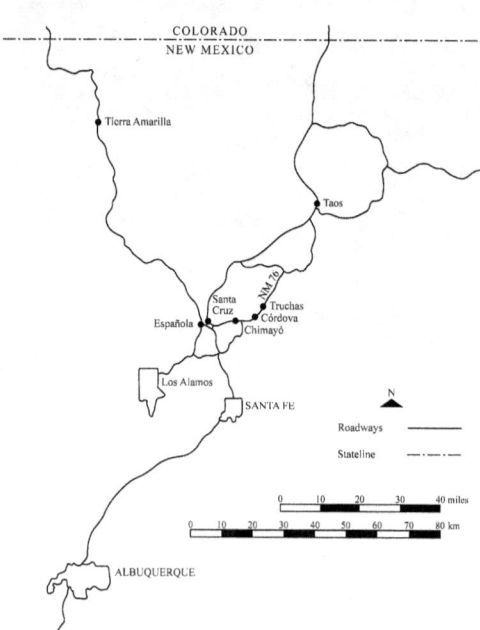

Figure 0.4. Córdova and Its surroundings

Spanish was hardly fluent. They were, nevertheless, intensively engaged. As George began each alabado, the remarkable musical features and the expression on his face and in his eyes seemed to transport him to a distant, sacred, and affectively charged realm. As a musician, my grandfather seemed to register each note in his facial expression, even if the alabados' acoustic parameters did not prompt a similar spiritual journey. My grandfather collected

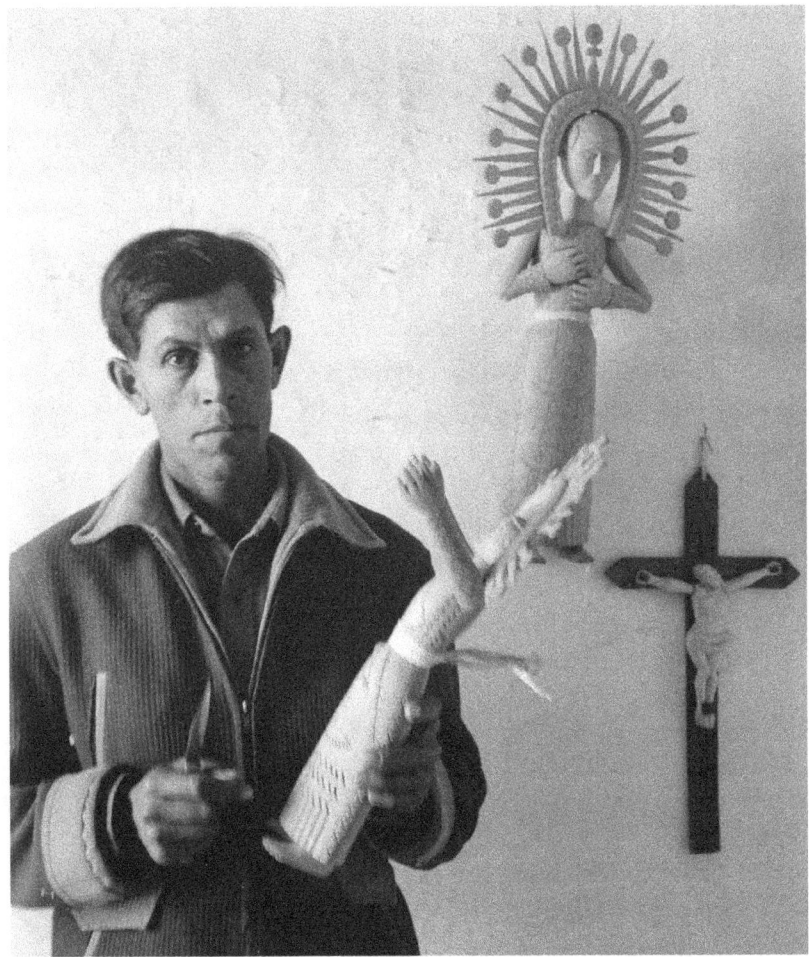

Figure 0.5. George López—Woodcarver of Córdova, 1945. (Laura Gilpin [1891–1979]. Gelatin silver print. Amon Carter Museum of American Art, Fort Worth, Texas, Bequest of the Artist. © 1979 Amon Carter Museum of American Art, P1979.134.335.)

some nine songs that day; several figured prominently in his massive tome *Hispanic Folk Music of New Mexico and the Southwest* (Robb 1980).

My return to Córdova six years later was influenced by a new mentor. During my first year in college, I fell in love. I was eccentric to the core—my affair was with an Austrian-British philosopher who died two years before I was born, Ludwig Wittgenstein. I was fascinated by the microphysics of language, how sounds and words get put together and enter into complex syntactic relations, but it was Wittgenstein's discussion of "language games" that opened my mind wider as I read each of the book's sections. Wittgenstein articulated how languages constantly come into being as they shape and are shaped by daily life. The voices of the beekeeper and Señor Olguín resonated within me: they had not just helped me learn New Mexican Spanish but allowed me to enter social worlds where words invited new relations to material objects, nonhumans, environments, history, and people. Old Man Hawkins taught me a language game that seemed to push beyond those analyzed by Wittgenstein, where fruit trees spoke to human beings and vice versa. Wittgenstein thus reanimated the words of the "vernacular" philosophers with whom I had grown up and led me back to the Lópezes. Planning for a week, I stayed fourteen years.

I slept on a cot next to the folding tables on which *los carvings* were displayed to visitors in the Lópezes' new home on the valley floor. The Lópezes seemed to dance behind the table; visitors lined up on the other side, picking up carvings or stooping to look more closely (see figure 0.7). I occupied neither space. The visitors' scrutinizing eyes suggested that I was matter out of place. The Lópezes were friends and mentors, but I looked more like the clients. Childless in a family-centered world, the Lópezes adopted a niece, Savinita, who married Cristóbal Ortiz. With the Ortizes and their five children, the Lópezes created a small enclave, its size increasing as each child married and built a house. Savinita and Cristóbal carved, and each Ortiz child became proficient at producing first trees and birds and then images of the saints, all in

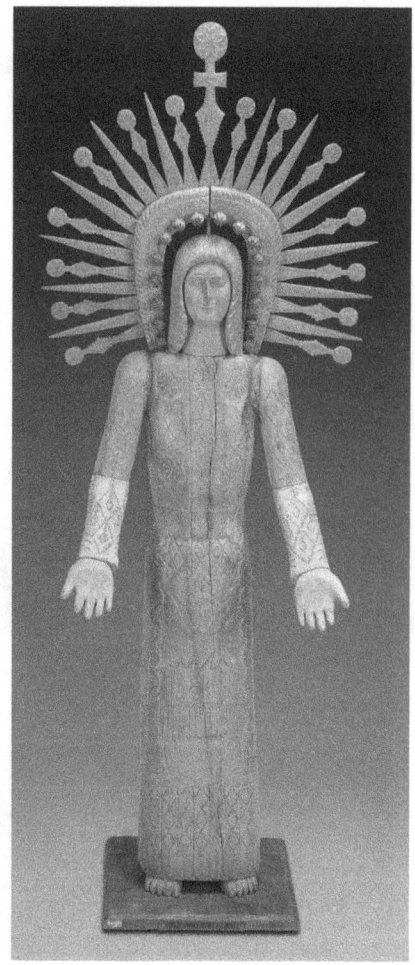

Figure 0.6. *Our Lady of Light* by José Dolores López, created through the Public Works of Art Program (photograph courtesy of the Colorado Springs Fine Arts Center)

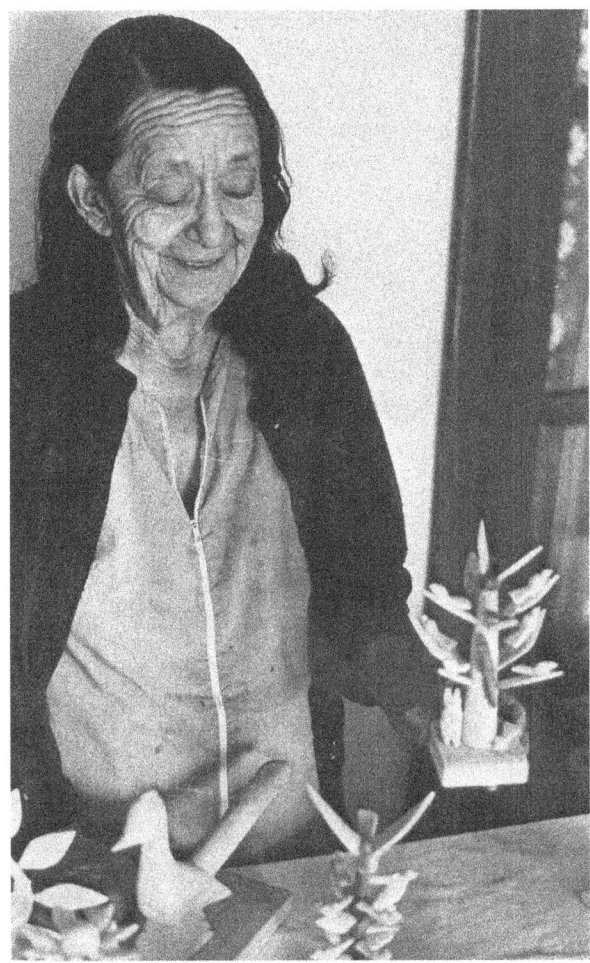

Figure 0.7. Silvianita López shows a carving to customers from her position behind the "table"

roughly the same style, and nearly all signed "George López"—"Otherwise the tourists won't buy them." We talked as I watched them carve. I especially befriended Alex Ortiz, who was my age.

Two things that happened in that initial week changed my life. First, I accompanied George on his daily walk to Córdova's post office. His visits were timed to coincide not just with the arrival of the mail but with that of some two dozen Córdovans who clustered outside, enjoying the April sunshine. This was, I realized, the folkloric nerve center of everyday life in the community. *La plática de los viejitos de antes* (the talk of the elders of bygone days) that unfolded there included proverbs, biblical allusions, jokes, and legends, folded in with commentaries on news and specials at the Piggly Wiggly supermarket in Española. For me the experience went beyond meeting a cross-section of residents; I realized that Córdovans and I were equally fascinated with the rhythms of conversation and how stories, histories, and personalities were woven into landscapes. Wittgenstein soon joined us there as the complex choreography of words, bodies, gestures, facial expressions, landscape, and mail, interrupted occasionally as a loud truck or vintage car passed by, illuminated his insight that "uttering a word is like striking a note on the keyboard of the imagination" ([1953] 1972:§6).

Second, the Lópezes had plans for me. When visitors asked to see the spectacular polychrome images in Córdova's San Antonio Church, George—as sacristan—obliged. Specialists sometimes brought books with photographs of work by José Rafael Aragón and other nineteenth-century artists, so George knew that "traditional" carvings had been the focus of countless museum exhibitions and publications. Although the Lópezes' carvings appeared in major US and foreign museum collections, no one had asked Córdovans for their stories of how they became carvers, why they carved, and what the carvings and interactions with visitors meant to them. George cast me as a mediator. I was a product of the urban, gringo world. Nevertheless, the Lópezes and Robbs had cultivated a relationship for over two decades. I was fluent in New Mexican Spanish, and they could see that my eyes opened wide and my head moved to the rhythm of older people's narratives. George pitched me the project: I should come back, spend more time listening, and write a book about Córdova's *contemporary* carvers, one that would tell *their* side of the story.

I was dumbstruck. Intellectual firecrackers had been going off in my head all week as the words of childhood mentors, Wittgenstein, the post office crowd, and the Lópezes' teachings about life, land, work, spirituality, and aesthetics collided. But I was nineteen years old. I felt inadequately prepared for the project. And I had other, more nineteen-year-old interests. I was becoming a highly proficient rock climber. I had fashioned a reputation as a popular radio disc jockey in high school and college. I went to the Museum of New Mexico to visit the leading authority on saint carving, the remarkable E. Boyd, hoping she would confirm my self-assessment, providing me with an escape route. Hearing me out, she told me what I least wanted to hear: "The Lópezes are right: scholars have only taken the 'traditional' carvings seriously." Dr. Boyd continued: "You are in the perfect position: you know Spanish and you know the Lópezes. You must do it." I protested, noting that I was just finishing my first year in college, I was ill-prepared, and that I needed to get on with my classes, but I could not dissuade her. "I'll help you, and so will a friend, Marta Weigle." Writing about the wood-carvers suddenly seemed like fate.

I had already accepted a summer internship in Gallup, New Mexico, but I spent two fall months in Córdova, enabling me to enjoy northern New Mexico during its most beautiful season, as aspens and cottonwoods turn gold and vines scarlet, residents harvest chile and other crops from small garden plots, and frost brings plumes of piñon and juniper smoke from wood stoves. I rented a trailer near the Lópezes' house. I spent most days with them. I had prepared: I borrowed a cassette recorder, purchased a small microphone, and typed up a dozen questions. The first evening we sat in their living room, positioned between the carvings table and a wood stove that provided warmth and a beautiful yellow glow. I turned on the recorder, grabbed my list of questions, and launched my career.

Having read up on interview techniques, I began with an easy, broad question designed to elicit a story: "Please tell me how you became a carver, how you began to carve." Instead of launching into the lengthy, detailed narrative I had assumed would be forthcoming, George tilted his head back, looked upward, and responded, almost musically, "Uuh, pues, quién sabe!" (Oh, well, who knows!). Dumbstruck, I just looked at him for some time, then retreated to my neatly typed list and tried the second question: "Could you please tell me how your father, José Dolores López, began to carve images of saints?" As if by instant replay, he looked up and intoned, "Uuh, pues, quién sabe!" You might think I am drawing on a vague recollection of our exchange, but that would be mistaken. I still have the recording of that abbreviated encounter. But frankly, I don't need it. Although nearly fifty years (horrors!) have passed, I can still hear the sound of his voice and see the way his head tilted upward. I sat still and looked down, but not at my list of questions. I was defeated. My scholarly career had ended almost before it had begun. We made small talk. I said that I was tired. I walked slowly back to the sanctuary of my trailer. For once in my life, I didn't even look up and wonder at the stars.

The next morning, I returned to the Lópezes' house. We acted as if nothing had happened. I sat across from them, enjoying the warmth of their wood-fire kitchen stove, sitting on a hard wooden bench. As I settled in, so did the feeling of profound discouragement that had emerged the night before. There was little talk. They carved as I vaguely watched. Finally, George grabbed a block of aspen and placed it in my hands, along with a penknife. It would be a lie to say that I had never carved. As a child, I explored numerous crafts. I learned to knit, driving my paternal grandfather to homophobic distraction: "Boys don't do that!" I bought a set of carving tools and tried my hand at wood carving. I became a fairly accomplished potter by the age of about thirteen, owning a kiln and wheel and even selling some of my work. Accepting George's offer, I therapeutically buried my desperation into how the knife cut though the soft layers of aspen.

After about an hour, George walked over, snatched the knife and wood away, made several demonstration cuts, and exclaimed: "You cut *with* the grain, not *against* it." Wood, knife, shock, and self-denigration merged anew. I persisted. A week passed, ever so slowly. I finished small birds and trees. Then I grew more ambitious, remembering George's beautiful image of St. Isidore that I had seen the previous Sunday during Mass in Córdova's church (see figure 0.8). Now *he* was watching *me*. "What are you carving?" "St. Isidore," I replied. He nodded. Perhaps an hour later, he suddenly burst forth with the *alabanza* (hymn of praise) for St. Isidore. Then George, as if talking to the world at large, told the legend of St. Isidore. A shorter pause. He recounted the time he first carved an image of St. Isidore and then, without a moment's hesitation, his father's first foray into the subject. No questions. No tape recorder. No desperation. A new beginning.

Confronting this initial failure—both emotionally and intellectually—did not prompt me to resurrect a preconceived research design: it transformed how I perceive, undertake, teach, and write about research, right through to the present. Still in my academic infancy, I had assumed that asking me to write a book automatically granted me rights to claim the role of researcher and positioned the Lópezes—and other carvers—as research subjects. Fieldwork came with a preset language game that all participants would know and would accept as legitimate: the interview. As the researcher, I would ask questions and they would answer them. Words, captured on tape, would enable me to produce knowledge. The concept of research and the presumed right to ask lots of questions had never limited my engagement with Old Man Hawkins, Señor Olguín, or the beekeeper and his wife, but it suddenly became a major obstacle to learning.

By refusing the interview language game and a subordinate role in the associated hierarchical structure, the Lópezes rejected the role of research subjects and claimed that of mentors. Part of the lesson they were imparting—and the power they were asserting—was to teach me how to learn; in terms of conducting research, I had to unlearn the "research techniques" that I was beginning to acquire. If it had not been for George's refusal to answer my questions, I would not be writing these lines today, nor would I be writing a book that traces the importance of mentorship in fieldwork and theorizing. I knew that images of the saints are more than objects, if the latter are seen as stable, bounded, passive entities defined by

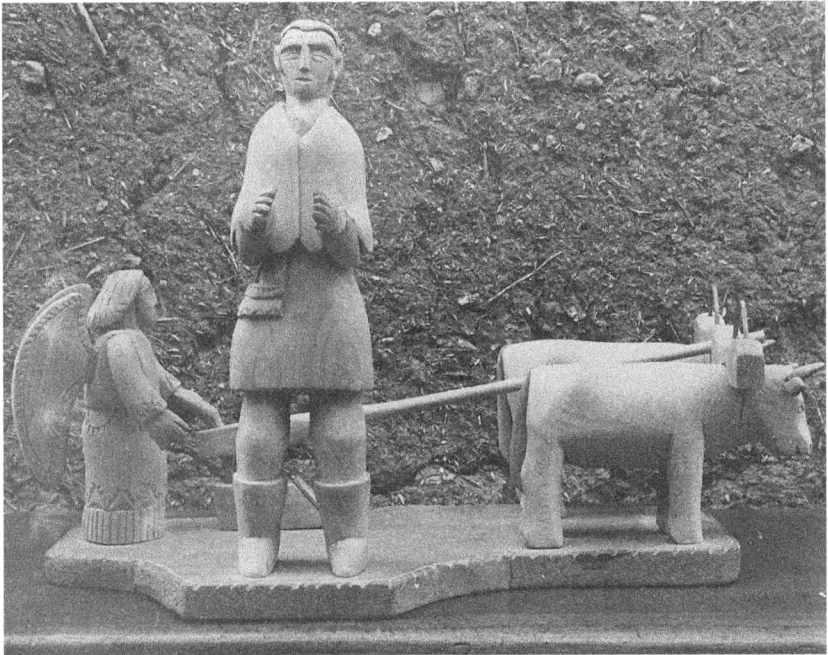

Figure 0.8. George López's first image of St. Isidore, 1949 (from a private collection)

human actions and imaginations. Growing up in New Mexico and visiting friends' homes and the Santuario de Chimayó had taught me that objects have not only social lives and biographies (Appadurai 1986) but spiritual lives too. But I had envisioned the study as a conversation between humans *about* objects. And Mr. López's "Uuh, pues, quién sabe!" demanded that I unlearn racialized assumptions about the politics of knowledge: nascent study of social science methodology entitled me—as a member of the urban, white middle class—to position myself as the knowledge producer and the Lópezes as requiring my ethnographic authority (Clifford 1988) to make their stories legible and significant.

Silvianita and George López taught me lessons that would be articulated decades later in the guise of the "new materialisms" and science and technology studies: objects have forms of agency that can shape human ways of knowing, acting, and relating. Gaining the ability and the right to write about carving involved holding a block of wood and learning to move a hand-knife assemblage in such a way as to find an artistic design and religious imaginary in the unique possibilities and forms of resistance offered by that particular chunk of aspen. It involved watching the Lópezes carve as much as examining the carvings on their table and in museums and, injuring my adolescent ego, having George snatch my block of wood out of my hands and show me what I was doing wrong. David Esterly (2012:64) wrote about carving: "The wood is teaching you about itself, configuring your mind and muscles to the tasks required of them. To carve is to be shaped by the wood even as you're shaping it." This process included aspen, words, songs, and stories—along with facial features, hagiographical attributes, decorative designs, and more than human ("spiritual") connections—as wood, knife, sandpaper, vocal cords, hands, arms, eyes, and imaginations continually intersected as if refracted in a kaleidoscope. Connections between craft and story became clearer to me later when I gained another mentor, German philosopher and cultural critic Walter Benjamin (1968), and read his essay "The Storyteller." The Lópezes pushed me to relate to scholarly research methodologies in more critical and experimental ways—to deny them any a priori authority; a decade later, I wrote a book entitled *Learning How to Ask* designed to pass along these lessons (Briggs 1986).

My initial acceptance of social science methodologies had prompted me to forget what living with my grandparents and my relationship with my neighbor Old Man Hawkins had taught me years before. In keeping with what Eduardo Viveiros de Castro (2004) calls a naturalist perspective, I perceived aspen in instrumental, abstract terms as a medium for revealing human imaginaries and histories and connecting carvers and customers. After the Lópezes slowed down my research, I traveled with them on trips to the mountains, learning to perceive aspen trees through a carver's eyes: which trees were of the right size and health and sufficiently free of knots to harvest, how long to dry the wood, and how to cut, split, and dry them in the sun.[3] Researchers rely on what science and technology scholars call affordances (Gibson 1997), aspects of the environment that enable particular ways of producing knowledge and action and impede others; affordances thereby significantly shape particular configurations of the politics of knowledge. The little social science I had learned led me to believe that books, tape recorders, microphones, lists of questions, and roles of interviewer and interviewee provided the only affordances I needed to learn how the Lópezes carved wood and worlds. The Lópezes had a different plan. For them, a block of aspen and a penknife provided the affordances required to begin to enter a multispecies universe in which trees were key players and their grains, irregularities, and textures played active roles in shaping human-human and, for blessed images, human-deity relations. The camera became a crucial affordance. I had to become a quasi-professional photographer, learning from such gifted artists as Laura Gilpin. Mastering use of a four-by-five-inch view camera and installing a tiny darkroom in the house I purchased in Córdova, I aspired to take photographs that conveyed the artists' vision of their work.

Working on the project over the next six years, I grew in other ways. E. Boyd's suggestion that Marta Weigle could help me was crucial. I often wondered why Marta was so generous with her time and knowledge with a young undergraduate who should have been bothering his own teachers. Marta was my first mentor in folkloristics. Her University of Pennsylvania training and deep knowledge of New Mexican folklore shaped frequent encounters that included a glass of wine (the legal age was eighteen at the time), reading lists, suggestions for building greater analytic sophistication, and a gentle scolding—always laced with good humor—when common sense and particularly gendered assumptions shaped my thinking. Marta took me back to the post office, challenging me to explore how proverbs, legends, folktales, jokes, gossip, hymns, and prayers were ingrained, as it were, in wood carving. She challenged me to let feminist approaches disrupt my thinking in ways that slowly induced two sets of realizations. First, I could see that women's performances were deeply gendered in relational terms. In other words, they critically engaged my gendered and racialized identity as a young white man, often performatively enacting stereotypes of older Latinx women—only to explode them (see Briggs 1988). Second, Marta's challenge to perceive how patriarchy shapes research prompted me to reflect on the problematic symbiosis that emerges as male fieldworkers often hybridize forms of male domination emerging in field sites with androcentric analytic perspectives.

The historical and political-economic scope of my research expanded. George articulated why he turned full-time to wood carving. Wage labor became a necessity for Córdovans when the US Forest Service and Bureau of Land Management and private landowners seized lands that Spain and Mexico had granted centuries before. Córdovans lost the right to graze goats and sheep in the surrounding hills and mountains. Many residents traveled daily across the Rio Grande Valley to work as janitors and maids at the Los Alamos National Laboratory or in the scientists' houses; traffic jams emerged weekday mornings as cars and trucks began a mad dash down the treacherous road toward Española and up the Pajarito Plateau. George did not like being stuck at the bottom of a racialized labor market or missing out on the collective daily life of the community. Wood carving enabled him to quit Los Alamos.

Córdovan carvers did not regard making images of the saints for sale to outsiders as a religious act, as their customers assumed. Some of their neighbors accused the carvers of "selling the saints to nonbelievers." Starting with José Dolores López, carvers developed a crafty dodge: they asserted that if images had not been blessed, they were just blocks of wood; their sale was thus not a sacrilege. Artists and buyers thus collaborated in positioning wood carvings on a racialized border that relationally defined working-class Mexicanos vis-à-vis middle-class whites. Buying carvings enabled the latter to decorate their modern, secular, often wealthy homes with what they deemed fragments of an exotic world inhabited by quaint, backward, simple people who were "close to nature" and exuded a "primitive religiosity." They preferred unpainted, "natural" wood surfaces to the bright colors of nineteenth-century polychrome and contemporary plaster of Paris images. Embodying the aesthetic values of patrons, the carvings became small-scale wooden models of the racist stereotypes held by white customers. The carvers thus reversed the attribution of naiveté, suggesting that tourists and connoisseurs were fooling themselves into thinking that they were buying an Other culture when they were actually consuming their own. Years later, I was pleased to see James Clifford (1988), Michael Brown (2003), Fred Myers (2002), and others explore how arts produced by Indigenous, Aboriginal, and other artists primarily for sale to whites constructed and complicated relations of race, class, colonialism, and nation. My disappointment in seeing that they failed to acknowledge the precedent set by *The Wood Carvers of Córdova* (Briggs 1980) was not personal; rather, they had missed the analytic insights generated by my mentors.

Córdovans changed my sense of identity as much as my scholarly instincts. Let's put it right out there—I was a Chicano wannabe. In high school, I spent a lot of time hanging out with my Chicano and Chicana friends and their families. An unconscious desire to be accepted as a Chicano deepened in Córdova, which I envisioned not as a "field site" but as my home. My dream job was commuting to the University of New Mexico, helping open up pathways to higher education and critical inquiry for students coming from under-resourced public high schools like mine. (Applications to UNM made over the next three decades never met with success.) I became increasingly engaged with the land struggle, joining community activists, progressive lawyers, and historians in organizing the Center for Land Grant Studies.[4] I became something of a celebrity in the region while finishing my doctoral fieldwork in 1978–1979. I went to the local Spanish-language radio station, Radio KDCE (*¿qué dice?*), to purchase a used desk. Having worked as a radio disk jockey, I asked about a sign advertising DJ positions. They hired me. I took my show's name from how friends made fun of me. One person would ask: "What is a *gabacho* doing here?" ("Gabacho" is a more derogatory term for gringo.) Another friend would ironically respond: "¡Debe estar perdido!" (He must be lost!), implying that

I was lost in body, mind, and spirit. I thus named my show "El Gabacho Perdido" (The Lost Gringo).

Chicano/a activist friends convinced me that I would be more useful if I stopped playing defective Chicano and embraced my location along a racial borderline and my status as a border thinker (Anzaldúa 1987). I thus had to transform my race, class, and gender privilege into a means of contributing to efforts to identify and challenge racism and its effects. I deepened the carving project by asking white, upper-middle class patrons why they bought carvings and what they meant to them, and I studied how images were displayed in homes and museums. For the land grant struggle, I complemented my research on the politics of knowledge in Mexicano historical narratives by scrutinizing the "rules of evidence" that shaped why oral history was largely excluded from courtrooms—as hearsay (Briggs 1987).

I learned to listen, in short, to people who defined me by relationally projecting historical and contemporary links between our opposing racial identities. By 1978, I was in full swing with a broader study that was shaped by ethnography of speaking (Hymes 1974) and performance-centered perspectives (Bauman 1977; Hymes 1981). I had the luck of finding another mentor, who similarly became one of my best friends and interlocutors as well as a coauthor—Dick Bauman. Although I was a new kid on the block and he a scholar celebrated in several disciplines, we shared fundamental misgivings about foundational scholarly truths. By the 1990s, syntheses of John Austin's (1962) insights on performativity, Bronislaw Malinowski's (1935, 1948) positioning of language and folklore as central to daily life, Kenneth Burke's (1941) take on literature "as equipment for living," and Roman Jakobson's (1960) approach to poetics had become fixed frameworks that were often unreflexively imposed on cultural forms. Getting together at annual meetings, conferences, and each other's homes, we tried to figure out where received theoretical presuppositions and modes of analysis got in the way. We thus launched a joint unlearning project, working our way back to seventeenth-century foundational separations between language, tradition, science, and politics. Where Richard Dorson (1968) found disciplinary heroes, such as John Aubrey, we located ways of thinking and researching that relegated folkloristics to a provincial, subordinate scholarly corner. We shared an attraction to what Dick called vernacular philology (Bauman 2008), attention to how performers who produce aesthetically elaborated forms also devise insightful ways of thinking about them. Our collaboration in crafting a framework that emphasized entextualization, decontextualization, and recontextualization—even as it probably tested the morphological limits of the English language—helped me attend to ways that Córdovan performers created pasts, presents, and futures and how they were teaching me to think about them. Conversations with Beverly Stoeltje about women and horses in West Texas (1988) and queen mothers in West Africa (Obeng and Stoeltje 2002) resonated with Marta's warnings about taking men, male perspectives, and male-dominated cultural forms as preconceived research objects and analytic perspectives.

Some folklorists and anthropologists were then interpreting performance-centered approaches in scientistic fashion as requiring erasure of traces of the fieldworker's presence. Linda Dégh's account of studying Hungarian legends is a classic: "The text below does not involve the collector... The tape recorder was outside of the room, and the microphone was camouflaged with a shawl; only the hostess knew of its presence" (Dégh and Vázsonyi [1969] 1976:103). Joel Sherzer proposed a "discourse-centered" framework that privileged "naturally occurring and recorded speech" (1983:10). I remember a prominent folklorist at the American Folklore Society's annual meeting asking me if I was present when the recording was made and if my presence had affected what unfolded. I responded affirmatively. He then informed me that my example "was not really a performance," suggesting that such contaminated materials were of little value.

When life gives you lemons, make lemonade! His dismissive comment motivated me to forge a distinct, reflexive approach. Trying to erase my presence would have produced an *un*natural discourse, missing the basic thrust of these performances and their role in shaping naturalcultural life. Performances of proverbs, legends, and personal narratives did not transparently reproduce the sort of pasts that Raymond Williams (1977) called archaic but rather created pasts, presents, and futures and connected them in dialogic and dialectical ways. For example, one night a group of Córdovan youths invited me on one of their all-night excursions. The next day things were different when I walked the quarter mile to the Lópezes a bit later and—shall we say?—more slowly than usual. The three of us began to carve wood. Silence alternated with small talk about the signs of fall. Silvianita began speaking about youths she referred to pejoratively as *la plebe*, their misdeeds, and how they drew the unsuspecting into what she projected as their lack of respect for collective well-being. I was, to repeat, nineteen, and I did not accept the role of the *inocente* readily. I attempted to extricate myself by suggesting that the youths seemed a lot like many kids in my predominantly working-class, Latinx high school, meaning that I thought I knew what was going on and could take care of myself.

Then Silvianita hit me between the eyes with a rhetorical two-by-four: a proverb. She repositioned our discussion from Albuquerque to neighboring

Truchas by invoking *un viejito de antes*, an elder of bygone days (thereby signaling a switch to performance). The somewhat enigmatic proverb suggested that even though Truchas's local ecology favored horsebean cultivation, this crop was part of broader ecological systems. (Here Silvianita anticipated current folkloristic interest in how plant-human relations are often used to performatively restructure human-human relations.) The relations in question were distally between miscreant youths and yours truly and, quite proximally, my attempt to challenge her authority. What had I learned? The proverb performance left me speechless, with no choice but to join George in accepting how Silvianita had cemented her position. I never hung out with the kids again, and I henceforth watched more carefully how my actions would affect their reputation and Córdovans' willingness to accept a gringo. Performances of treasure tales and other narratives similarly positioned me precariously along a racialized border.[5] Was I one of those gringos who came to steal Córdovans' few resources? Or would I reject claims to race and class privilege, distance myself from the gringo bosses, bureaucrats, and swindlers who enforced racialized labor hierarchies on Córdovans, and help build collective futures not undermined by racism and expropriation? If I had hidden my role in these performances, I would have missed the opportunity to convert the positionality they forged for me into an analytic that could produce insights into the politics of knowledge, performance, racialization, and inequality.

VENEZUELA

Over a decade and a half, I tried to honor my Córdovan mentors' insights in a number of books and efforts to turn racial inequalities into social justice. I got the sense that I had done what I could as a scholar and activist in northern New Mexico. Growing up around speakers of Navajo and Puebloan languages and subsequently studying Navajo, I was fascinated with the way words, grammar, and poetics that had resisted linguistic oppression for half a millennium struck the keyboard of the imagination. Nevertheless, my childhood friends had impressed upon me that their language and ceremonial life was not something they wanted to share with outsiders. I was also deeply interested in Latin America and wanted to spend more time there. I first thought about going to Colombia, but in 1985 I heard President Betancourt give a speech in which he elegantly cited Plato and Nietzsche and remarked that he planned to kill each and every guerrilla. I traveled around Venezuela instead, asking one question of representatives of Indigenous communities, scholars, and officials: where might my training be of value?

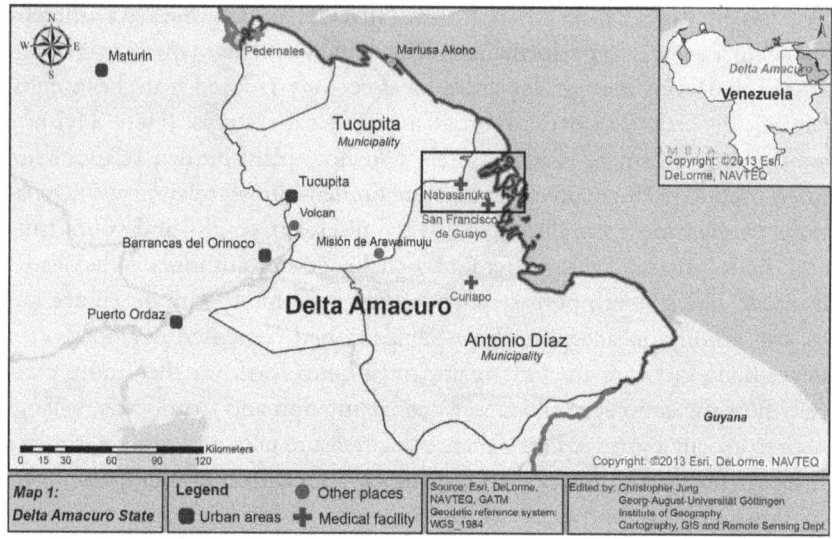

Figure 0.9. Delta Amacuro State, Venezuela

I almost ended up working with Kariña people in Monagas State. I was fascinated by their cante fables, beautiful narratives with embedded songs. They introduced to the community by interviewing me on their radio station, which made me feel right at home. Nevertheless, the place made me feel sad. After oil was discovered on their ancestral lands, Kariña people had been forced to live on small asphalt-covered islands. The painful effects of land expropriation and environmental degradation were still too fresh from my experience in New Mexico.

Neighboring Delta Amacuro State, on the other hand, was perfect (see figure 0.9). The Delta, approximately 40,000 square kilometers, was formed by the vast Orinoco River where it entered the Caribbean, creating swampy islands accessible by navigating myriad tributaries and the smaller waterways that connect them (see figure 0.10). For a kid from New Mexico, which has almost no water, the fluvial landscape was fascinating. Missionaries prompted many residents to establish permanent settlements on riverbanks and to supplement fishing and hunting with agriculture, particularly taro (*Colocasia esculenta*) cultivation. Others continued to live in the forest, moving seasonally to sites where moriche palms, fish, game, and other resources abounded. Some 35,000 people were classified as "indigenous members of the Warao ethnic group," and nearly all spoke the Warao language.[6] The phonology and morphology had been analyzed, but no linguistic anthropology or sociolinguistic work had explored its social dimensions.[7] Anthropologists

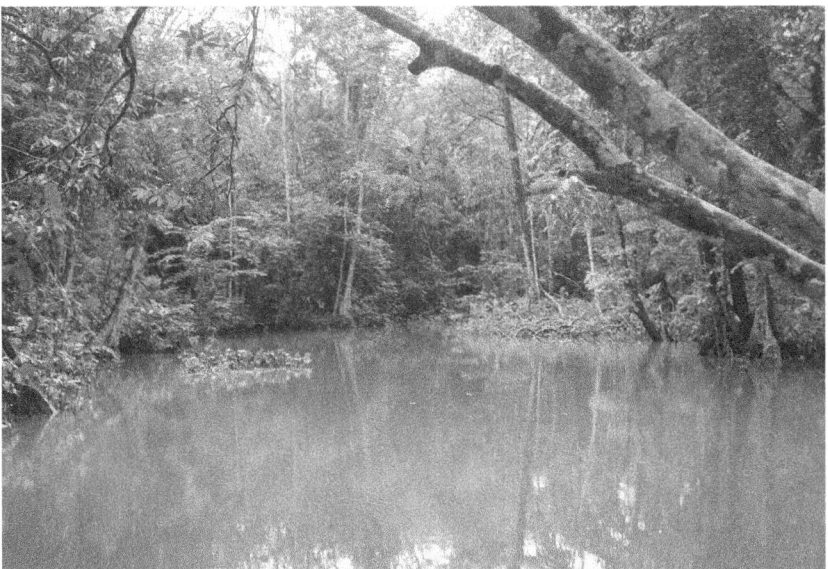

Figure 0.10. Hana Hubasuhuru, a stream that connects two Orinoco tributaries, Delta Amacuro, Venezuela

had documented Warao ritual and healing. And missionaries and anthropologists had compiled extensive collections of myths and folktales, presented largely as decontextualized, objectified texts; they had not studied them ethnographically.[8] Many areas lacked schools and health facilities. Given the absence of potable water and sewage facilities, health conditions were abysmal. Malaria, tuberculosis, measles, and pertussis were common, and between 26 and 36 percent of children died before the age of five.[9] People I met during my 1985 trip to the area told me that documenting the social life of language, oral genres, and the interface between biomedical and vernacular healing might be of value for strengthening educational and health programs. So I returned in 1986 and stayed for a year. Purchasing a fifty-foot dugout canoe and a forty-horsepower outboard motor, I learned to find my way through mazes of tributaries without getting lost—and thus possibly ending up as crocodile food (see figure 0.11).

My first mentors were members of the Moraleda family in Nabasanuka, a town of 453.[10] Teodoro (see figure 0.12), then in his seventies, taught me both about life in the forest, where he grew up, and the experience of being "recruited" to live in a Catholic boarding school.[11] He was a leading member of the local Catholic congregation and a practicing healer. I became close to three of Teodoro and his wife Tomasa's sons: Librado, Conrado, and

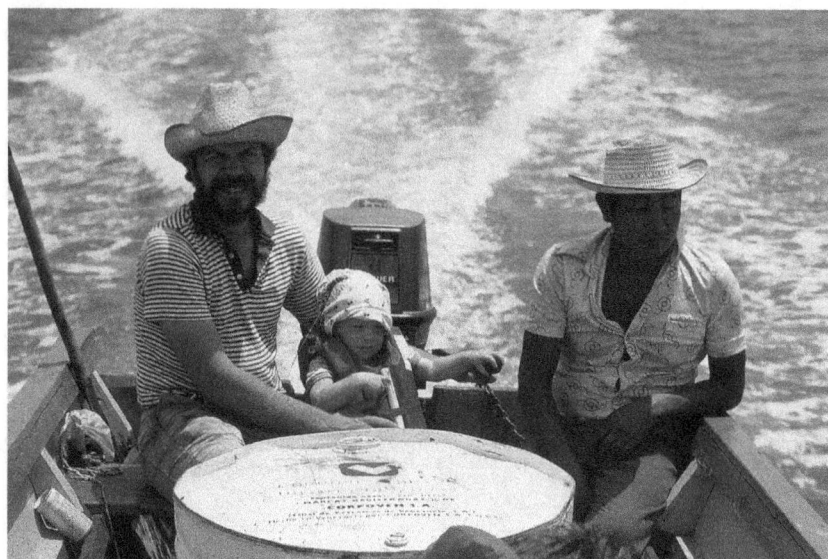

Figure 0.11. The author and son Gabriel operating their motorized dugout canoe (photograph by Barbara E. Fries)

Enrique. Librado and Enrique, two of the Delta's most visible and respected leaders, had joined the socialist party (Movimiento al Socialismo) as teenagers. Librado, a schoolteacher with tremendous charisma and intelligence, became the first president of the Delta's Indigenous social movement (see figure 0.13). Before President Hugo Chávez Frías launched the Bolivarian socialist revolution in 1998, Librado founded Muaina, a coastal community, as an experiment in Indigenous socialism. He spearheaded efforts to outlaw politically powerful palm heart factories and sawmills, arguing that they damaged the rainforest and brutally exploited workers. Despite death threats, he succeeded. Enrique helped the Delta's first Indigenous elected municipal official form a government. Conrado (see figure 0.14) became the president of the health committee, working with physicians and nurses in the local clinic; he played a crucial role in resolving a mysterious epidemic (which I describe in chapters 6 and 10) that killed scores of children and young adults in 2007–2008.

I was staying with the Moraledas when they received an invitation to attend the elaborate *nahanamu* festival in Mariusa. Preparations for the nahanamu center on cutting moriche palms, extracting the starch, and placing it in a giant basket under a temple structure. There *wisidatu* healers invited *hebu* spirits, which are deemed responsible for many respiratory and other illnesses, to bathe in the palm starch and enjoy the singing and dancing

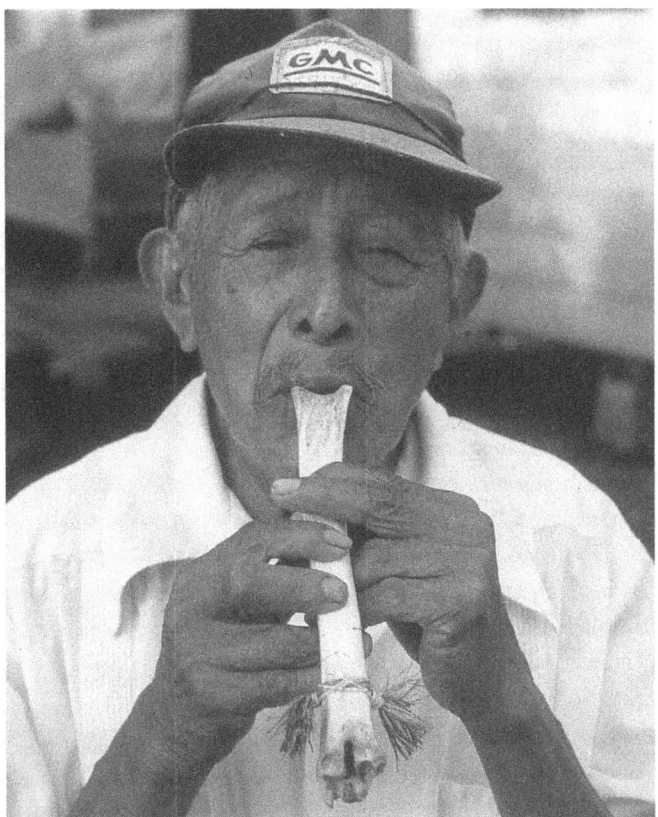

Figure 0.12. Teodoro Moraleda playing a bone flute

performed on a nearby dance platform, exhorting them to refrain from causing illness. The Moraledas invited me—and my canoe—along. There were no stores, missions, schools, or clinics in Mariusa. Rather than practicing agriculture, Mariusans alternated between fishing on the coast and living deep within the moriche palm groves, gathering palm starch and other forest products and hunting. At the festival I met Santiago Rivera, a remarkable healer and leader who became a key mentor—and my student. Frankly, my first experience in the rainforest wasn't easy. There was little food, mainly tiny swamp fish, palm starch, grubs, moriche fruit, and palm hearts; I lost fifteen pounds in two weeks. Trying to stay awake as healers chanted and people sang and danced nearly all night and then worked in the forest during the day was exhausting. My Warao language skills grew rapidly.

Seeking entertainment, leader Santiago Rivera called a woman up to the dance platform one afternoon, then commanded me: "Ihi, hotarao, nao! Hoho!" (Hey you, white guy, come here! Dance!)[12] He handed me the healer's sacred rattle, probably expecting me to stand there waving it. Little did he know that I had taken ballet, modern, and jazz dance classes, or that my interest in performance had prompted me to watch closely the wisidatu healer who served as the nahanamu's father (see figure 0.15). I replicated his actions, right down to how he rotated his eyes and head. Santiago stopped the dancing and called me over. "Do you know Spanish?" he asked. Having learned Warao speech styles, I replied, "A little." "Do you know English?" "A very little," I replied. "Then you will come back and live in my house; you will teach me English and I will teach you Warao." Given that Trinidad lay seven miles across the Caribbean, a major source of cash for Mariusans was selling crabs to Trinidadians, who spoke only English; the two parties could barely communicate. Santiago wanted the language skills to negotiate a better price.

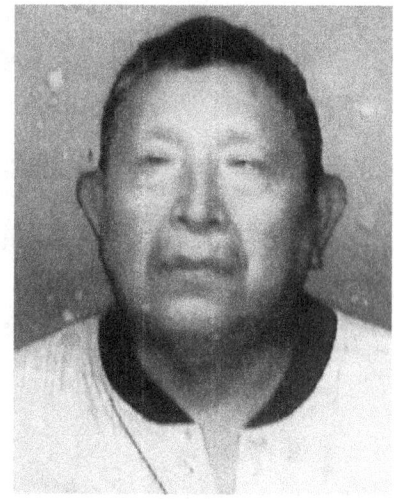

Figure 0.13. Librado Moraleda (photographer unknown)

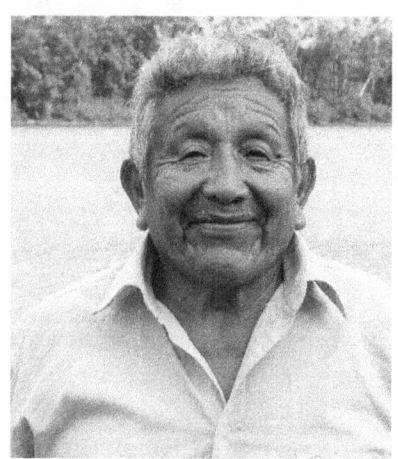

Figure 0.14. Conrado Moraleda

I lived with Santiago and his three wives in the forest and on the coast off and on for several years. It is hard to sketch all he taught me. The universe was suddenly enlarged for me as I watched and listened as his voice, hands, face, and body brought unseen worlds into being by performing myths. His renditions taught me that the same myth can be performed in radically different ways (Briggs 1993a). One night, Santiago challenged me with "your myth, the myth of the *hotarao*" (non-Indigenous people); he used the performance to insert me into the struggle for Mariusan land, rights, and dignity (Briggs 2000). He also performed the myth of Daunarani, Mother of the Forest, that figures centrally in chapter 10.

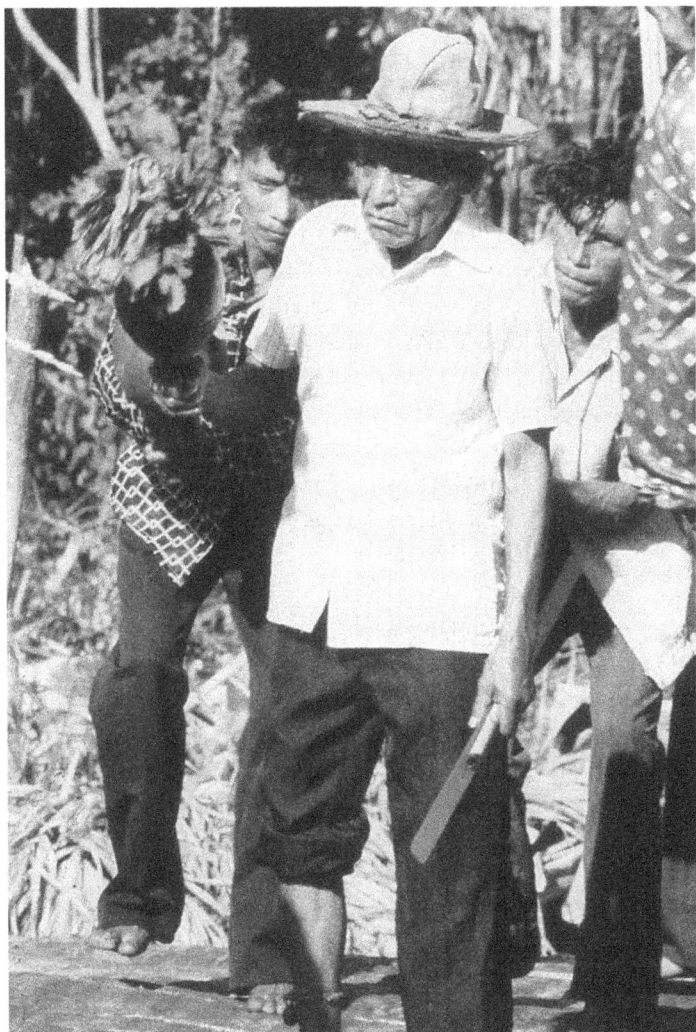

Figure 0.15. A wisidatu healer performing in the nahanamu festival

One afternoon Santiago visited his close friend Manuel Torres. They sat, gossiped, and told a myth. My relationship with Manuel that began that day would change my life. A *hoarotu* healer who outranked even Santiago, he called me his son and decided to train me as a healer. Distrusting the motives of white North Americans who traveled to South America "to become shamans," I declined. He insisted. I eventually gave in. Manuel blew healing spirits into my chest, causing me spiritual consternation. He taught me scores of exquisitely beautiful healing songs. And he prepared cigars of pungent local tobacco rolled in palm leaves, often two feet in length and over half an inch in diameter. Having never been a smoker, I became so intoxicated that I could only crawl back to my hammock at night. Becoming a hoarotu requires dreams that enable candidates to visit spirits who impart songs and knowledge. I may have had such dreams, but the intoxication was so intense that I could remember nothing. Each morning Manuel whispered the same question in my ear: "Did you dream a little?" I was not inclined to lie, to fake it. He became increasingly disappointed by his failing student.

Finally, I had one of those dreams and then my repertoire grew. Manuel began to position me beside him, pushing me to ask diagnostic questions of patients and, laying them in a hammock, use my hands to search for pathogens. I cannot adequately convey how I felt the first time I sang a song that embodied my diagnostic hunch and felt a mass in the patient's abdomen "stand up" when I intoned its magical name; it departed when I ordered it back to its home. Like the times I heard Santiago bring invisible but co-present worlds inhabited by mythic beings close and palpable through performance, this experience provided an analytic challenge to stretch John Austin's notion of performativity, Wittgenstein's work on language games, Bauman's and Hymes's work on performance, and my ontologies of disease to where I could begin to comprehend what I was experiencing. I've gotten closer, but I'm not there yet.

Santiago's sister María Rivera also became my mentor, teaching me about phytotherapy. A remarkable woman, she was renowned for the skill she gained through looking at, smelling, touching, and harvesting plants and watching, listening to, and smelling human bodies. In both Mariusa and Nabasanuka, I watched and listened to her as she gathered plants and treated patients. María challenged gender barriers, as did the two transgender siblings with whom she lived. Women are only allowed to learn the powerful techniques for treating patients with *hebu*, *hoa*, or *bahana* sickness when postmenopausal; male healers avoid menstruating women altogether. Even postmenopausal women confront great obstacles recruiting a teacher and establishing a reputation. In her mid-fifties when I met her in the 1980s, María was training as a hoarotu healer. It was fascinating to see her combine plant- and hoa-based systems, ordinarily separated by ontologies of healing and by gender. She was the only woman I met who became a *deherotu*, a performer of myths; I watched several times as she began to perform a myth, only to be drowned out by a male deherotu. Chapter 10 draws on experiences with María and other phytotherapists.

Life in the Delta seems to be precariously positioned on the border between life and death. In 1987, I watched people wrapped in blankets in 100-degree weather shiver violently during an outbreak of malaria. Murako and Kwamuhu were particularly struck by tuberculosis, and I was there when several young adults died.[13] The area has an unconscionably high rate of child mortality; I was present as many babies died. I watched mothers, grandmothers, and aunts gather around corpses and collectively perform ritual laments. The effect was overwhelming as their words constituted poetic evocations of their relationship to the deceased, speculation as to what might have killed them, and the depth of the pain and rage the mourners were experiencing. The musical features amplified the affective charge in such a way that the laments seemed to rise up from within the bodies and psyches of the performers and enter my own. I recorded laments in Kwamuhu in July 1987. Two years later, María Fernández asked me if she could hear the recording of the laments she performed for her son José. Soon the entire community had gathered in her house—so many that its muddy foundations partially collapsed—to listen to my small cassette recorder.

I spent a week with María, her mother, and other women as they taught me about the poetics of mourning. Remarkably, they could still remember their laments. This experience brought me back to two of my mentors, Sigmund Freud and Mrs. Griego. In the laments, I heard echoes of Mrs. Griego's rosary, the iterative words that seemed to call on the Virgin Mary and Jesus to bring her Peter back. Like the healing songs I sang and the imaginative power of mythic performances, psychoanalytic theory helped me think about ways that sounds, words, gestures, and images circulate between bodies—living and dead—and minds, linking them through multiple semiotic, corporeal, and political modalities. I extend these reflections in chapters 6 and 7.

Death seemed to have completely overwhelmed life in the Delta when I arrived in November 1992. Traveling to Caracas for the defense of a PhD student of mine, I decided to take the overnight bus to Tucupita, the capital of Delta Amacuro State. There I found that thousands of rainforest residents were living on the streets in appalling conditions. The cholera epidemic that had begun in western Venezuela the previous December had caused hundreds of deaths, including that of Santiago Rivera. I returned the following summer for a month, trying to figure out if there was anything I could do to help. There I met a Venezuelan public health physician, Dr. Clara Mantini (see figure 0.16). I decided that if my scholarship were ever to be of value, that was the time and place. I took a year's leave and returned in 1994–1995. Clara and I visited all parts of the vast Delta, working with local residents to determine why some 500 people had died from

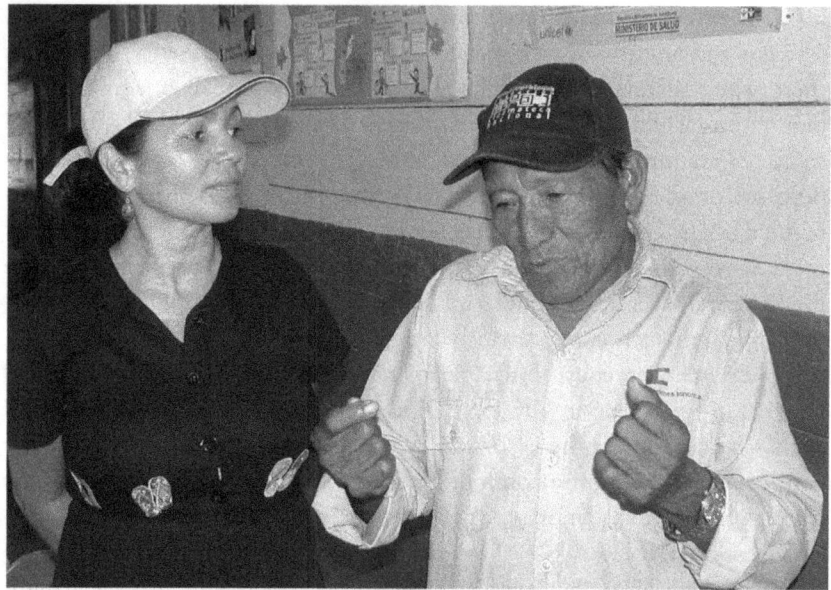

Figure 0.16. Clara Mantini-Briggs with healer Paulino Zapata at the Arawabisi Clinic

a preventable and treatable bacterial infection, doing health education, providing healthcare. In Mariusa, Clara trained a bilingual nurse and established a nursing station. We documented the circulation of narratives told by public health officials, physicians, nurses, and politicians about the epidemic to rationalize unhealthy public health policies and of the counter-narratives told by residents that sought to disconnect what were being construed as natural relations between race, space, and germs and explore decolonial, anti-racist alternatives (Briggs and Mantini-Briggs 2003). The 2020 COVID-19 pandemic is unfolding as this book goes to the printer. The much higher rates of infection, serious illness, and death among US Black, Latinx, and Native American populations have provided a grim reminder of the lesson that cholera taught me: epidemics X-ray society in such a way as to not only reveal deep fractures and inequities but—altogether too frequently—render them lethal.

During this period, I would encounter another mentor under quite different circumstances. I met Herminia Gómez in July 1994 in a jail cell on the outskirts of Tucupita. The context was not research or health intervention; rather, Clara and Héctor Romero, a progressive lawyer, recruited me as a translator for Herminia, who was accused of killing her newborn daughter. I was asked to help her retell a narrative. "Herminia is 'indigenous,'" they informed me, "so she didn't understand what the police and judge told her"; her conviction on infanticide charges was thus the result of a misunderstanding. If I could elicit her story in Warao, problems of language and translation would vanish and the real story would set her free. She was to provide a simple, linear narrative of her daughter's birth and death. This simplistic account of the politics of bilingualism and racial inequality made me uncomfortable, but I trusted my friends' political commitments. I thus sat in a prison cell on a metal chair opposite Herminia, surrounded by her aunt and uncle (whom I had known for years), Héctor, and Clara. Outside this circle, menacingly, three guards watched.

But Herminia did not want to supply content for yet another imposed narrative form. Denying the premise of linguistic Otherness that predicated the encounter, she noted: "I understood perfectly. How could I not know Spanish? I went to school, and I worked [as a maid] in *criollo* [non-Indigenous] houses for more than two years." Refusing to accept the narrative temporalities imposed by police, prosecutor, defense attorneys, and supporters alike, her story began not with her child's death but with her own birth and her mother's death. Expressing her inability to tell the solicited narrative, hers became a story about other people's stories, her own constraints as a narrator, and the profound consequence of these stories—her conviction on a count of first-degree murder, for which she faced eighteen years in prison. She had no illusions that a gringo anthropologist who could shift inexplicably into a language that stigmatizes its speakers could magically end her nightmare; rather, she used Warao to talk about her mistreatment by the glaring but uncomprehending guards. Crucially, she asked me to help her figure out how the narrative used to convict her had been constructed and to devise a different way of talking about violence that could enable her to gain her freedom, including from sexual violence, labor exploitation, and dehumanization.

I never saw Herminia again. The prison door was soon shut to us. We learned why. Herminia had been repeatedly raped by one of the three overhearing guards who then tried to cover up the crime by forcing an illegal and nearly fatal abortion. When she landed in the hospital, rumors proliferated, enabling a supporter to find her and denounce what had taken place, leading to a grant of clemency—for the rapist—and a shortening of Herminia's sentence and her release into a stigmatized life as "that crazy Indian girl who killed her baby daughter." After wandering the streets of Tucupita, she disappeared.

It may seem odd to refer to Herminia as one of my mentors, given the brevity of our encounter. For people on both sides of the racialized Warao versus non-Indigenous chasm, she symbolized not power and wisdom but abjection and stigma. But she changed my life, not so much on a single day as through years of reflection on our conversation. The plethora of stories about her that circulated as gossip, journalism, police records, court documents, and pro-Indigenous activist discourse were all incarcerated within the narrative forms, temporalities, spatializations, and actor networks that structured each site of knowledge production. Herminia forced me to think about the politics of translation, of how the seemingly practical need for translation permits ideological constructions of bounded and opposed races, languages, cultures, spaces, and forms of cognition and action to be produced, naturalized, and policed. She deconstructed narratives of violence, leading me to see how they presuppose problematic understandings of what sorts of acts of violence require narratives and what sorts of narratives are deemed adequate means of representing violence, not to mention the ways they incarcerate particular types of people. The questions she posed just wouldn't let go of me, and I began to trace the lives of other Venezuelan women who had been convicted of infanticide, exploring how these narratives shape national imaginaries of motherhood, stigma, violence, and ethics even as they dehumanize the individuals they turn into monsters. More than a quarter century later, I am just beginning to get a sense of how we can develop strategies for disrupting these problematic connections.

Clara and I worked elsewhere in Venezuela for a number of years, documenting the public health system created by President Hugo Chávez's socialist government and how revolutionary news media reported health issues. We returned to the Delta in July 2008. Sadly, Manuel Torres, María Rivera, and Teodoro Moraleda had died. The book that Clara and I wrote about the epidemic, *Stories in the Time of Cholera*, had won several awards and garnered royalties (Briggs and Mantini-Briggs 2003). We decided to use these funds to work with residents in devising a new kind of healthcare delivery model. But Conrado Moraleda stopped us in our tracks. He was waiting for us in Nabasanuka, where we had traveled to ask the doctor about some strange deaths: Conrado told us that a mysterious epidemic had been killing children and young adults for a year, but doctors had not succeeded in diagnosing it. After failing to get health officials to act decisively, Conrado and his brother Enrique launched their own investigation; they asked us to join. They also recruited Tirso Gómez (see figure 0.17), a healer who worked with us during the cholera epidemic, and his daughter Norbelys Gómez, a nurse (see figure 0.18).

In order to succeed where clinicians and epidemiologists had failed, we needed a wide spectrum of evidence. Having studied narratives, dispute

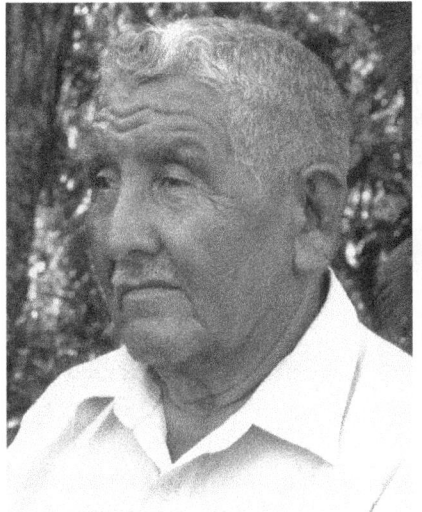
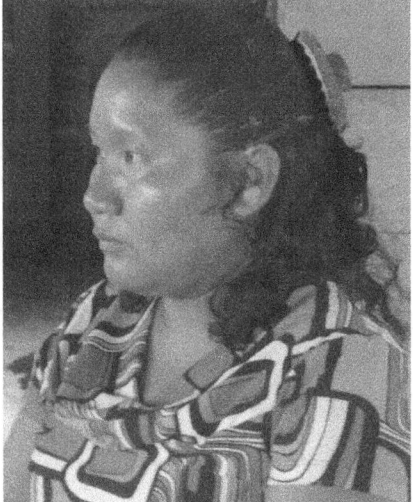

Figure 0.17. Tirso Gómez

Figure 0.18. Norbelys Gómez

mediation, oratory, healing, laments, clinical medicine, and epidemiology, I realized that each was associated with different ways of producing knowledge. We used what residents jokingly refer to as "Warao Radio," the oral circulation of narratives about recent events, to locate communities in which the strange deaths had occurred. We held meetings in fourteen such communities, giving parents the chance they had demanded to tell publicly the story of their children's illnesses, how they sought to obtain the care that might save their lives, how they died, and the impact of their loss. Healers and nurses related how they lost one patient after another, sometimes leading them to question their skills. Narratives elucidated the broader social and political context, including problems with government officials and businesses operating in the area. On two occasions, we listened to laments sung over the corpses of young adults. Enrique and the parents asked me to draw on the skills I had developed as a photographer while researching Córdovan wood-carvers: "We want lots of people to know about our children!"

Soon a common set of symptoms—fever, headache, generalized pain, hypersensitivity to touch, tingling in the extremities that turned into paralysis, hallucinations, inability to swallow first food then water, hydrophobia, excessive salivation, and death—became apparent. Clinical examination of a patient, Elbia Torres Rivas, prompted Clara to provide a presumptive diagnosis of rabies. The parents' testimonies revealed that most patients had been bitten by vampire bats one to two months before symptoms began, providing a likely route of transmission.[14] The team drew up a report and took it to national health officials. Political controversy and international attention by journalists erupted as four Indigenous people—commonly stereotyped as too incarcerated by culture to understand what doctors tell them and unable or unwilling to follow guidelines—took the lead in diagnosing a mysterious epidemic and demanding justice in health.[15] Decades of fieldwork and community-based collaboration proved crucial in creating an open-ended, horizontally organized process of knowledge exchange and collective action.

This experience was not framed as research, and Clara and I did not initiate or direct the investigation. Listening to the parents' stories and watching Elbia die from a preventable disease was one of the most difficult experiences of my life; it took awhile to recover. Community-driven throughout, the team's work was oriented toward confronting stereotypes, demanding justice, and shaping health policies. Conrado, Enrique, Norbelys, and Tirso wanted to share their experience and their vision with people who also face structural violence. Transforming the creative and collaborative nature of the investigation into a writing strategy, we recorded more than sixty hours of conversations over three years, transcribed them, turned them into narrative that was structured as a dialogue about the epidemic and our work, and published it in a leading critical public health (*salud colectiva*) series in Argentina (Briggs et al. 2015). Clara and I wrote a book (Briggs and Mantini-Briggs 2016) that attempted to bring what we had learned from parents, leaders, nurses, healers, doctors, and epidemiologists to academic audiences. I return to these experiences in chapters 6 and 10.

DRAWING IT BACK TOGETHER

In some sense, the trajectory I traced here is not unique: learning to create dialogues between lessons garnered from mentors within and beyond the academy is, I think, a hallmark of knowledge production in anthropology and folkloristics and its greatest source of creativity. What is less common, I suspect, is how many of these relationships unfolded and the ways they shaped me as a scholar and person. From my meeting with Señor Olguín right through the 2008 experience in a rabies epidemic, I did not inaugurate or control most of these experiences. I did not sign up to work in cholera or rabies epidemics; once I stumbled into the middle of them, however, I could not simply turn my back on requests to contribute my modest skills to efforts to save lives and achieve justice in health. These experiences, as well as working with communities in New Mexico that were devising ways to recover lands and livelihoods that had been stolen from them and my encounter with Herminia, were unexpected and disconcerting, producing forms of vulnerability that pushed me beyond my personal and intellectual limits. I want to stress here not the personal effects of these encounters, which were sometimes acute, but the way they disrupted business-as-usual research techniques. Take the failed initial interview with the Lópezes. It was supposed to launch a long series of encounters between human beings that would be structured by the unequal roles of researcher and subject, interviewer and interviewee. By refusing to be interviewed and inviting me to develop a relationship with aspen wood and a penknife, Mr. López turned the tables on assumptions about knowledge production and the hierarchical ordering of relations between participants. What made the difference in my process of becoming a scholar is that years of reflection placed experiences and mentors located on and beyond the borders of research at the center of my own particular approach. These experiences' refusal to stay within easy borders was tied to the fact that they had real-world stakes for people, stretching from the Lopezes' ability to reshape the racialized borders that determined how their customers treated them to Herminia's fight for freedom and dignity to efforts by cholera and rabies patients to confront death, social and biological.

As I have suggested, these experiences had profoundly transformative effects on me in personal and scholarly terms, but none of these occurred overnight. Indeed, it took years for me to allow them to uproot the business-as-usual research concepts and techniques I had learned. They also unfolded synergistically as each new experience interacted dialogically with the disruptions and insights that had emerged from past encounters, linking vastly different types of events in quite different settings. Crucially, my mentors have included people trained as folklorists, anthropologists, philosophers, nurses, physicians, epidemiologists, and art historians; others skilled as healers, beekeepers, and agriculturalists; and others—like Herminia—who lacked such special skills. They interacted within me, as exemplified by the way Wittgenstein shaped how I listened to the Lópezes and how their teaching inflected my reading of Wittgenstein. Freud's essay "Mourning and Melancholia" ([1917] 1957) similarly equipped me to listen to laments in Kwamuhu, Muaina, and elsewhere and to what women like María Fernández, Florencia Macotera, and Anita Rivas were teaching me, even as their laments and reflections left me with the questions I ask Dr. Freud in chapter 6.

As I draw this introduction to a close, I think that the particular, somewhat quirky experiences and relationships I describe here might be of value to others, particularly those who are just beginning to shape their own paths. Since I myself am getting to be one of those viejitos, although not quite yet de antes, let me recast my reflections in the form of advice; let's call it "Briggs's Principles for Unlearning":

- Don't limit yourself to safe, predictable situations that are under (your) control.
- When you find yourself in an edgy, disconcerting situation, including one that may feel like a colossal failure, embrace it—don't run away.
- Surrender to the uncertainties, the doubts; let them sink in deep.
- Keep asking yourself, "Why does this disconcert me? What is this situation trying to tell me?"
- Turn these reflections into sources of theoretical and methodological creativity by allowing them to call standard assumptions and operating procedures into question.
- Keep a chorus of your mentors' voices going inside your head, thereby permitting different perspectives and insights to come together in novel ways.
- When such experiences offer forms of resistance as you attempt to submit them to conventional rhetorical forms, devise experimental forms of writing that enable you to more adequately (if never perfectly) bring the disparate and sometimes clashing voices of mentors and the call of contrasting experiences into dialogue.
- Repeat the above steps for a few decades.

Given that the neoliberal university exerts more and more pressure on us to shorten "time-to-degree" and both it and many nonacademic organizations impose metrics for generating research "products," I certainly don't want to give the impression that I am suggesting you should reflect on such experiences for decades before writing about them. Indeed, my point is more that all fieldwork is long term in the sense that its capacity to uproot sedimented ways of thinking can continue to emerge over long periods of time and in unpredictable ways—if you let it. And even as you produce texts that respond to the complexity, power, and disconcerting qualities of such conversations and experiences, keep some in your back pocket for a few years or a few decades, letting their disruptive effects continue to operate on you as new conversations and encounters unfold.

PLAN OF THE BOOK

I have greatly enjoyed recounting the experiences that brought me to write this book and shaped the perspectives it presents, and I hope that you have enjoyed reading about them. For those of you who have kindly followed my work over the years, I hope that these words have given you a better sense of the unlearning process that informs what I have written about poetics, pandemics, and the politics of knowledge. And for students, my reflections may help illuminate the tremendously complex process of choreographing dances between ethnographic experiences and theory.

But now it's time for the more mundane task of telling you what you will encounter in this book. The chapters draw on what my mentors have taught me in attempting to intervene in scholarly conversations in particular ways. Although my concerns are multiple, they center around three themes.

One focus, which I develop in part 1, pertains to issues of what science-technology-society studies scholar Thomas Gieryn (1983) refers to as boundary-work, designs for separating scholarly (or scientific) from "popular" ways of knowing, for keeping members of a particular discipline in and others out; chapter 1 focuses on this issue. Chapter 2, written in response to essays by linguistic anthropologists who were rethinking ethnopoetics, prompted me to reflect on how cultural forms come to be seen as intrinsically mobile or immobile. I question core beliefs about mobility, ideas that represent cultural forms as imbued with immanent capacities to move, scrutinizing often-unquestioned assumptions in arguing that performers and scholars alike imbue some cultural forms with features that make them seem intrinsically mobile at the same time that other features and forms are fashioned in such a way as to make them seem trapped in "local" spaces. This chapter sets up issues that I address in later chapters. In chapters 3 and 4 I join respectively Américo Paredes and Sadhana Naithani, the first as perhaps my most important scholarly mentor and the second as coauthor, in challenging the foundational Eurocentrism of folkloristics, anthropology, and related fields. The two essays reflect on the course that scholarship might take if culture and folklore were defined in terms of difference, borders, and colonialism, rather than assuming that they consist of shared ideas and forms that exist within bounded social groups.

Part 2 focuses on my long love affair with psychoanalysis. Even as I advance Alan Dundes's claim that psychoanalysis has much to offer folkloristics, I embrace, as it were, a different relationship with psychoanalysis. Chapter 5 engages a broader range of psychoanalytic works and ideas, looking at some of Sigmund Freud's foundational texts through the lens of poetics and performance and incorporating other psychoanalysts, such as Jacques Lacan, Melanie Klein, Julia Kristeva, Jean Laplanche, and Juan-David Nasio. Dundes fashioned psychoanalysis as a stand-alone theory, even explicitly at times walling it off from contamination by other theories that folklorists have found productive (see Dundes 2005), including feminist and performance-centered approaches. This was, I think, one of the sources of folklorists' resistance, as it were, to psychoanalysis, about which Dundes frequently complained. To the contrary, here I use poetics and performance to rethink psychoanalysis, and I use psychoanalysis as a prompt for reconfiguring scholarly approaches to the study of cultural forms.

Chapter 6 uses an experiment in ethnographic writing to cut to the heart of the project I developed in this introduction. It joins my efforts to create synergies between what I learned from different mentors with the task of the preceding chapter—creating new sorts of dialogues between psychoanalysis and performance and poetics. For several years, this project had met with massive resistance within me. I tried to bring together a mentor whom I had never known but who influenced me deeply, Sigmund Freud, with several Delta women who taught me so much about the pain of losing a child. My initial efforts created a terrible imbalance, given that Delta mourners impacted me greatly through their laments, narratives, comments on the process, and their friendship, not to mention their demands that I join their efforts to figure out what killed their daughters and sons and help them keep their remaining children alive. Freud's role, on the other hand, was more distant, reduced to a discussion of his famous essay, "Mourning and Melancholia" ([1917] 1957). I only grew increasingly frustrated with myself, knowing that within me their relationship was more balanced and intimate than my writing was capturing. It suddenly struck me: "I'm going to write Freud a letter!" Leaving the constraints of academic genres aside and embracing the more personal and evocative style invited by this epistolary form enabled me to reconnect emotionally and intellectually with the essay and opened up new analytic possibilities. Rather than writing experimentally for the sake of experimentation or in an effort to project creativity, in that chapter I struggle to break through the analytic and ethnographic constraints that often thwart attempts not only to acknowledge but to take account of the impact of diverse sources of inspiration.

Part 3 centers on attempts to unlearn assumptions that shape how three scholarly topics are addressed. The first two chapters, which are analytic in focus, break with ways that "folk medicine" and the study of "folklore and the media" have been framed. After a brief history of research on "folk medicine," chapter 7 draws on ways that medical anthropologists have moved from an ethnomedical focus on the health-related "beliefs" of subaltern populations to join medical sociologists and historians and scholars of science-technology-society studies in researching how medicine, healing, bodies, physicians, patients, and technologies are constructed in clinics, laboratories, marketing firms, the homes of patients and healers, and other sites. The essay proposes a set of principles for what I call "the new folkloristics of health," suggesting how it can contribute to concerns of scholars who have never been interested in "that medical stuff." Chapter 8 addresses foundational assumptions that underlie work on "folklore and the media." I bring together traditionalization and mediatization, frameworks drawn respectively from folkloristics and media studies, in suggesting how media ideologies and sets of practices for producing and interpreting media forms lie at the heart of both folklore and folkloristics.

If my discussion stopped there, I would leave received boundaries between media- and medical-oriented analytics in place. I rather use the frameworks that I develop in these chapters to experiment with new ways of approaching, respectively, the study of pandemics and nonhuman-human (and specifically plant-human) relations in the following two chapters. Chapter 9 thus juxtaposes concerns with media and health through a focus on news coverage of health issues. It scrutinizes a highly visible genre of mediatized health narrative—news stories of pandemics. Ethnographic work with public health officials, journalists, clinicians, and others permits detailed analysis of how they collaborated in co-producing the story of "the swine flu pandemic" in just twenty-four hours in April 2009; it ends by comparing H1N1 with the 2020 COVID-19 pandemic. Chapter 10 returns to the rabies epidemic, looking at how discrepant and often conflicting perspectives on the deaths played out through plant ontologies expressed by engineers, healers, and phytotherapists. Creating a dialogue with plant philosopher Michael Marder, it traces how Delta residents went beyond confronting a disease to offer the Bolivarian government of Venezuela a new vision of socialism, based not on the environmentally destructive extraction of fossil fuels by large corporations but a "phyto-socialism" in which plants are not only respected but help create more ecologically, socially, and politically sustainable designs for life. This chapter finally brings me closer to actually getting what Old Man Hawkins, Señor Olguín, the Lópezes, and Delta women and men have been teaching me for over half a century about ways that humans and nonhumans become co-creators and co-performers in crafting new ways of thinking about life and death.

This introduction should provide you with a sense of how these essays are informed by a common set of deeply rooted experiences and analytic concerns. Although I have reworked most of the essays in such a way as to extend their logics and develop common threads, I have not attempted to impose a single totalizing approach. I have tried to minimize what might seem like distracting overlaps of, for example, quoted material; nevertheless, I hope that remaing points of intersection will indicate how I keep thinking through events, issues, and provocations. My hope is that this book will inspire both seasoned scholars and those just starting to develop their own perspectives to unlearn accepted points of departure and conjure new futures.

NOTES

1. According to the US Census, *Number of Inhabitants, New Mexico* (https://www2.census.gov/library/publications/decennial/1950/population-volume-2/26082967v2p31ch1.pdf).

2. I addressed them, in accordance with local usage, as Mano George and Mana Silvianita (from *hermano* and *hermana*, meaning "brother" and "sister").

3. See Stengers 2005 on slow scholarship.

4. See Briggs and Van Ness 1987.

5. See Briggs 1988; Briggs and Vigil 1990.

6. This population figure is taken from the Indigenous Census of 2001 (Instituto Nacional de Estadística 2003).

7. The key work on the structure of the Warao language is by missionary Henry A. Osborn, as presented in a doctoral dissertation at Indiana University (1962). For an excellent analysis of the politics of missionary Warao linguistics, see Rodríguez 2008. Barral (1979) compiled a dictionary.

8. I discuss much of this work and provide references in *Poéticas de vida en espacios de muerte* (Briggs 2008). For a few key works by missionaries on Warao folklore, see Barral 1961 and Lavandero 1991. The classic ethnographer of the Delta is Johannes Wilbert (1987, 1996); also see Dieter Heinen 1988; Dale Olsen 1996; and Ayala Laféé and Wilbert 2001, to mention just a few.

9. A study conducted from the 1950s to the 1970s by Miguel Layrisse, Johannes Wilbert, and their colleagues placed prepubescent mortality at 50 percent (Wilbert 1980). Research in the northwestern Delta in the late 1990s, led by Jacobus De Waard, calculated that 36 percent of children die in their first year of life (Servicio de Apoyo Local 1998). The most recent—and probably most reliable—study (Villalba et al. 2013) put this figure at 26 percent in 2011.

10. From the 2001 Indigenous Census (Instituto Nacional de Estadística 2003).

11. I use first names here. I was thirty-three years old when I began working in the Delta, and I was on a first-name basis with my Delta mentors, except where kinship terms or honorifics were required.

12. *Hotarao* actually means non-Indigenous person, but I opted for a more evocative translation here.

13. According to Maes et al. (2008), the Indigenous population of Delta Amacuro has the highest tuberculosis incidence in Venezuela and the lowest life expectancy. Abadía et al. (2009) estimate tuberculosis incidence among the population in general at 450 per 100,000. Tuberculosis specialist Jacobus de Waard of the Institute of Biomedicine confirmed that

Murako and Kwamuhu were tuberculosis hotspots where the incidence was much greater (personal communication, 1995).

14. Nocturnal bites by vampire bats often do not leave visible bite marks or blood and are thus commonly missed.

15. The phrase "incarcerated by culture" is Arjun Appadurai's (1988).

Part I
Unlearning Racialized Disciplinary Genealogies

1

Disciplining Folkloristics

> *But when one draws a boundary it may be for various kinds of reason. If I surround an area with a fence or a line or otherwise, the purpose may be to prevent someone from getting in or out; but it may also be part of a game and the players be supposed, say, to jump over the boundary.*
>
> —Ludwig Wittgenstein, *Philosophical Investigations*

LEE HARING (2008B) CURATED A SET OF ARTICLES that responded to Alan Dundes's provocation regarding what he assessed as "the continued lack of innovation in what we might term 'grand theory' in folkloristics" (Dundes 2005:387). This essay springs from Haring's kind invitation to provide my own response. I must admit from the outset that my excitement in contributing to a debate regarding the place of theory in folkloristics was tempered by lingering frustration. Forging more prominent spaces for theoretical work in folkloristics has been one of my central goals for several decades. Nearly three decades ago, Amy Shuman and I curated in *Western Folklore* a set of papers on theory (1993). But here's the rub: Shuman and I attempted to turn these articles into a collection for classroom use, but were repeatedly told by publishers that there is no market for books on folkloristic theory. Seeking to disprove this assessment, in 2003 Richard Bauman and I published a book exploring how the study of folklore has informed canonical epistemologies and political projects of the modern world for three centuries. I wish I could say that *Voices of Modernity* stimulated broad rethinkings of the politics and poetics of the discipline and sparked new attempts to insert folkloristics more centrally in interdisciplinary theoretical debates, but I am not sure that it has. Nevertheless, the text seems to have become part of the discipline's intellectual infrastructure, particularly for graduate students preparing to take PhD orals.

I thus could not have been more pleased to see my predecessor in the directorship of the University of California, Berkeley, Folklore Graduate Program, Alan Dundes, deliver a spirited call for theoretical debate to a packed ballroom at the 2004 American Folklore Society Annual Meeting, which he published the next year (Dundes 2005). I applaud the contributors to the special issued edited by Lee Haring for responding to Dundes's challenge (Haring 2008b). Starting with Mills's (2008) provocative questioning of the category of theory, the authors insightfully queried the theory/folklore relationship, examining how the constitution of these categories overdetermines their interrelations. I would like to further explore this reluctance to embrace theory.

I draw on science studies, especially Thomas Gieryn's (1983) notion of "boundary-work." In the mid-twentieth-century United States, Richard Dorson and other folklorists developed a largely atheoretical form of boundary-work that successfully delimited an autonomous folkloristics and expanded its resource base and academic authority. Subsequently, the ethnography-of-speaking and performance-centered approaches in folklore fostered an opposing rhetorical style that used theoretically engaged analysis to promote creative exchanges across disciplinary boundaries. Pointing out why these rhetorics seem less viable in the twenty-first century as discipline-building strategies and returning to the issue that inspired the introduction to this book, I suggest an alternative approach that fosters innovation by collaborating on theoretical issues with nonacademics who reflect deeply on the poetics and politics of vernacular culture—people scholars used to call "the folk."

Science studies critiques have become markers of academic importance, even for disciplines that also situate themselves in the humanities. But my goal is not just to put folkloristics on the science studies map but to reflect on folklorists' discipline-building practices and their viability within contemporary academic and sociopolitical contexts—and to imagine alternatives.

BOUNDARY-WORK AS DISCIPLINARY STRATEGY

Acknowledging Dorson's role in consolidating US folkloristics, Simon Bronner (1986) sagely shows that his influence emerged less from new theoretical visions than tireless efforts to promote folkloristics, particularly by creating academic controversies in which he himself featured centrally. Science studies can bring Dorson's contribution clearly into focus. As Gieryn elucidates in his classic article, boundary-work is a rhetorical style that constructs social boundaries, demarcating intellectual activities accorded the prestige of science from nonscience or pseudo-science. It is most commonly used "to enlarge the material and symbolic resources of scientists or to defend professional autonomy" (1983:782). It builds individual reputations and expands disciplinary boundaries by claiming authority and resources from other professions.

In *The British Folklorists*, Dorson tells the story of John Aubrey's discovery of a preexisting object—folklore: "With the sure instinct of the tradition-hunter, he recognized the rupture in society caused by new inventions and new political forms, and the damaging effect of these innovations on the old peasant culture" (1968:5). Discovering folkloristics' object required a distinct set of methods, collecting "at first hand, from his own immediate world" (8). The precarious, evanescent nature of folklore required boundary-work that distinguished the true object from superficially similar forms. As Bruno Latour (1987) suggests, a key feature of scientific work is the generation of textual-cum-social-cum-material networks. Modes of collecting, classifying, and comparing empirical objects and transforming them into texts thus created networks or communities, first termed antiquarian and later folkloristic. Dorson traces connections from Aubrey's foundational instincts to their institutionalization in a science of folklore, professional societies, a specialized literature, and increasingly explicit, standardized methods adopted by scholars—a network that seemed to grow continually through space and time. Boundary-work is hardwired into Dorson's origin story of folkloristics, seemingly required by the nature of folklore and the folk. The dissemination of this genealogy reproduced boundary-work globally. (I take up the colonial aspect of Dorson's genealogy centrally in chapter 4.)

When he turned to the United States, Dorson similarly fought to consolidate folkloristics as a discipline, to demarcate and defend its boundaries. Such military metaphors provided the language for Dorson's boundary-work, undertaken in the context of the Cold War. He opened "Folklore, Academe, and the Marketplace" by bemoaning the way that folkloristics has been misunderstood: "my academic life has been largely spent in attempts to combat these misunderstandings" (1976:1). Echoing the militaristic rhetoric of the early Cold War, Dorson coined the term "fakelore" in 1950, which he defined as "a synthetic product claiming to be authentic oral tradition but actually tailored for mass edification" (5). Reflecting that "fakelore" was crafted as "a battle cry," Dorson argued that "the study of American folklore was being invaded by commercializers and could not as yet be protected by scholars, since specialists in American folklore had not yet been trained"

(1971:7). His attacks on amateurs, popularizers, the mass media, and academic interlopers helped to professionalize the discipline, defining folklorists through the ability to recognize a distinctive object, develop distinctive methods, and form professional networks. The production of legitimate knowledge about American folklore thus required departments of folklore and professorial positions. Just as scholarly authority over "folklore" marked the disciplinary boundary from within, Dorson's explicitly polemical concept of "fakelore" drew it from without, demonizing commercialization, the mass media, "frivolous" folklore investigations, and scholars from other disciplines who "dabbled with folklore" (7) as possessors of mere fakelore. The key marker of the disciplinary boundary was fieldwork, which other scholars did not undertake (at least properly), even as professional training prepared "the academic folklorist [for] zeroing in on a specific target" (1976:13).

The power of boundary-work in mid-twentieth-century folkloristics helps us understand why theory played a limited role in North American folkloristics until recent decades. The fate of folkloristics depended, Dorson claimed, on laying exclusive claim to distinct objects, methods, professional societies, texts, and departments—not theories. The papers in which Dorson claimed theoretical ground, "A Theory for American Folklore" (1959) and "A Theory for American Folklore Reviewed" (1969), are exceptions that prove the rule. Dorson argued that "students of American folklore must find common theoretical ground if they aspire to be more than random collectors or public entertainers" (1959:212). In the 1960s, anthropology, linguistics, sociology, literary studies, and other disciplines were redefining themselves in theoretical terms. Dorson distanced himself from "a modish cult—say of symbolic structuralism, or sociopsychodynamics, or linguistic folklife, or computerized mythology" (1969:227). Echoing American exceptionalism, Dorson rejected foreign theories in favor of a construction of theory that starts with examples of American folklore and proposes definitions as precursors to theory. Professionalizing training in folklorists, he argues, will transform folklore scholarship into "a cooperative inquiry into the behavior of folklore within the American environment" that will "illuminate the American mind" (1959:213). Even this self-proclaimed turn to theory extended Dorson's boundary-work by adopting a narrowly inductive, not to mention nationalist, understanding of theory that was explicitly defined in opposition to the definitions of theory that were galvanizing and redefining other disciplines. US folklorists could not simply become part of the global expansion of British folkloristics. Building a discipline from made-in-the-USA folklore created a boundary vis-à-vis European folkloristics: high theory was to remain on the other side of the Atlantic.[1]

I suggest that the question is not just whether folklorists produce or use theory but theory's marginality to discipline building. Placing boundary-work at the core of discipline-building strategies produced a strong sense of commitment and esprit de corps; nevertheless, as Fine (2008) points out, theory plays a crucial role in providing intellectual cohesion and coherence. Uniting around objects, methods, and a zealous commitment to protect the discipline against usurpers is less successful in fostering broad participation in intellectual debates.

Here I note a contradiction in Dundes's role in the field. Dundes became the major successor to his teacher in continuing Dorson's role as folkloristics' primary boundary worker.[2] Most folklorists attribute Dundes's inability to promote theory to his having bet on the wrong theoretical horse (leaving his earlier explorations of structuralism aside here). Nevertheless, the tremendous importance of psychoanalysis in history, literature, feminist studies, and other fields in recent decades would suggest that the case is not so simple. Indeed, bringing new interpretations of Freud, Jacques Lacan ([1966] 1977), and other psychoanalysts into folkloristics could have created theoretical dialogues across disciplines. I would, rather, argue that Dundes's difficulties in generating more interest in theory emerges from his persistent efforts to press boundary-work as the sine qua non for discipline-building—or, increasingly, discipline-preservation—strategies for folkloristics. By definition, central reliance on boundary-work produces, in Noyes's (2016) terms, provincial intellectuals, defined through their (self)exclusion from what they characterize as metropolitan sites of high theory production.

During the Cold War expansion of scientific ideologies and resources in the mid-twentieth century, Dorson and some of his students passionately expanded disciplinary autonomy, scholarly authority, academic departments and programs, grants, and public recognition. The unstable "poetics of disappearance" (Kirshenblatt-Gimblett 1998b:300–302) that defined a continually vanishing object helped create and naturalize new forms of modernity (Bauman and Briggs 2003). In a post–Cold War, postmodern, fragmenting, and rapidly shifting world, the market for modernities collapsed and then became restructured as a critical, reflexive enterprise. The juxtaposition of closely guarded boundaries and claims to scholarly authority with the erosion of resources and prestige sparked a proliferation of declensionist disciplinary narratives—folklorists' dysfunctional tales of woe. Following up on a point by Bauman (2008), communicative technologies were often used as means of demarcating the boundary of folklore—through their placement on the other side. Accordingly, practitioners could not claim shifting and productive relationships to new technologies as scholarly sites—even as Hermann Bausinger ([1961] 1990) was convincing European folklorists of their productivity.[3]

THEORETICAL BOUNDARY CROSSING AS DISCIPLINARY STRATEGY

The experience of the 1960s and 1970s suggests, however, that folkloristics can generate substantial academic authority creating analytical models that generate dialogic zones with adjacent disciplines—in short, in theoretically inspired boundary *crossing*. Dell Hymes (1974) placed folklore and folkloristics at the center of the "ethnography of speaking," infusing a new analytic perspective that galvanized research in anthropology, communication, linguistics, and folkloristics with such central notions as genre, repertoire, community, and transmission.[4] Hymes (1981) and Bauman (1977) then used the notion of performance in redefining and reinterpreting folklorists' objects of study.

Two features are crucial here. First, whether or not one wants to call these frameworks "theory," they generated broad textual networks through shared analytic principles. Second, rather than defending boundaries, folklorists drew on concepts and modes of analysis from anthropology, literary studies, linguistics, and history, and they convinced other scholars that folkloristics was valuable for their own fields of inquiry. The cross-disciplinary dialogue that took place in the 1980s in the *Journal of American Folklore*, the cross-disciplinary popularity of folklore courses, the demand for folklorists in other departments, and the emergence of symposia and special issues on performance in adjacent fields indicate the success of this opposing mode of discipline building. Theoretically oriented folklorists seemed to have been clearly aware during this period that theory is, as Fine (2008) suggests, productive of social-textual networks.

Nonetheless, my goal, to brutalize Shakespeare, is not to praise Bauman and Hymes and bury Dorson. Indeed, more theoretically or analytically based strategies have their drawbacks, too, and these are tied to the epistemological and social underpinnings of the very notion of theory. As Mary Poovey (1998) shows, the theory/fact opposition is a quintessentially modern artifact, reflecting an Enlightenment conviction that facts can exist apart from interests, opinions, and epistemological positions and that general propositions occupy a privileged sphere that is not contingent on history or politics. What gets defined as "theory" is what can best dress itself up as rational, general, disinterested, abstract, and universal—that is, as quintessentially modern and "Western." As Mills (2008) observes, theory is markedly interdiscursive, explicitly tied to other academic texts; it is also metadiscursive, defining, limiting, and regulating what counts as scholarly discourse within a particular field. What is perhaps most crucial for folkloristics is that the social location of the author helps decide what gets classified as "theoretical": the words of white, male senior professors from leading US or European universities are much more likely to be dubbed theoretical (I write self-reflexively) than those of women of color, scholars in schools that lack graduate programs, or nonacademics.

Notions of "high," "middle," and "low" presuppose this privileging of seemingly decontextualized, abstract discourse, project spatial/social relations in epistemological terms, and reproduce the scale-making claims of theory—the idea that it can enable us to jump from universalities to particularities and back without losing our balance. I would locate the politics of theory less in *theories* as epistemological objects than in *theorizing*, in discursive practices that both produce certain types of formulations and frame them as theory. Theoretical discourse is thus potentially exclusionary, expelling merely empirical, classificatory, or methodological work and creating hierarchically ordered textual networks—with the generators of theories on top, their authorized interpreters next, those charged with "applying" them to data just below, and researchers seemingly ignorant of or incapable of citing theory on the bottom. Hierarchies of prestige between universities, within nations and between them, get naturalized in the process. Ever since the seventeenth century, claiming privileged access to spaces constituted by seemingly abstract, general, interest-free knowledge and immunity from forms of situatedness that seemingly constrain the aspirations to universality (Tsing 2005) of projects framed as theoretical has formed a crucial infrastructure for white supremacy and the production of racial hierarchies.

Roberts (2008) indicates how closely theorizing reproduces racial inequalities. The continuing force of three centuries of identifying the speech of white, elite, Euro-American males with rationality, abstraction, and the unmarked subject, and of projecting women, the working classes, and people of color as "local" and marked subjects whose speech is concrete and provincial (Bauman and Briggs 2003; Shapin 1994) is painfully captured by the marginalization of work on African American folklore as well as the fate of Américo Paredes's *With His Pistol in His Hand* (1958). As I detail in chapter 3, half a century ago, Paredes reconceptualized folklore as politically charged expressive forms that define the shifting borders of conflict, difference, and oppression. Some of Paredes's colleagues and students incorporated these insights (see Bauman 1971; Bauman and

Abrahams 1981; Limón 1994), but most folklorists continued to embrace a consensus model built around a reified, depoliticized notion of folklore. If folklorists had followed Paredes's lead, I suspect that the field would be enjoying a much stronger position in the contemporary academic landscape which, as Roberts (1999, 2008) suggests, is centrally concerned with cultural pluralism. Rather, as José Limón notes, Paredes has been expunged from most genealogies of folkloristics (2007).

Theory-based modes of disciplining folkloristics can thus be as exclusionary as boundary-work–centered strategies. Although one or the other tends to predominate at particular times and within specific textual-social networks, they intersect and overlap in complex ways, reproducing social and epistemological hierarchies and obstructing creativity. According to boundary-making perspectives, only professional folklorists can discover a ready-made object and then collect, classify, entextualize, analyze, and compare it. From the theory-centered perspective, analytic principles are generated in academic settings and used in determining which phenomena are "theoretically relevant." These strategies converge in generating scholarly narratives that cast nonacademics as makers of folklore and academics as producers of folkloristic knowledge.

Missing here are some of the key sources of theoretical or analytic creativity. As I outlined in the introduction, I have worked on the expressive culture of Spanish-speaking areas of New Mexico and a region in Venezuela where Warao (an Indigenous language) is spoken. In both, I could only begin to comprehend the vast amount of knowledge that shaped everyday life after I apprenticed myself to intellectuals, individuals recognized as reflecting actively and creatively on social life and its discursive representation. George and Silvianita López in New Mexico and Santiago and María Rivera in Venezuela had contemplated for decades the aesthetic features and social/political impact of the discursive genres they performed and the material forms they produced.[5] In researching proverbs, legends, curing songs, laments, and other forms, I spent years with them, participating in daily life, recording and transcribing performances, and collaborating in interpretive work. The Lópezes had attended elementary school, but the only formal education open to the Riveras (brother and sister) were the English classes that I provided. With all four, I entered into discussions of quite abstract and complexly interdiscursive formulations that explicitly served metadiscursive functions, seeking to define, interpret, and regulate everyday discourse. Trying to understand Mrs. López's proverb performances, for example, involved a radically different way of defining proverbs and tracing their rhetorical effects (Briggs 1988). I did not *find* discursive objects—these and other mentors *told* me what I should document. I am not suggesting that my analyses flowed directly from their perspectives; my interpretations rather emerged by bringing their words into dialogue with philosophy, history, folkloristics, anthropology, ethnic and racial studies, ethnomusicology, and other fields.

Both anti-theoretical boundary-work and folklorist-as-theorist perspectives teach us to approach "informants" as purveyors of cultural forms who lack the ability to consciously analyze them—and who are therefore positioned outside scholarly boundary. Scholars who follow these ideologies commonly draw on their collaborators' analytic reflections but fail to acknowledge their role in the work of theorizing. In doing so, they reproduce racial, national, class, and professional hierarchies and commit serious lapses of professional ethics by failing to acknowledge intellectual debts. Noyes (2008) may indeed be correct in asserting that folklorists suffer from an "inferiority complex" vis-à-vis other scholars, but both Dorson's (1976) rejection of "amateurs" and "popularizers" and the general failure to acknowledge "folk" collaborators would suggest (to adopt psychoanalytic terms) a form of compensation that results in a superiority complex in relation to nonacademic theoreticians.

Both boundary-work and theory-driven approaches also fall short by failing to grasp how "the object" often contains "the theory." Bauman and I have drawn on Bakhtin (1981, 1986) in suggesting that performances are not snapshots of a particular moment in time but complex cartographies of the movement of discourses, subjectivities, and politics between contexts, genres, and texts (Bauman and Briggs 1990; Briggs and Bauman 1992). As Margaret Mills presciently suggests, "our data—anecdotes, gossip, incidents where we were present—are *always already* speaking 'theory'—somebody's theory, theory in the everyday—and it's our job to sort out *whose* theory" (1993:174, emphasis in original). Texts themselves are thus both interdiscursive and metadiscursive, attempting to shape how participants will "read" prior discourse and how they will project what is said or written into the future. In many cases, these interdiscursive and metadiscursive cartographies achieve a high level of scope and traction. In short, "the theory" can be right there in "the data." Folklorists, as Dell Hymes (1981) reminds us, are taught to look closely at texts not just as aesthetic or ethnographic objects but also as sources of insight into social life and ways of interpreting it (see also Abrahams 2005). A recent book by Alex Chávez (2017) provides a model here. Chávez, himself a performer, includes extensive transcriptions of texts from *huapango arribeño* performances, in which two groups of musicians engage in competitive and dialogic exchanges that last most of the night. Rather than simply fodder for Chávez to demonstrate his theoretical prowess, however, the texts themselves introduce key dimensions of the book's analytic. *Sounds of Crossing* is thus as dialogic as the performances it documents, as Chávez exchanges analytics with the performers, creating a challenge for readers who have learned to look only to the author's words (and the scholars she or he quotes) in locating theory.

BEYOND BOUNDARY-WORK AND THEORY-BASED HIERARCHIES: A PROPOSAL

I would like to provocatively lay out some proposals:

1. *Theory is dead! Long live theory!* Insofar as "theory" is defined in Enlightenment terms and is tied to a means of generating and naturalizing practices of exclusion and subordination, folklorists should rightly reject "grand theory" and its less pretentious equivalents. Here I stand with Haring (2008a) in echoing literary theorists who reject the use of theory as a means of regulating scholarly writing axiomatically.
2. Nevertheless, I am not arguing against theorizing. Without powerful interdiscursive and metadiscursive principles we must rely on boundary-work to generate debates that renew disciplinary objects and methods. Nor do I wish to rule out discipline-building practices altogether, strategies for refashioning folkloristics and efforts to secure resources and authority. I think rather that we should develop new disciplinary practices that depend neither on boundary-work nor standard theory-building modes.
3. One way that folklorists can take the lead in redefining and repositioning the category of theory is to document *practices of vernacular theorizing*, metadiscourses that are excluded from the communities that are created, as Fine (2008) suggests, by academic theorizing; here we can follow up on Abrahams's (2005) and Bauman's (2008) attention to vernacular understandings of cultural forms. We must tread carefully here, because reified understandings of theory's opposite, whether defined as "local," "lived world," or "vernacular," are just as much products of modernity as are "theory"; embracing them uncritically thus involves presupposing and privileging theoretical concepts (see Shuman 1993; Goldstein and Shuman 2016). Vernacular is

defined in opposition to something else; vernacular *versus* cosmopolitan distinctions reproduce local *versus* global, concrete *versus* abstract dichotomies that have sustained the opposition between modernity and traditionality for over three centuries (Bauman and Briggs 2003). In order to keep from reproducing social and epistemological hierarchies, we will need to extract the term *vernacular* from its opposition to *cosmopolitan* and the entailed denial of generality, abstractness, and explanatory capacity to vernacularity (Briggs 2005).

4. The question remains as to the relationship between *vernacular theorizing* and *theorizing the vernacular*. Rather than viewing their differences and similarities in relativist or comparative terms, I suggest tracing the intersections and exchanges that take place between them. If we examine folkloristics, anthropology, performances, and vernacular theorizing as practices for producing, circulating, and receiving knowledge, we can examine how they differentiate themselves as well as how they intersect and interact. Once we bring other disciplinary (academic) and institutionally based knowledge-making practices (such as developed by public folklorists) into the debate, we will have powerful new ways of articulating what folklore and folkloristics can offer other disciplines and sites beyond scholarly boundaries—which is crucial for the future of the profession. Fostering exchanges between knowledge-making practices across the lines of discipline, class, race, nation, and professional status will generate novel approaches and contribute centrally to decolonial, anti-racist, and justice-oriented agendas.

If "theory" is identified by its social location and its ability to present itself as abstract, rational, and general, then Noyes (2008) is probably right that folklorists will find it difficult to compete with psychology or sociology. Nevertheless, if, as Haring (2008a) argues, the Chartists and 1960s folklorists strove to democratize the notion of creativity, perhaps it is our major calling now to democratize the notion of theory, to acknowledge the crucial theoretical insights that we gain from vernacular intellectuals. Mills (2008) interestingly asks who gets credit for generating interdisciplinary ideas; I would like to extend this question to interlocutors classified as nonacademics.

I have not offered "a new theory" of theory here. My goals are more modest, at the same time that they are not simply "methodological." I hope to have identified a major impediment to theory building—too great a reliance on boundary-work—and suggested why this practice is partially responsible for disciplinary setbacks, especially in the United States. I pointed to the centrality of participation in interdisciplinary theory building in giving rise to junctures during the twentieth century in which folkloristics enjoyed scholarly visibility and access to academic resources. Suggesting that conventional understandings of "theory" and who gets recognized for doing it can also be exclusionary and hierarchicalizing, I urged recognition of a broader community of theorists. Such a community would include practitioners in other disciplines and thinkers heretofore barred from academic networks. I argue that links should be created through detailed attention to how different theoretical communities produce knowledge, how discourses and practices move between them, and the differences of power and political economy that shape who gets credit for theorizing and gets to claim their formulations as intellectual property.

Here we can fruitfully bring Wittgenstein into our network. Knocking down all boundaries—folding folkloristics into anthropology, cultural studies, performance studies, or cross-disciplinary programs—would undermine its intellectual locus as a unique crossroads between vernacular theorists and theorists of the vernacular. We need new theories, and making and debating them will require new spaces for theorizing, for creatively rethinking concepts, practices, rhetorics, and objects and imagining how they can inform and be informed by the profound transformations of culture and capital, bodies and labor taking place in the contemporary world. This project will require recognition and support from foundations, states, agencies, and nongovernmental and international organizations as well as from universities, which, in turn, will require boundaries: there needs to be a there *there* for researchers to be taken seriously. Rather than creating boundaries based on discrete, fixed objects and methods and spending our time defending them, trying to keep folklorists in and intruders out, folkloristics might take a clue from Wittgenstein's words in the epigraph and focus on maintaining a flexible, playful relationship to boundaries, jumping over them in such a way as to link and enrich the games being played on both sides.[6]

NOTES

1. Here Dorson replays Henry Rowe Schoolcraft's textual nationalism (Bauman and Briggs 2003, chapter 7).

2. See Dow's anecdote (2008:60) in which Dundes repeatedly asks German scholars, "Where's the folklore?" Dundes's boundary-work often took the form of a statement: "That's not folklore!" He begins his essay with a declensionist story in which the erosion of clear disciplinary boundaries has resulted in a "sad situation" in which "there is no longer

a purely separate, independent doctoral program in folklore per se anywhere in the United States" (2005:385).

3. Dundes (1980:17) provides an important exception here.

4. Hymes's ability to cross disciplinary boundaries and reconfigure work within them is signaled by his election to the presidencies of the American Folklore Society, the American Anthropological Association, and the Linguistic Society of America.

5. Doctors, epidemiologists, lawyers, and politicians have also been my collaborators in theorizing cultural forms over the years.

6. Elizabeth Kelley kindly brought this quote from Wittgenstein to my attention.

2

Contested Mobilities
On the Politics and Ethnopoetics of Circulation

LIKE FRANZ BOAS AND EDWARD SAPIR, DELL HYMES connected linguistic anthropology with social/cultural anthropology and folkloristics. The terms he coined and the perspectives he advanced drew on wider perspectives, thus bringing linguistic anthropologists into larger conversations and enabling work in linguistic anthropology to gain greater visibility among colleagues with different disciplinary allegiances. I would argue that this is precisely the move that has long fostered new spurts of creativity within the subdiscipline and greater visibility for linguistic anthropologists. Work on performance inaugurated in the 1970s by Hymes (1981) and Richard Bauman (1977) energized not only anthropology but also linguistics, communication, and literary studies; the cross-fertilization between linguistic anthropology and folkloristics at this juncture was crucial, as has been true at other points as well. Studies of ideologies of language (Kroskrity 2000; Schieffelin, Woolard, and Kroskrity 1998) suddenly transported linguistic anthropology from the relative doldrums of the 1980s to a period when new faculty positions opened up and anthropologists came to see that linguistic anthropologists had a great deal to offer to studies on such topics as colonialism (Hanks 2010; Irvine 2001; Keane 2007), media anthropology (Spitulnik 2002), and more. A crucial feature of these points of intersection is that they did not simply "borrow" from adjacent fields but critically revised foundational concepts.

We are, I would argue, at precisely another juncture where a shot of epistemological energy would be particularly valuable. A number of linguistic anthropologists have recently taken on issues that are of interest to other scholars by focusing on race, racism, and anti-immigrant discourses (Blommaert and Verschueren 1998; Chávez 2017; Hill 2008; Mendoza-Denton 2008; Rosa 2019), therapeutic regimes (Briggs and Mantini-Briggs

2003; Carr 2011; Dick and Wirtz 2011), globalization (Blommaert 2010), and how languages, linguistic practices, and constructions of language get commodified in neoliberal market schemes (Duchêne and Heller 2012; Heller and McElhinny 2017). Rather than take up objects framed as "new," articles by Gerald L. Carr and Barbra Meek (2013), Sean Patrick O'Neill (2013), and David W. Samuels (2013) engage ethnopoetics in ways that open up different strategies for building dialogues among folklorists, anthropologists, and other scholars. Recently, a great deal of work by social scientists has focused on circulation and mobility, and here, I think, is a way to extend ethnopoetics and articulate what it can offer to scholars of other stripes.

PROBLEMATIZING CIRCULATION AND (IM)MOBILITY

It would be easy to point to stimuli for a shift in emphasis from how cultures inhabit spaces to how they travel, to use the terms posed in James Clifford's (1997) *Routes*. Certainly Arjun Appadurai's (1996) work on globalization and influential reformulations by Saskia Sassen (2006), Aihwa Ong (Ong and Collier 2005), and Ana Tsing (2005, 2015) have been important here. For people who think about language and performativity, Jacques Derrida's (1988) critique of what he characterized as the analytical limits of J. L. Austin's (1962) "total speech situation" was important. Derrida sought to locate performativity not in originary acts of speaking but in iterative movements in which "something new takes place" (1988:40). Discourse, he suggested, is neither free-floating nor locked in contexts. John Urry (2007) argued that casting particular technologies and practices as intrinsically mobile required profound changes in ideologies, practices, landscapes, and modes of embodiment, adding that making some phenomena seem mobile simultaneously casts others as inherently immobile.

Geoffrey Bowker and Susan Leigh Star (1999) suggested that in the case of diagnostic categories and statistics, producing mobility involves two contradictory processes. First, unique configurations of "expert" knowledge, objects, and practices enable categories and statistics to circulate and multiply in particular sites. Retaining their mobility requires, however, that the indexical traces of these complex constellations be stripped off to enable them to circulate and retain their authority.[1] Some actors, interests, languages, conflicts, technologies, and the like must disappear; of the stuff that circulates, some features become figures and others part of the ground, some get referentially coded while others are lodged in nonreferential features. Reception, of course, further complicates this process, as some people who get interpolated down the line know enough of the indexical histories to infer elements that have been erased while others are unable to decode even foregrounded elements.

Work in anthropology, science-technology-society (STS) studies, and other areas on circulation thus suggests a number of points. First, scholars often seem to imbibe a sort of naive neoliberal Darwinism of cultural forms and objects, including languages, narratives, and texts—the sense that people always want them to move as far, as fast, as freely, and as long as possible, which Greg Urban (2001) refers to as a metaculture of modernity. Second, mobility is not intrinsic but imbued through complex processes that involve forms of silencing and erasure. Third, forms, objects, and the like do not move evenly or naturally, like water flowing downhill but, as Tsing (2005) suggests, travel through particular sorts of grooves or channels and often encounter resistance along the way. Fourth, making mobility involves creating immobility; as with secrets and gossip, people are sometime more interested in limiting or stopping circulation than in inducing it. Fifth, people construct cultural or ideological models of circulation at the same time that they engage in complex circulatory practices. Although we may reify our models as faithful maps of how things are actually moving, the two are never identical; here we encounter anew the questions of metapragmatics and pragmatics and of language ideologies that linguistic anthropologists have analyzed so extensively. One final point: scholars have no privileged or disinterested position here; when we construct cartographies of circulation and mobility, we are just as caught up in these processes as anyone else, just as much at the mercy of our own models of mobility and techniques of (im)mobilization.

RECIRCULATING ETHNOPOETICS

Whence ethnopoetics? In a word, its study has long revealed the complexities of how processes of indexical embedding and making mobile are invested in narratives. Exploring these two dimensions in a richly ethnographic modality, Carr and Meek (2013), O'Neill (2013), and Samuels (2013) critique ways that received, generally implicit models of circulation impede our understanding of how narratives, texts, and languages circulate. They go on to suggest how narratives and translated sermons and language revitalization projects involve complex intersections between competing models and practices. My goal here is to use the insights they offer in opening up broader questions of circulation and mobility, thereby hoping to increase their potential for contributing to ways that folklorists, anthropologists, and other scholars discuss these issues.

O'Neill (2013) usefully repositions the translation of narratives from northwestern California into the context of relations between Native American nations. His article seems to suggest that some of the most famous work in the Americanist tradition was informed by a shallow model of circulation that led such scholars as Alfred Kroeber and Edward Sapir to overestimate "the *uniformity* of the regional culture" rather than to see how the people they studied were as interested in imbuing cultural forms with immobility as with fostering their broad dissemination (224; emphasis in original). O'Neill points to the Boasian roots of what he terms a "fidelity ideology" (221), which culturally constructs a trajectory from "the original text" (220) through inscription, translation, and publication, which sounds to me rather like what I have called the ideology of intertextual transparency (Briggs 1993b). This model would lead us to expect that translation practices at least strive to maximize circulation.

O'Neill's ethnographic skill is revealed in the way he listened to his collaborators' refusals—both to translate entire texts as well as to "preserve" such details as the gender of characters. What emerges is a complex construction of circulation that refuses the dictates of a free market of cultural forms, if you will. O'Neill turned what must have been tense moments when translators transformed their assigned tasks into pedagogical events in which his collaborators could teach him a variety of models and practices of circulation. These seemed to range from "wholesale adoption" to "parodic mimicry" to transformations of the gender identifications of characters to outright rejections of narratives (226). Reflecting on the way his consultants opened up competing models of circulation, O'Neill looks at other perspectives that problematize what we could call open-source, unrestricted-intellectual-property perspectives on the translation and the circulation of texts, especially those framed as religious or spiritual (see Povinelli 2016).

The origin stories for tales, songs, and "visible features of the world" (O'Neill 2013:244) that O'Neill's consultants provided were also origin stories of circulatory models, as embodied in such powerful characters as Coyote and Across-the-Ocean Widower. One might suspect that the grammatical properties he identifies, such as tense/aspect forms that projected the temporal contours of narrative events, might also have been modeling circulation as "ongoing, without a clear beginning or end" (233) or, in other cases, as cutting off circulation in the distant past. At times, translators stopped the circulation process right in front of O'Neill's eyes. His discussion of how "speech taboos" posed obstacles to translation is perhaps the most suggestive in this regard. Here translators encountered boundary objects (Star and Griesemer 1989), which seemed to suggest how selves, narratives, spaces, and languages were positioned on borders, a theme I will revisit below and in the following chapter.[2] And then comes the sucker punch: even as narratives sometimes become immobile, it is songs composed of what are often referred to as "nonsense syllables" that seemed to be designed for circulation across cultural and linguistic borders, "allowing members of each speech community to understand some of what is going on in any given performance" (242).

Echoing the proposition that poetics provides "an implicit schema for the organization of experience" (Hymes 1996:121), Samuels (2013) takes us into a realm of experience that might be acutely uncomfortable for most anthropologists—Christian missionization. Here he traverses the bridge between poetics and social/cultural anthropology that Webb Keane (2007) opened up in *Christian Moderns*. Scholars may participate in Urban's (2001) metaculture of modernity yet at the same time have a bias for stable replication in the circulation of signs classified as traditional. This dual fetishization of circulatory motion can lead to too easy a jump from poetics to ethics, to viewing the imposition of obstacles to circulation as ethical violations; efforts to promote circulation thus become ipso facto confirmations of ethical sanctity. Linda Tuhiwai Smith argues that "the word itself, 'research,' is probably one of the dirtiest words in the Indigenous world's vocabulary" (1999:1), adding that it is always "embedded in multiple layers of imperial and colonial practices" (2). Positioning oneself as a champion of traditional circulation thus seems to confer an ethically positive aura on situations where, as Smith suggests, any research project—even when carried out by Indigenous researchers—is suspect. Here we can usefully juxtapose Sherry Ortner's (1995) concept of ethnographic refusal: consultants and/or ethnographers can decide that *not* allowing particular topics to circulate through ethnography, recordings, interpretion, or publications is the best ethical course.

Herein lies, in my view, the potential of Samuels's work for stimulating rethinkings of both ethnopoetics and circulation. He traces practices of translation that many of his readers would probably like to see *fail*, bringing up the problematics of relationships between linguists and missionaries working in the same sites—and sometimes being one and the same person. By drawing attention to "poetic and rhetorical forms undergoing the stresses of postcolonial expropriation and missionary influence" (2013:274), his article raises the specter of another form of relativity, which, adding to Whorfian and Hymesian notions, I might term *colonial relativity*. I use this term to help us think about how different interpretations of the same forms may reflect their embeddedness in distinct experiences of colonial violence and expropriation. These indexical connections are not "post" (postcolonial) for many Indigenous peoples, as Smith (1999:98) suggests.

Colonial relativity emerges in how missionaries preaching to San Carlos Apaches also embraced, like anthropologists, notions of fidelity or intertextual transparency, similarly framing faux translations as ethical problems. Their focus was not, however, on the transformation of oral texts into written transcriptions and translations but of positioning Scripture in oral performances of sermons. Here transparency went hand in hand with the sort of anti-poetic poetics and anti-rhetorical rhetoric that would have made John Locke happy. Samuels explores medieval theories that tied ethics to achieving the proper relationship between poetics and truth, form and content. This discussion also points, I would suggest, to how these histories similarly tie ethical positioning and the politics of performativity to debates about circulation and mobility, about which discursive forms should circulate and which dimensions should be infused with mobility—poetics, logical content, or perfect proportional relations between the two.

In comparing missionary Alfred Uplegger's 1964 Easter Sunday sermon and its translation by Fergus Sneezy, Samuels examines the juxtaposition of competing practices for circulating Christian texts. Suggesting that "Hymes consistently emphasized the culturally embedded nature of intersubjectivity in verbal practice" (2013:225), Samuels draws attention to the "circulation of culture" by detailing what Lee and LiPuma (2003) refer to as cultures of circulation. Samuels notes Hymes's statement that "the way that a mother speaks to a child contains as much poetry as the most elaborate ceremony" (2013:255). Hymes's (1981) analysis of the Clackamas narrative "Seal (and) her younger brother lived there" might suggest that how children talk back can reveal the importance of competing models of circulation, where insisting on unquestioning replication of the voice of custom and the shushing of efforts to disrupt it can have lethal effects. In the end, Hymes emerges less as an analytical voice that stands outside of history than as an advocate—alongside the Uplegger family, Sneezy, and medieval commentators—for particular perspectives on poetics and truth, practices of translation, and models of circulation.

Carr and Meek (2013) point to another site for enacting conflicting models of circulation. They extend Hymes's efforts to shift the camera angle, here actually turning it around, focusing less on "language loss" by Yukon Aboriginal peoples than the ideologies of language, text, and circulation that shape interventions by linguists and educators into Aboriginal language education and revitalization. Here, we might say, a confrontation between object-centered and process-centered models of circulation is evident. In the "rule of experts," to use Timothy Mitchell's (2002) phrase, the circulation of language over time and between generations requires the production of an object that can be exchanged—a text—resulting in a form of text fetishism, extending Karl Marx's ([1867] 1967) "commodity fetishism," that seemed to dominate in many of the language revitalization projects they describe. What was missed in overlooking "the interactive dimension of storytelling" (Carr and Meek 2013:201)? Might Hymes's (1981) distinction between report and performance enter in here? Might the elders have been onto something?

The Yukon elders seemed to grasp problems of scale (see Carr and Lempert 2016) better than the "experts": modeling circulation in interaction might seem to project how circulation occurs over the *longue durée*, over lifetimes and generations. Real-time simulations might provide an aura that is lacking in reporting the existence of temporally and socially distanced narrative worlds. In invoking Walter Benjamin (1968), I want to juxtapose two of his essays—"The Work of Art in the Age of Mechanical Reproduction" and "The Storyteller." Benjamin warns about what happens to narrative transmission when it is severed from the material practices in which both the transmission and the performance of stories are embedded. In the eyes of language pedagogy experts, the mobility of language from place to place and generation to generation was centered in the materiality of easily transportable objects, texts; if everyone could just focus on these objects, their intrinsic mobility would guarantee circulation.

Elders, from what I can see, were highly attuned to the processes of erasure required by the production of texts and who controlled their circulation. They rather insisted on the centrality of performance—that is, on imbuing discourse with mobility by the online, real-time creation of new indexical histories. This, in turn, required metapragmatic calibration (Silverstein 1993) of a very specific sort, calibration of relationships between indexical histories and how narratives are embedded in them. Weaving displays of words and knowledge into preschool activities or tanning moose hides required calibrating how the circulation of cultural forms was woven into a succession of indexical histories, not just a single, reified proximal context. Materiality was not exhausted by a text, by spoken words, or by moose hides and blocks; it rather entailed relating these materialities to those concerned with caring for younger siblings or other features of daily life and labor. The elders privileged performance as a site not just for exhibiting narratives but for enacting models of circulation, for putting on display acts that imbue cultural forms with mobility through the collaborative creation of new indexical histories and recovering remembered histories.

BACK TO CIRCULATION, VIA ETHNOPOETICS

These issues invite us to reflect anew on what I would call, following Gregory Bateson (1972), the foundational double bind of Americanist linguistics. In researching Kumeyaay language pedagogy, in which he participated, Kalim Smith (2005) documented how linguists declared their firm belief in linguistic diversity at the same time that they were often blind to the wide range of language ideologies in which it was situated. Combine the ethical positioning I cited above and this foundational double bind and what do you get? "Hi. I have come to help you save your language. But *we* can only succeed if *you* accept *my* definition of language (as embodied in grammars and dictionaries) and materializing strategies, as centered on the production of grammars, dictionaries, and other texts and their use in structuring projects and interactions." Language "preservation" seems to come at the cost of symbolic violence, in Pierre Bourdieu's (1991) terms, of displacing a complex array of language ideologies and related models of circulation in favor of singular, totalizing, seemingly scientific models. Carr and Meek (2013), O'Neill (2013), and Samuels (2013) articulate how this violence has been inflicted and how Native Americans have placed obstacles in its path.

Imbuing objects with mobility entails encountering obstacles to circulation and restrictions as well as creatively inventing tactics for navigating the channels or grooves through which particular cultural forms travel in specific directions. Urry's (2007) analysis of the simultaneous production of mobilities and immobilities and Bowker and Star's (1999) scrutiny of the indexical stripping required to make categories and numbers circulate point to the problems that arise when anthropologists and folklorists embrace naïve teleologies for the circulation of cultural forms and use them as means of ethical self-posturing. As these authors reveal, past generations of scholars may have succeeded less in salvaging natural circulatory circuits than in buying into rather shallow, monologic models that led them to miss—or even sometimes to suppress—the diversity of practices people were attempting to use in inoculating languages and cultures against successive plagues of colonial violence or, perhaps more humbly, just imbuing translations of sermons with parallelism and other poetic resonances.

What, then, do we make of Native Americans who are generously granted the status of privileged circulators by anthropologists, missionaries, educators, funding agencies and, one might add, tribal councils, but who then seem to obstreperously impose impediments by refusing to focus exclusively on written texts, pointing out that kids are not listening, or by just saying no—not only to whites (no, you may *not* record that story) but to narratives from neighboring nations as well? Ethnopoetics, as usual, looks closely at these processes, discerning how grammatical forms, the gender of a name, a tabooed word, or a cacophonous cascade of blocks can disrupt hegemonic models and practices of circulation. "Just technical issues," many scholars may say, but these Native American interventions might suggest to them, if they are listening, how the materiality of objects like high-priced mushrooms (Tsing 2015) or global pharmaceuticals (Petryna, Lakoff, and Kleinman 2006) might be imbricated with such silly things as morphemes, discourse particles, nonsense syllables, and rhetorical patterns.

The return, with Carr and Meek (2013), to performance provides a particularly important lesson here. Bauman and Briggs emphasized the centrality of entextualization to performance; fashioning "a stretch of linguistic production into a unit—a *text*" can foreground gaps between indexical histories as well as attempts to minimize them, thereby modeling circulation in quite different ways (1990:73; emphasis in original). What Bauman (2008) referred to as vernacular philology (see chapter 1) involves collaboratively recovering what seemed to have been erased and thinking about how to create mobile forms that do not reproduce colonial models of circulation. Drawing attention to intertextuality, heteroglossia, and mixed genres complicates notions of indexical erasure and points to how embedding and disembedding do not stand in complementary distribution. The forms of collaboration in which most of us engage these days involve us directly in the making of indexical histories, the production of texts (often digital), the staging of performances, and the creation of events centered on cross-generational circulation; we thus help shape forms of entextualization that erase or background some indexical features and foreground others. In 2009, Warao communities in eastern Venezuela asked me to use curing songs taught me by people who are now deceased on patients *and* for a copy of my archive. The challenges involved in complying with both requests have increased my awareness that participation in the production of indexical histories spans generations and can make our own roles uncomfortably visible.

Thinking dialogically, there is also an important lesson here for scholars about being willing to listen to their colleagues. A rich anthropology of documents (Riles 2006; Brenneis 2006) and recent work on the intimate place of inscription in bureaucratic practices (Gupta 2012; Hull 2012) might help us think about why written texts so quintessentially embody mobility and modernity, far beyond the constraints of the outmoded opposition between orality and literacy. Linguistic anthropologists and folklorists often fail to attend to how colleagues in other areas have critically retheorized the material, medical, legal, environmental, or other objects that constitute the mere referents of the forms they scrutinize. When dialogue is not only reciprocal but critically transformative, as Hymes suggested, creativity and renewal can proliferate.

One of my favorite narratives is a Hopi I'isaw story told by Helen Sekaquaptewa (1978) to her grandchildren, filmed by Larry Evers, which has been analyzed by David Shaul (2002), Andrew Wiget (1987), and Dell Hymes (1992). Observing the birds from a distance, I'isaw, a figure generally (but, according to Risling Baldy 2015, incorrectly) translated as Coyote, tries to get close enough to turn them into "a snack" (Wiget 1987:302). He watches them winnow grass seeds, blow away the husks, and then fly above Old Oraibi. Trying to beguile the birds, I'isaw is himself beguiled as he learns their song:

> Pota, pota, pota,
> pota, pota, pota,
> yowa'ini, yowa'ini,
> ph, ph, ph, ph.

Adorning him with their own feathers, the birds then lure I'isaw into flying up with them higher and higher, at which point they take back their feathers one by one. He falls to his death.

This narrative suggests what ethnopoetics can offer to the study of circulation and mobility—and also constitutes a cautionary tale. Ms. Sekaquaptewa masterfully models the circulation of cultural forms here in multiple ways simultaneously. In showing us how I'isaw learned the birds' song, she is also modeling how her grandchildren can learn both song and story. Here models of circulation imbue cultural features with mobility in particularly forceful ways, drawing bodies and voices as well as heads and ears into the process. As Carr and Meek (2013) and the elders with whom they worked observed, this process operates as much in performances as in circulating texts. Ms. Sekaquaptewa's use of her own voice, face, head, and hands points to the crucial role of intersubjectivity as she moves frequently between a variety of positionalities—a narrator who draws her grandchildren into becoming co-performers as much as an actor who assumes the shifting spatial-temporal-behavioral-linguistic positionalities of I'isaw, birds, narrator, and grandmother. (I return to this point in chapter 5.) The expressive potential of features of the narrative are doubled through use of cante fable (a mixed genre, to use Bakhtin's 1986 term), enabling Ms. Sekaquaptewa to infuse the story with drama, bring her characters to life, expose their ethical and subjective complexities, imbue them with possibilities for ethical reflection, juxtapose a world in which birds can speak and coyotes can fly with the contemporary world confronted by Hopi children, and open up powerful forms of interaction with her young, shy interlocutors.

A different sort of model of circulation is also apparent here, one whose production involved the participation of not only producer Larry Evers but Ms. Sekaquaptewa's son Emory—a lawyer, judge, jeweler, University of Arizona faculty member, editor of a Hopi dictionary, and principal consultant on the film project. Originally a videotape, the recording now circulates via the internet, and English speakers can read the subtitles and learn the song, like Ms. Sekaquaptewa's grandchildren, through the various repetitions. We thereby seem to enter directly into the experience of the mobility of culture. The performativity attached to the circulation of a hybrid cultural form, a song embedded within a story, relying (as O'Neill 2013 might have predicted) on semantically empty vocables, seems to imbue it with such mobility that it can cross species and engender remarkable forms of physical mobility—a coyote can learn to fly. And this multispecies pedagogical exercise seems to engage us directly in learning the possibilities, limits, and dangers of circulation.

My simple summary of a wonderful narrative is meant to invite scholars to reflect on how they are learning complex and heterogeneous models of circulation and transporting them into scholarly realms. Nevertheless, Ms. Sekaquaptewa's story provides a strong warning. Just when we think that we have become the master cartographers of the circulation of cultural forms, we may, like poor I'isaw, be taken in by the very illusions that we help create.

NOTES

1. Indexicality is Charles S. Peirce's term. He defined it as "a sign which refers to the Object that it denotes by virtue of being really affected by that Object" ([1940] 1955:102). In his trichotomy, indexes do not signify by code-like, relatively context-independent relations between a sign and its object (symbols) or perceived similarities between the sign and its object (the icon) but emerge existentially through sharing temporal, spatial, intercorporeal, or other "contextual" relations.

2. Star and Griesemer define the term as follows: "an analytical concept of those scientific objects which both inhabit several interacting social worlds . . . *and* satisfy the informational requirements of each of them. Boundary objects are objects which are both plastic

enough to adapt to local needs and constraints of the several parties employing them, yet robust enough to maintain a common identity across sites . . . They have different meanings in different social worlds but their structure is common enough to more than one world to make them recognizable means of translation. The creation and management of boundary objects is a key process in developing and maintaining coherence across intersecting social worlds" (1989:393, emphasis in original).

3

What We Should Have Learned from Américo Paredes

The Politics of Communicability and the Making of Folkloristics

IN THE FALL OF 2007, AS I TAUGHT Américo Paredes's *With His Pistol in His Hand* to several hundred Berkeley undergraduates, I realized that the following year would mark the book's fiftieth anniversary. I soon came to the conclusion that the occasion should be marked by an event that would not only detail Paredes's many contributions to the discipline but also explore why, as José Limón (2007) has pointed out, Paredes has been virtually erased from dominant genealogies of American folkloristics.

As early as 1958, Paredes articulated a radically different agenda for folkloristics, providing insights that could have fundamentally reoriented the field's epistemological, methodological, and political points of departure. He redefined the basic object of study, offering a principled challenge to the legacy of Eurocentrism, colonialism, and racism in shaping the view that folklore consists of shared cultural elements that exist apart from modernity. Recent scholarship on Paredes has illuminated how he transformed understandings of folklore, culture, and the politics of race, both within the academy and beyond, anticipating later revolutions in ethnography and postmodern scholarship. As the lethal effects of whiteness, racism, and violence directed against racialized populations as well as long-standing demands for racial justice became the national conversation in the United States in 2020, digging more deeply into Paredes's insights and exposing the complicity that marginalized his work—along with that of other Latinx, Black, and Native American scholars—is more crucial than ever.

This task confronts us with some important questions. How can we account for folklorists' general failure to respond to the challenge presented by Paredes's work? Should folklorists concern themselves with rewriting intellectual genealogies in order to accord Paredes his proper role, particularly in light of the way that genealogical narratives—not as objects of deconstruction but as positive acts of constructing memory and scholarly canons—are often disparaged these days? Addressing this question will initially raise the issue that is central to chapter 4: the need for multiple genealogies of folkloristics. What are the implications of this injustice, not simply for Paredes's legacy but for folkloristics and anthropology more generally?

Américo Paredes posed the fundamental challenge that this book seeks to address: unlearning scholarly infrastructures and challenging the problematic politics of knowledge that animate them. This chapter accordingly acknowledges Paredes's mentorship in shaping this project, attempts to deepen and sharpen our understanding of the analytical and political contours of Paredes's provocation, asks what would have happened if his insights had become disciplinary foundations, and ponders what kinds of futures they might still conjure.

Here, I address Paredes's work from a new angle, one that requires a theoretical intervention. Science studies scholars argue that modes of representation shape objects of scholarly analysis not only in terms of their content but also how they are produced and circulate (Knorr-Cetina 1999; Latour 1987; Rabinow 1996). Just as Paredes anticipated shifts in ethnographic representation and in the politics of culture, he pointed to a different way of thinking about how diverse actors, including folklorists, anthropologists, and laypersons, produce knowledge. I argue that Paredes's research challenged a notion that had guided the study of folklore since its inception in the seventeenth century, the assertion that the social life of folklore constitutes a sui generis circuit of circulation for cultural forms that are naturally occurring elements of the social landscape—folklore—a circuit that is defined through its autonomy from and opposition to other modes of knowledge production and circulation. Moreover, Paredes presciently offered an alternative formulation, one that is very much in line with contemporary understandings of power, difference, and the creation of publics and counter-publics.

The major thrust of the contribution I hope to make here is to identify foundational assumptions about poetics, performance, and the politics of knowledge. I build on the alternative that Paredes opened up, outlining a framework, based on the notion of communicability, that can enable us to draw on his insights in gaining new perspectives on how folkloristics developed as well as some complex and pressing problems in contemporary scholarship.[1] My goal is to help bring about the revolution in folkloristics—still timely—that Paredes's work could have sparked over a half century ago.

FOLKLORE, CONFLICT, AND THE POLITICS OF BORDERS

The wide-ranging scholarship in *With His Pistol in His Hand* seems to coalesce around two central foci. One, of course, is the figure of Gregorio Cortez. The second is a direct challenge to a foundational assumption of folkloristics, the notion that folklore springs from shared culture. According to this view, the existence of culture is contingent on the existence of a "folk group." Alan Dundes seemed to express a radical view when he argued famously that "the term 'folk' can refer to *any group of people whatsoever* who share at least one common factor" (1980:6, emphasis in original). Gone is the Romantic Nationalist perspective that a "people" shared a deeply rooted "organic" bundle that included language, history, literature, territory, and so forth. Gone is the notion that "the folk" must be rural and illiterate and that folklore must stand apart from technology. Nevertheless, folklore still rests on commonality, common membership in a "sphere of consensus" (Hallin 1986) created by sharing a worldview and a set of cultural forms.

Rather than locating folklore within zones of shared culture, Paredes situated it along the border, which he defined as not simply the Mexico–United States border but a shifting, complex "sensitized area where two cultures or two political systems come face to face" (1993:19–20). Folklore, for Paredes, was not made within a sphere of sameness and then transported across a racialized boundary but was forged in cultural, economic, political, and physical conflicts associated with inequalities, injustice, and violence. Unlike either Enlightenment or Romantic Nationalist understandings of folklore (Bauman and Briggs 2003; Bendix 1997; Cocchiara 1981; Ó Giolláin 2000), Mexican American folklore did not preexist modernity but rather sprang precisely from modern forms of political violence—an imperialistic appropriation of a large portion of Mexico's land mass and the forced imposition of racial domination, particularly at the hands of the Texas Rangers.

To be sure, Paredes envisions two opposed Mexican American and Anglo cultures and political systems.[2] Nevertheless, Mexican American and Anglo folklores are not constituted in autonomous isolation but through dialogues, often acrimonious. Moreover, the boundaries are not hard and fast. Paredes notes that the same *corrido* (or ballad) can both laud a Mexican American uprising against Anglo-Texan rule and, in other variants, ridicule Mexican American "Seditionists" and cast the Texas Rangers in a positive light (1993:18). His classic essay "Folk Medicine and the Intercultural Jest" analyzes how jests emerged at the intersection of two borders—a class difference between middle-class narrators and working-class, especially rural dupes and a racial border between Mexican Americans and Anglos (1993:49–72). Rather than embracing a romantic and nostalgic affective stance, Paredes located these forms in a politics of ambivalence and social distance. This complexity involves not only individuals' occupations of distinct social and political locations but also their shifting positionalities springing from "the Mexican American's bilingual/bicultural makeup, which allows (or forces) him to occupy somewhat different viewpoints at different times, depending on the language he happens to be using as an instrument to calibrate his experience" (37). These words, first published in 1978, anticipate work on the politics of bilingualism, race, and racism (Hill 2008; Mendoza-Denton 2008; Rosa 2019; Urciuoli 1996; Zentella 1997) and contradictory logics of social identity (Balibar 1995).

José Limón (1992, 2012) and José López Morín (2006) have argued that Paredes's work anticipated critical and experimental strategies of ethnography in using multiple voices, irony, humor, inversion, and forms of textual heterogeneity that mirror social conflict. Limón (1992:75) suggests that "as a multiple-voiced performance, *With His Pistol in His Hand* is just such a polyphonic ethnography, a dialectical juxtaposition of identities, traditions, and cultures." Renato Rosaldo points to Paredes's foreshadowing of postmodern trends in cultural anthropology in his development of "a sophisticated conception of culture that attends to history, politics, and relations of inequality" (1991:87; see also Rosaldo 1985). López Morín (2006) suggests that Paredes's emphasis on cultural performance, his literary talents as a writer, and his cross-disciplinary perspectives helped make these later scholarly reorientations possible; he goes on to argue that Paredes's control of multiple genres of writing and performance and his reflexive explorations of his own location along various borders enabled him to surpass much later experimental work. Indeed, Paredes revealed how anthropologists construct subject positions of ethnographer and "informant," depicting the latter as one-sided, simple subjects (Gordon 1997) who can only embody homogeneous cultural patterns, not complicate, critique, or play with them—let alone critically engage ideologies of racial dominance. Unfortunately, Paredes's analysis of how ethnographers construct their authority and naturalize power relations was no more visible in the literature on ethnographic critique than in folkloristics; his work does not even appear in the bibliographies of *Writing Culture* (Clifford and Marcus 1986) or *The Predicament of Culture* (Clifford 1988).

Nevertheless, Paredes himself limited the transformation of his insights into a new agenda for folkloristics in a number of ways. Several writers have commented on Paredes's lack of attention to issues of the location of folklore along borders of gender and sexuality and the way he slips at times into a declensionist narrative, expressed in a longing for a rural, less complicated social world that seemingly once stood outside modernity and capitalism (Herrera-Sobek 1990; Limón 1994, 2007; Rosaldo 1989; Saldívar 2006).[3] Just as significantly, Paredes constructed Mexican American social life, including folklore, through a politics of exceptionalism, emphasizing time and time again its uniqueness, its fundamental difference from other social and cultural worlds in both Mexico and the United States. In answering his own rhetorical question as to why he devoted so much attention to US-Mexican relations, Paredes suggests that "the reason is that the shock of cultures and peoples in a continuing situation of cultural conflict has given Mexican American folklore the traits which distinguish it from other folklores, including that of Mexico" (1993:13). In rightly stressing the particular historical, social, and political features of Mexican American folklore in Texas, Paredes seems to suggest that the constitution of folklore through social, cultural, and political conflict is peculiar to Mexican American folklore.

I would surmise that part of the reason he stressed the theme of uniqueness is related to the political location that he fashioned for his scholarship. In answering criticisms that he had romanticized Mexican Americans and left out patriarchy, Paredes told Ramón Saldívar (2006) that he viewed his scholarship as a sort of legal brief, a political intervention on behalf of an oppressed and denigrated people. Nevertheless, studies of African American folklore by such writers as Zora Neale Hurston ([1935] 1978) and the growing militancy of the American Indian Movement did not lead Paredes to connect his vision of social conflict on the border to the realization that connections between folklore and conflict might have been central for African Americans and Native Americans as well. If Paredes had linked his insights into the role of power, conflict, and borders into a general understanding of folklore, as does Bauman (1971) in his "Differential Identity and the Social Base of Folklore," it might have been harder for generations of folklorists to turn their backs on the broader implications of his work.

ETHNOGRAPHIC AUTHORITY AND THE CIRCULATION OF MEXICAN AMERICAN FOLKLORE

Recent studies of Paredes's oeuvre have beautifully captured the way that Paredes constructed a counter-hegemonic discourse that destabilized ethnographic authority through a poetics that reflected his own strategic locations in Mexican American culture (Limón 1992:77). I wish to draw attention to the way that Paredes created a critical model of how the circulation of folklore simultaneously shapes and is shaped by politics of culture and cultures of politics, including both the way cultural forms move and how such movements become objects of representation.

Much more than most anthropologists, folklorists have long attended to the circulation of cultural forms. James Clifford (1997) criticized anthropologists for depicting the culture of the Other as *dwelling*—in other words, as emerging from and stuck within particular places—until an ethnographer stumbles along and enables it to travel; Arjun Appadurai (1988) wryly suggests that such moves represent Others as being "incarcerated by culture." Since the nineteenth century, however, folklorists have been just as interested in how cultural forms *travel* as in the ways they dwell. Nevertheless, as I argued in chapter 2, folklorists and other scholars have often claimed credit for being the ones who are conscious of circulation, depicting "the folk" as only aware of culture forms when they are sensuously embodied in local, face-to-face traditional social worlds.

Paredes, I suggest, turned this conception on its head. In discussions of corridos and legends related to them, he depicted knowledge about events of border conflict as circulating through a range of circuits, including English- and Spanish-language newspapers, courtrooms, gossip, legends, oral history, corridos, and various types of scholarly accounts, including work in both history and folkloristics. Corridos, he argues in "José Mosqueda and the Folklorization of Actual Events," initially offer rich details that satisfy a desire for news (1974), before being transformed into more general statements regarding Mexican American resistance. Far from being disqualified, cast into the realm of "fakelore," in Richard Dorson's (1976) terms, by crossing from print to oral performance, from oral transmission to print, or back and forth repeatedly, it was this circulation across the borders associated with genres and technologies that *created* Mexican American folklore and imbued it with social force. One of the strongest features of *With His Pistol in His Hand* is the way Paredes documents how legends of Gregorio Cortez were told by both Mexican and Anglo Texans and how their accounts were shaped through exchanges of images and interpretations—as well as of gunfire and horses. Indeed, the corridos he analyzes often move between multiple subject positions, sometimes taking the position of Anglo publics and officials, only to go on to highlight heroic Mexican American personae and perspectives.

Paredes brilliantly revealed that this complex circulation was less part of an implicit "political unconscious" (Jameson 1981) than evidence of sophisticated forms of conscious awareness of the politics of the circulation of cultural forms on the part of working-class and middle-class

Mexican Americans. In a Chicano studies classic, Paredes (1993) insightfully returns in his essay "On Ethnographic Work among Minority Groups: A Folklorist's Perspective" to texts by Anglo anthropologists (Madsen 1964; Rubel 1966) that had been widely criticized by Chicano and Chicana scholars (such as Romano-V. 1968). Paredes reflects on how and why these anthropologists reproduced dominant stereotypes. He suggests that when white anthropologists asked Mexican Americans to comment on their culture, playful respondents attempted to locate themselves and the fieldworkers collaboratively in relationship to the public circulation of denigrating stereotypes. Their critical commentaries took the form of joking performances that invited the anthropologists to join in deconstructing mainstream representations of Mexican Americans and in creating alternative circuits of circulation. When anthropologists' questions touched on images that figured in popular stereotypes (such as rejecting biomedicine in favor of "folk" medicine, living for the present, fatalism, and privileging familial solidarity over individual achievement), Mexican Americans recontextualized such tropes as caricatures. They anticipated that anthropologists would use their own privileged positions in dominant publics in fostering the future circulation of these deconstructions and providing more sensitive cultural portraits. Instead of laughing at these intercultural jests, however, Paredes suggests that the ethnographers took them seriously, wrote them down, and enshrined them as Mexican American culture.

Paredes thus argues that the Anglo anthropologists' respondents located cultural forms in a broad process of circulation that jumped scales between interactions, collective constructions of identity, and broadly circulating public discourses. The anthropologists, according to Paredes's analysis, saw Mexican Americans as incarcerated by culture, unaware of dominant epistemologies and discourses and thoroughly invested in occupying a subordinate subject position. Fieldworkers thus missed or misconstrued these powerful examples of double consciousness (Du Bois [1903] 1990)—their consultants' ability to see how they are represented racially by Anglos as well as through their own multiple lenses. The idea that Mexican Americans could only imagine their own cultural forms as circulating within their own local, oral, social worlds is thus part, Paredes reveals, of the hegemonic racial attitudes that were scientized by anthropologists. Accordingly, what fieldworkers "discovered" were core features of the politics of knowledge emerging from whiteness and racial domination, not Mexican American culture. When their interlocutors presented them with a mirror, they mistook the images they saw for what they perceived to lie on the other side of a racial divide. Even as consultants invited them to participate in collaborative, community-based modalities of research, ethnographers were incarcerated within extractive, monologic claims to ethnographic authority.

COMMUNICABILITY AND CIRCUITS OF TRADITIONAL CIRCULATION

Paredes's work thus provides an excellent example of the issues regarding circulation that I discussed in the previous chapter. First, culture, in this view, is not an object that is simply deposited on the social landscape, growing in particular places and waiting to be found and imbued with mobility by ethnographers. It is rather actively made through the circulation of social representations and aesthetic forms through time and space and across borders, including those of race, genre, and mode of transmission (newspapers, oral history, ballads, etc.). Representing these processes of circulation is a crucial dimension of folkloric performance, as illustrated by the way that corridos often project their own place in the circulation of news about an event (see McDowell 2000) or, as Bauman (2012a) points out in discussing Paredes's work, how *décimas* map communicative practices of everyday life. These representations of the circulation of cultural forms are just as actively contested as their symbolic content.

In other words, Paredes showed how Mexican American performers of corridos, legends, jokes, and other forms contested the politics of knowledge that granted Anglos privileged rights to construct news and history, placing their own accounts in dialogue with dominant discourses. Paredes commented critically on how folklore enters directly into these processes, both building on preexisting modes of circulation (journalism, popular media, history, rumor, ballads, and so forth) and playing a role in shaping them. Thus, Paredes analyzed decades ago the importance of circulation to the emergence of folklore, including both the complexity and breadth of these circulatory processes and the complicated ways that representations of circulation were written into poetic features of the cultural forms themselves—and also sometimes written out (in the case of Anglo anthropologists).

Rather than suggesting that these features are unique to Mexican American folklore, let us consider the notion that they are constitutive of folklore in general—even if the particular forms, circuits, borders, and practices of contestation that Paredes traced are themselves historically, socially, and culturally specific. He grasped decades ago some of the points I raised in the previous chapter about such scholarly notions as mobility (Urry 2007), circulation (Latour 1999; Lee and LiPuma 2003), and the constitution of publics (Warner 2002). Cultural forms, like forms of capital, technologies, epistemologies, and so forth, can be socially constructed in such a fashion as to picture them, in Clifford's (1997) terms, either as dwelling or traveling in particular ways. In analyzing these processes, much can be gained by distinguishing the complexities of how signs circulate from the way that people represent signs and attempt to regulate their uses. Michael Silverstein (1976) refers to these dimensions respectively as pragmatics and metapragmatics. Paredes points to the complexity, heterogeneity, and contested nature of the *pragmatics* of the circulation of cultural forms, the practices that move folklore across scales, genres, and borders of various sorts, placing it in dialogue with cultural forms that purport to refer to the same objects (such as Gregorio Cortez) that circulate in newspapers, popular culture, legal and political discourses, literature, and so forth. A parallel process, *metapragmatics*, represents pragmatics selectively, picking out particular features and organizing them in specific ways, as well as seeking to regulate them. Metapragmatics, essentially, is talk about talk, discourse about discourse. Beyond the ability to selectively represent the complexity of pragmatics, the power of metapragmatics lies in making projections of circulation just seem to be accurate reflections of how cultural forms are actively circulating—that is, in reifying them.

So, if Paredes clued us in to the importance of how people culturally construct the circulation of folklore, the conceptual framework of communicability can help us generalize beyond the cases he developed in order to see how constructions of circulation enter into folklore more generally. In building this framework, let me distinguish two facets. First, good ballad scholarship, such as that undertaken by Paredes on Mexican American ballads and McDowell (2000) on Afro-Mexican ballads, attends carefully to the pragmatics of circulation, the movement of cultural forms through legends and other prose narratives, newspapers, courtroom testimony, and other genres, as well as through ballads; social media now enter centrally into this mix. The pragmatics of folklore circulation are complex and multifaceted—no matter how hard folklorists or historians try, it is difficult to pin down all the routes of circulation and transformations that even a single form will take. A second facet consists of cultural representations of this process, which we use in imagining how circulation is taking place; these representations are always simpler and less nuanced than the pragmatics of circulation. Purporting to map how particular cultural forms are moving, some representations are embedded in the cultural forms themselves and others in discussions of them. The variants of the "Ballad of Gregorio Cortez" that Paredes examined are filled with references to reported speech, projecting how one character relayed an account of the events to another or to a broader collectivity, investigative questioning by the Texas Rangers, the role of the telegraph and newspapers in carrying news about Cortez, and the circulation of "wanted" posters. In several variants, Cortez bids his interlocutor, "Tell me the news"; in variant X, he provides this information himself, recounting what people are saying about him (Paredes 1958:157). The penultimate stanza of a Mexico City broadside that Paredes (154) includes projects how the poet represents his own work of circulation:

Participo esta noticia
a gente culta y honrada . . .
los de lista enumerada,
la suerte la sea propicia.

I make this news known
to cultured and honest people;
those on the numbered list—
may fortune be propitious to them.

There are, of course, genres where the attention directed to how cultural forms circulate—and the social consequences attached to such assessments—are much more focal, as Amy Shuman's (1986) account of he-said-she-said gossip would suggest. Folklorists, in turn, construct their own accounts of how traditional cultural forms circulate, often in dialogue with the models offered by other scholars, the media, and "the folk." Chapter 8 takes up one of the most influential models of the circulation of traditionalized cultural forms, Jacob and Wilhelm Grimms' collection of folk narratives, which has shaped both conceptions of the distinct communicability of traditional cultural forms and how they are inscribed onto the surfaces of poetic forms to this day.

Let me build here on the discussion of circulation I launched in chapter 2 through use of the term *communicability*. I use it to refer to such understandings of the production, circulation, and reception of cultural forms (Briggs 2005). Communicability always involves processes of simplification of the complex pragmatics of circulation, amplifying some dimensions and erasing or downplaying others. Two types can be analytically distinguished: communicability emerges in general *models* of circulation as well as in communicable *cartographies* of particular cultural forms, of the type that I illustrated for the "Ballad of Gregorio Cortez." Communicable models and cartographies are no less contested than cultural forms; performers and audiences contest versions of the origin and route of transmission of a song, for example, as much as folklorists have disputed throughout the discipline's history models of how folklore is produced, circulates, and is received. Moreover, the power of communicable models and cartographies springs from the way that they generally present themselves as direct reflections of how cultural forms are actually traveling. Paredes taught us about both of these facets in his discussions of intercultural jests, ballad legends, and interviews with anthropologists—disputing the pragmatics of circulation and communicable models and cartographies is an important part of contesting the politics of knowledge. The problem is that folklorists, particularly when they claim that "the folk" lack awareness of how folklore circulates, present their own models and cartographies as definitive accounts, thereby turning other accounts of circulation into mere folk distortions. Bauman and Briggs (2003) argue that this was precisely Franz Boas's characterization of the genesis and nature of folklore—the misrepresentation of how cultural forms actually circulate.

COMMUNICABILITY AND THE SHIFTING BASIS OF FOLKLORISTIC AUTHORITY

The power of Paredes's work arises in the way it challenges models of communicability that have shaped research on folklore for several centuries, thereby providing us with a means of rethinking genealogies and foundational frameworks. In seventeenth-century England, John Aubrey envisioned two opposing models of communicability. One, associated with traditionality, views cultural forms as moving through purely oral channels and face-to-face interaction, largely through countrywomen. Cultural forms were circulated unconsciously, he claimed, not submitted to conscious reflection, and they reflected interest, irrationality, sexual desire, and superstitious logics such as magical attempts to obtain a husband.[4] Modernity, on the other hand, revolved around knowledge obtained directly from nature, not from other people. It emerged as individual men (and I do mean men) reflected rationally on the world. Rather than circulating as poetic forms, as was seemingly characteristic of traditional communicability, modern cultural forms consisted of plain speech that transparently communicated disinterested knowledge. Speaking for traditional communicability, Aubrey suggested that "when I was a child (and so before the Civill Warres) the fashion was for old women and mayds to tell fabulous stories nightimes, of Sprights and walking of ghosts, &c. This was derived downe from mother to daughter, &c." (1862:15). He similarly suggested that "in the old ignorant times, before women were Readers, the history was handed downe from Mother to daughter . . . So my Nurse had the History from the Conquest down to Carl. I in Ballad" (1972:289–90).

When books and other modern technologies entered into traditional circuits of communicability, however, the latter fell apart: "Before Printing, Old-wives Tales were ingeniose: and since Printing came in fashion, till a little before the Civil-warres, the ordinary sort of People were not taught to reade: now-a-dayes Bookes are common, and most of the poor people understand letters: and the many good Bookes, and variety of Turnes of Affaires, have put all the old Fables out of dores: and the divine art of Printing and Gunpowder have frighted away Robin-good-fellow and the Fayries" (Aubrey 1972:290). Nonetheless, the way that Aubrey positioned himself in relation to traditional communicability was complex and contradictory. Moreover, Aubrey positions members of the elite at times within traditional communicabilities, such as in describing magical cures performed by and for the aristocracy and even the king.

Romantic Nationalism expanded models of traditional communicability. Johann Gottfried Herder distinguished *Naturpoesie* from *Kunstpoesie*, and he used them in defining opposing and seemingly autonomous models of communicability. Folklore emanated from the "patriarch's hut," which constituted a small republic of social and cultural life ([1774] 2002:323). There the patriarch transmitted folklore by word of mouth through forms filled with affect, energy, immediacy, and a sense of presence to all family members, thereby producing a homogenous familial cultural repertoire. From there, folklore was passed by word of mouth outward toward the community, region, and finally to the borders of the nation—at which point it halted abruptly. As it traveled, folklore created affect and a sense of community that emanated from shared cultural forms; even as it varied increasingly in detail as it moved outward from the patriarchal ground zero, Naturpoesie retained its passionate embodiment of the spirit of the people (*volksmässig*), grounded in the collectivity (Herder [1877–1913] 1967:189). Even as it obscured forms of sexual domination and violence that organized relations within the "patriarchal hut," this sexualized and racialized communicability constituted a chronotope for nationalism in which patriarchy and whiteness provided the purported sense of commonality and connection through which folklore could define a people and delineate its borders. Kunstpoesie, on the other hand, differed in all of these respects, springing from and directed toward individuals—lacking passion, presence, and immediacy—and circulating through the mediation of the written word. (By pointing out the key role of communicable models in Herder's construction of traditional cultural forms, I do not want to suggest, however, that his work was monolithic or consistently anti-Enlightenment, romantic, and nationalistic.)

Jacob and Wilhelm Grimm, of course, challenged Herder and other contemporaries for not adequately appreciating the depth of the difference between traditional and modern communicabilities and particularly for hybridizing them in their own texts, such as in Herder's influential collection of *Volkslieder*, published in 1778–1779. The Grimms claimed that becoming a scholar of traditionality involved identifying objects (such as folktales or legends) that had been untouched by modern communicability—particularly by literacy—and then tracing how they traveled through circuits of traditional oral communicability. This process involved crossing the cultural boundary dividing the subject positions that separated the two communicabilities—modern subjects who dedicated themselves to folklore study, like the Grimms, thereby gained an intimate appreciation for traditional circulation. This process involved particular forms of extraction: "One must quietly lift the leaves and carefully bend back the bough so as not to disturb the folk, if one wishes to steal a furtive glance into the strange yet modest world of nature, nestled into itself, and smelling of fallen leaves, meadow grass, and fresh-fallen rain" (Grimm and Grimm [1816] 1981:11).

Entextualization strategies required preserving the poetic features that traditional communicability inscribed on the surfaces of folkloric forms. Folklorists must pursue a politics of textual transparency, somehow preserving the essential features of traditional communicability as forms are written, edited, and published (see Briggs 1993b; Bauman and Briggs 2003). The Grimms extended the pragmatics of the circulation of scholarly discourse about folklore beyond the nationalist restriction that limited how folklore itself circulated, according to their communicable model, in promoting what I term *folklore cosmopolitanisms*—international exchanges of texts and textual models. Quite a number of writers have challenged the Grimms for not rigidly pursuing their communicable roles, leveling charges that they collected material from literate contributors and engaged in unscientific editing practices, adding such features as proverbs, elements of repetition, quoted speech, and the like, at the same time that they eliminated other features (Ellis 1983; Kamenetsky 1992). In other words, the pragmatics associated with their work did not perfectly match the communicable models that they both explicitly projected and inscribed on the surfaces of texts by infusing them with elements that seemed to provide direct evidence of their oral, folk transmission. Such criticisms, however, simply reproduce doctrines of traditional communicability, the notion that folkloristics *should* focus exclusively on the oral circulation of traditional objects and that scholarly practices and traditional communicable models *should* match perfectly.

Historical-geographic approaches have probably developed the most systematic means of turning traditional communicability into formal methodologies that ring of scientific objectivity. Kaarle Krohn identified two fundamental principles for mapping traditional communicability: "folklore migrates through time and space" ([1926] 1971:57), he argued. The justification for the primordial status of time and space was articulated precisely in terms of a traditional communicability, which envisioned folklore as always on the move—but as traveling through particular circuits: "Of great importance, however is the steady influence of the constant movement within a neighborhood. Up until the modern age, the country peoples of Europe were bound to the soil. The diffusion of their traditions took place orally through the folk mouth, traveling from farm to farm, village to village, parish to parish, in a continuous chain of neighborly contacts. Like coins passing from hand to hand, traditions migrated from mouth to mouth" (59).

The equation of oral transmission with monetary transactions, which evokes the materiality of discourse as much as capitalist exchange (see Keane 2007), is intriguing. In short, "the folk" are dwellers, and their consciousness of folktales involved the manner in which forms were rooted in local social spaces. Nevertheless, these acts of dwelling unwittingly made tales move. Traditional communicability thus wove features of time and space onto the textual surfaces of folktales. The ability to render these features conscious was reserved for folklorists, who created their science by learning to extract these time-space features from texts. Thus, the sine qua non of folkloristics was to recover the very features that folklorists' own communicable model had imbued in tales and reified as intrinsic! Krohn ([1926] 1971:142) argues that folklorists are like mathematicians, tracing "the same chain of thought in a reverse direction" in viewing how folktales travel along communicable routes. If folktales provide the distinctive object for the creation of a new science, "the flora and fauna of folklore" (80), tracing the "mechanical laws" (98) of their movement would provide the means of creating a distinctive disciplinary methodology. The Aarne-Thompson (Aarne and Thompson 1961) schema for classifying and mapping folk narratives permitted an endless production of individual cartographies of traditional communicability through a discourse of scientific specificity, all the while restricting models of circulation largely along Eurocentric lines.

Richard Dorson was probably the most influential codifier of traditional communicability in twentieth-century folkloristics, at least in the United States. In *The British Folklorists*, he lauded Aubrey for having discovered traditional objects and their distinct routes of circulation and for developing folkloristics' fundamental methodology—entering spaces of traditional communicability, recognizing their autonomy vis-à-vis modern communicabilities, extracting forms "at first hand" (Dorson 1968:8), and entextualizing them in such a way that their communicative and cultural Otherness could be appreciated by modern audiences. In short, Dorson asserted that Aubrey discovered one communicable model, traditionality, and created another, which later came to be enshrined as folklore fieldwork. Dorson's characterization of Aubrey was highly selective, reifying particular dimensions and erasing other facets of his collection and entextualization practices and the shifting class and racial position of folklore in his work, a point I develop in chapter 4. Dorson consolidated the role of the folklorist as providing a unique bridge between autonomous and opposing models of communicability, traditional and modern. He required that folklore be mediated by traditional, oral communicabilities—elements of mass media and print transmission must be expunged and commodification clearly avoided—lest cultural forms be cast into the denigrated realm of "fakelore" (Dorson 1976). Dorson's folklore/fakelore interventions attempted to coerce folklorists into accepting a single model of the circulation of folklore—whatever did not fit simply was not folklore. To extend a point I made in chapter 1, it was traditional communicability that enabled Dorson to constitute folkloristics through a practice of boundary-work (Gieryn 1983), preventing folklorists from straying outside this communicable realm and keeping popularizers, other scholars, and laypersons from daring to enter it. Imposing this regime of communicability was hard work, because the complex pragmatics of the circulation of cultural forms could never be reduced to such a simple communicable model, and new gaps emerged each time a major revolution in media technologies and popular cultural practices emerged.

To be sure, the idea that folklore is located within a traditional, oral realm of communicability that is rigidly separated from its modern, literate equivalent has been challenged in a number of ways. Dundes (1980) argued that technologies do not kill folklore but expand its production and extend its transmission. Bausinger ([1961] 1990) viewed particular technological formations as shaping types of folklore and their position in society. Bauman and Feaster (2005) have shown how both the pragmatic practices and the communicable models associated with oral performances were transformed as phonographic and gramophone recordings were commodified, advertised, and disseminated. Other scholars, such as Weidman (2006), have inserted mechanical reproduction through radio and television into the picture. (See also Martín Barbero [1987] 2003.) Folklorists laid to rest some time ago the notion that orality and literacy are separate and autonomous cognitive and social domains. Regina Bendix (1997) argued that the notion of authenticity was central to constituting folkloristics as a discipline and infusing it with scholarly authority; authenticity is a communicable construct par excellence, projecting routes of transmission for cultural forms that keep them within spaces that are certifiably "traditional." Scholars have traced how the construction of traditionalities and modernities goes hand in hand (García Canclini [1990] 1995, 1995) and how their production has helped constitute shifting notions of the modern and modes of constructing and empowering modern subjects since the seventeenth century (Bauman and Briggs 2003). A great deal of research at present focuses on global regimes for the commodification, circulation, and regulation of objects that supposedly circulate via traditional communicability (Bendix 2018; Hafstein 2004, 2018b; Scher 2002). Public folklorists have challenged the notion that folklore becomes contaminated when it circulates through institutional contexts, as mediated by public folklorists (Feintuch 1988).

Recent scholarship has thus moved us closer to responding to the far-reaching challenge to persistent models of traditional communicability that Paredes offered over a half century ago. What Paredes presented was a radically different communicable model. He argued that folklore does not reside in an autonomous realm of traditional communicability that exists prior to and autonomously from modern communicability. He contended that the circulation of folkloric forms is deeply entwined with that of the mass media, official pronouncements, legal discourse, and other circuits. It does not emerge within a realm of cultural sharing and sameness and then proceed through a process of natural, gradual variation until it reaches the limits of the nation, constituting a people who share a set of core cultural characteristics. It does not emerge exclusively within one racialized population but rather emerges from the violent borders that constitute them—and then crosses and recrosses them. Folklore does not jump scales gradually and unidirectionally, from patriarchal huts to local to regional to national realms; rather, discourses that constitute dominant and counter-public spheres on both sides of borders are thoroughly entangled with intimate exchanges of songs, legends, and jokes between friends and family at every point, as Richard Flores (1995) and José Limón (1994) have detailed. Where I think we have fallen short, however, is in fully incorporating Paredes's insight that the politics of circulation, including both pragmatic strategies and communicable models, are central to the constitution of folklore and its role in producing and contesting social and political-economic categories and relations.

Folklorists, according to Paredes, do not insert themselves into preexisting realms of traditional communicability but enter in complex and multiple ways into the politics that constitute circuits of circulation and their representations. He is clear that modes of circulation are multiple and competing—and that their relations are constituted in political-economic terms. Whereas Anglo Texans and especially Texas Rangers had power to impose on Mexican Americans the subordinate subject positions and social relations that were mapped by their communicable models, Mexican Americans were less able to use their models in undermining Anglo control of dominant public spheres; exercising greater control over how discourse circulated through newspapers, telegraphs, courtrooms, and legislative bodies was certainly crucial. Paredes clearly notes that communicable projects, Mexican American and Anglo alike, never transparently mapped how cultural forms and power circulated—and he shows how this gap helped to constitute both white supremacy and Mexican American resistance. As with the Anglo anthropologists whose work Paredes analyzed, folklorists could either contribute to imperialism (as he suggested Frank Dobie did) and the reproduction of denigrating stereotypes (like anthropologists Madsen and Rubel) or, as Paredes said of his own research, their scholarship could constitute a legal brief in support of an oppressed people (Saldívar 2006). Paredes thus critiqued scholarly constructions of a distinct, self-contained realm of traditional communicability as a crucial building block for authorizing a racialized politics of knowledge that (re)produced inequalities of race and class—even if (for Paredes) not so squarely of gender—rather than, as for Dorson, an accurate reflection of cultural facts on the ground.

CONCLUSION: PAREDES'S LEGACY AND NEW SCHOLARLY AGENDAS

Américo Paredes argued that folklorists' and anthropologists' failure to attend to conflict as a social base of folklore is probably due to "a certain mistaken delicacy, or the desire not to offend, not to bring up painful matters which we all know have existed and which we all want to remedy" (1993:18). And then the prescient punch line: "But this is to deny folklore study its place as a scholarly discipline." Paredes was clearly denied his proper place in the scholarly discipline of folklore. A crucial question thus confronts us: what is the appropriate response to this sort of genealogical exclusion? Derrida ([1967] 1976) would warn us, of course, of the problems that follow from attempting to construct a supplement to what is already a surplus of discourse (a genealogy), thereby extending its discursive and political effects. I myself find the anti-genealogical perspective of Deleuze and Guattari ([1980] 1987) quite appealing, as I do their notion that ideas might be more productively projected in rhizomic terms, organized through unpredictable and shifting sorts of horizontal connections, rather than in arboreal terms—as roots, trunks, branches, and leaves in a fixed hierarchical structure. Nevertheless, it seems apparent that genealogies are powerful tools of canonization; even if we critique them, they help shape patterns of citation, syllabi for core graduate seminars, and scholarly and textual networks. This issue is particularly important in the face of demands to dismantle genealogies and canons structured by whiteness and to challenge the racism and sexism that denied visibility to work by Black, Latinx, and Native American scholars.

That Paredes's vision had a lasting impact on folklore, anthropology, Latinx studies, and literary studies is clearly evident in the work of his former students and colleagues and that of other scholars, including myself. The question I would ask is, now, more than fifty years later, is it finally time to recognize his contribution more broadly? Again, my Deleuzian and Derridian tendencies draw me in an anti-genealogical direction. Nevertheless, to say that we are now beyond genealogies would remind me of Michel-Rolph Trouillot's (1991) offhand comment in his "Savage Slot" essay that postmodernism has now doubly excluded Haitians: if being postmodern entails rejecting modernist master narratives, what is to become of subjects who were always already excluded from those narratives, either as narrators or as protagonists? Similarly, now that we have recognized more clearly the devastating impact of racialized but supposedly race-free (universal) approaches to the study of folklore and anthropology in racializing the reception of Paredes's insights, we declare: game over! Critical, theoretically oriented scholars do not construct genealogies! Following on the argument I advanced in chapter 1, this conclusion would leave that task to the boundary workers and their projects of disciplinary consolidation.

To take this position, would, I fear, just lead to the marginalization of Paredes's work all over again. Nevertheless, simply writing Paredes into established genealogies as a mode of recuperation is not an adequate response, I think, to the task that confronts us. The strategy that I have adopted here is to try to unlearn the assumptions that underlie scholarly foundations in order to further our understanding of Paredes's insights and embrace their transformative potential. As I noted above, a number of scholars have reflected on the way that Paredes resituated folklore as a product of difference, borders, border crossing, conflict, and power. I went on to point to another dimension of Paredes's prescience, his critical scrutiny of knowledge making and circulation practices and their political significance. Given the centrality of notions of dwelling and travel to folkloristics and anthropology, I have argued that constructions of the way that cultural forms emerge and travel, which I have termed communicability, are crucial. These models—and the individual cartographies that are projected for particular forms—are ideological, not in the sense that they are false or ipso facto tools of domination but because they are constructed, positioned, interested, and partial. They do not diverge from the pragmatics of folkloristic research just when something goes wrong: communicability and pragmatics always dance a tense tango—always closely intertwined and mutually constitutive even as they are always separated by constantly changing gaps and fissures.

Projecting how cultural forms circulate is not intrinsically evil—anthropologists and folklorists could not do their work without projecting communicabilities. But Paredes can help us analyze a number of crucial problems, which, I have argued, are tied not only to communicable models of traditional discourse, but also to how scholarly analyses often derive their power by pretending to be simple reflections of the way that cultural forms are actually produced, circulated, and received. I have tried to build on Paredes's insights in advancing a distinct scholarly agenda, which can be summarized as follows:

1. Folklorists should continue to follow their traditional, as it were, dedication to tracing in detail how particular cultural forms circulate. Attention should focus on multiplicities and contestations, on the existence of competing routes, on how potential circuits are obstructed or denigrated, and on the friction (Tsing 2005) that channels how and where cultural forms travel. Forms of circulation that define themselves as scholarly, whether as folkloristics or as part of other disciplinary trajectories, should be scrutinized alongside vernacular ones (see Bauman 2008), as well as the full range of sites (including museums, tourist attractions, old and new media, etc.) that are evident, not placed in separate epistemological or social spheres. Kirshenblatt-Gimblett's (1998a) work on metaculture, on ways that heritage subjects come to develop a reflexive and ironic—and potentially distant—relationship to the very practices that are projected as their own is particularly interesting. I do not claim to break new ground here; this seems to be precisely the thrust of much recent scholarship in the field.
2. At the same time, however, folklorists should ethnographically explore the full range of communicable models and

cartographies that claim to chart these forms of production, circulation, and reception. Here it is important to look at ways in which communicability is lodged in cultural forms themselves as well as discourses that seek to represent them, be they claims made by competing performers, scholars, national or international bodies, or what have you.

3. By analytically separating pragmatics and communicability, scholars can then grasp their complex interplay. Particular attention should be devoted to cases in which competing models and cartographies claim to map the same pragmatic contours and the way that a single (often hegemonic) communicable model or cartography elides differences between competing pragmatic trajectories. Folklore seems to lie precisely at the intersection between attempts to reify links between pragmatic and communicable dimensions and efforts to pry the two apart, especially to reveal the inadequacy of hegemonic communicable models.

4. Rather than continuing the work of reification by constructing a single communicable model or cartography and attempting to reduce competitors to the status of the folly of amateurs, the malfeasance of fabricators of fakelore, the lack of conscious awareness on the part of "the folk," or the influence of competing (and therefore mistaken) scholarly models, scholars should use these analyses of the distinct parameters of pragmatic and communicable dimensions to denaturalize reifications, promote awareness of conflicting strategies and models, and explore alternatives. This is, of course, precisely where I locate Paredes's work.

5. Neither pragmatic nor communicable models are simply discursive, if that term is used in the impoverished sense of linguistic representations that seem to exist apart from material realities; rather, they are both shaped by, and in turn shape, materialities and broader political-economic dimensions. Another way of stating this point is that the reason both pragmatic strategies and communicable models are multiple and competing is that they involve real stakes.

With regard to the latter point, the reservation that I have always had about the literature on the "invention of tradition" (Hobsbawm 1983; Handler and Linnekin 1984) is that it seemed to stop at the point of showing that a particular set of communicable cartographies of tradition does not adequately map the pragmatics of circulation. Surprise—they never do! My critical engagement of scholarly work on "the invention of tradition" has sometimes been read as suggesting that researchers should simply repeat or even celebrate—but never deconstruct—representations of traditions (Briggs 1996). It is certainly true that the communicable models presented by both dominant sectors and oppressed populations involve crucial reifications that attempt to consolidate claims over the circulation of cultural forms. Nevertheless, the resources that different parties bring to the reification game are often unequal and, as Indigenous critics have pointed out, the effects of deconstructing them are quite different for national governments, corporations, and community activists (see Jaimes and Noriega 1988; Trask 1991). My goal was thus not to induce scholars to turn off their deconstructive skills but to provoke them to extend their critical, analytical gaze—by turning it on themselves and the positions of privilege they sometimes enjoy as much as on those performing (ethno-)nationalist traditions. Moreover, Paredes made it very clear that we should attempt to anticipate the effects of our research projects and pedagogy on the politics of knowledge, even if we can never guarantee that they will come out the way we hope. The Texas Rangers and their supporters, after all, responded to Paredes's deconstructions with death threats.

Folklorists are now taking on some powerful "folk," such as United Nations Educational, Scientific and Cultural Organization (UNESCO) and World Intellectual Property Organization (WIPO) bureaucrats, major recording artists and companies, and the representatives of nation-states who attempt to regulate how "intangible cultural heritage" is defined, possessed, preserved, and globally circulated. (See Bendix 2018; Feld 2000; Goodman 2002; Hafstein 2004, 2018b; Kapchan 2007; and Scher 2002 for just a few examples of this exciting work.) The demands of documenting and analyzing these processes, let alone of scaling up ethnographic models to accommodate them, are enormous. I think the communicability framework and the five strategies that I outlined above will help scholars address these complex, globally distributed issues. International bodies, nation-states, corporations, nongovernmental organizations of varying sorts, scholars, activists, artists, and others now engage in pragmatic strategies and assert communicative models and cartographies that are co-produced, collide, collaborate, and conflict in complex and rapidly shifting ways. As these authors and others have argued, the stakes are high, and both scholars and practitioners are deeply implicated in processes and outcomes—without, to be sure, being able to determine them. Here, I have attempted to add modestly to these efforts by building on Paredes's insights into the fascinating and precarious implications of ways that we construct and attempt to regulate the circulation of culture.

NOTES

1. I first applied the communicability framework to folkloristics at the 14th Congress of the International Society for Folk Narrative Research in Tartu, Estonia, in July 2005, and I wish to thank participants for helpful questions and comments.

2. I use the terms *Mexican American* and *Anglo* in deference to Paredes's own usage.

3. In an interview with Saldívar, Paredes suggests that "Greater Mexico begins at the border of Guatemala and extends all the way to the Great Lakes, to New York, or where there are *mexicanos*. They vary from one place to another, but to my mind, they're basically the same. The differences are in degree of acculturation" (quoted in Saldívar 2006:141–42).

4. The pragmatics of Aubrey's own texts, however, often wove oral and textual sources together in complicated ways, as I explore in chapter 4.

4

The Coloniality of Folkloristics
Toward a Multi-Genealogical Practice

with Sadhana Naithani

IN THESE PAGES WE CHALLENGE GENEALOGIES OF FOLKLORISTICS by according a central place to the relationship between folkloristics and colonialism, which we refer to as the *coloniality of folkloristics*. The establishment of folklore has long been located in relation to the emergence of modernity in northern Europe, including both its negative relationship to Enlightenment rationalism in the seventeenth and eighteenth centuries and its positive role in the appearance of Romantic Nationalism in the late eighteenth and nineteenth centuries. As I outlined in the preceding chapter, histories of folkloristics often stress the centrality of research by John Aubrey in the English countryside in constructing a traditional "Other" that helped define a perceived gap between premodern and modern worlds, along with the roles of Johann Gottfried Herder and Jacob and Wilhelm Grimm in projecting a "German nation" that provided a political and textual model for a German nation-state.

These pivotal moments provide four stories that structure many genealogies of folkloristics. First, Richard Dorson's *The British Folklorists* credits Aubrey with providing "probably the earliest statement in English of the value in recording folk traditions" (1968:7) and with having discovered traditional subjects and cultural forms in the English countryside and saving them—at least in textual form—from modernity, literacy, and technology. Second, in *Voices of Modernity*, Richard Bauman and Charles L. Briggs (2003) challenge this logic, suggesting that Aubrey was just as centrally involved in constructing a new object, traditionality, as Boyle, Locke, and Newton were engaged in producing an opposing set of new subjects and objects associated with science, rationality, capitalism, and the modern state—and that both elements of this process were crucial in making modern projects possible. Third, generations of folklorists followed the Grimms in positing the existence of illiterate, premodern folk populations in the countryside of Germany, France, England, Spain, and other countries; they similarly defined folkloristics as using scholarly practices to rescue traditional cultural forms before literacy, technology, and cosmopolitanism rendered them extinct. Fourth, Regina Bendix (1988b:235–46), Michael Herzfeld (1982), Sadhana Naithani (2006, 2010), Diarmuid Ó Giolláin (2000), William Wilson (1976), and other scholars turn this narrative on its head, pointing to the role of folklorists in constructing "the folk" and other social, cultural, and literary categories that, along with political-economic transformations, made nationalist and colonial cultural politics possible.

These four types of narratives suggest the degree to which folklorists have recently multiplied and complicated disciplinary narratives. At the same time that our account builds on a number of critical genealogies, we provide a different sort of narrative of folkloristics—one that takes colonialism as its point of departure and its constitutive contradiction. Our effort to rethink and reposition folkloristics draws on a shift in how we think about modernity and its Others associated with work in postcolonial studies by Dipesh Chakrabarty (2000) and perspectives emerging from decolonial studies by Enrique Dussel ([1992] 1995, 1998), Aníbal Quijano (2000), Walter Mignolo (2000), and others. We engage scholars in postcolonial and decolonial studies not to suggest that they have all the answers, or that folkloristics has no relevant insights of its own to offer. On the contrary, folklorists can provide important correctives to the elitism, distance, and nostalgia that sometimes characterize perspectives on vernacular cultural forms that emerge in the writing of Chakrabarty, Mignolo, and other authors. If Mignolo suggests that we should always think of modernity as modernity/coloniality, we introduce the notion of *traditionality/coloniality* to suggest that it is equally problematic to think of a traditionality that existed apart from colonialism and colonial power. Rather than simply extending postcolonial and decolonial studies, the notion of traditionality/coloniality can help destabilize some of the more romantic notions of the nature of Indigenous and other subaltern identities that underlie some work in both postcolonial and decolonial studies.

One goal of this chapter is to reposition colonialism in genealogies of folkloristics. Colonial folkloristics is often seen as a detour of nineteenth-century European folkloristics, which placed the study of narratives, proverbs, "customs," and so forth at the service of colonial officials in India, Africa, the Pacific, the Americas, and the Caribbean. The fascination of

Spanish and British colonizers with Indigenous belief, religion, and ritual has been well known to scholars in South Asian and Latin American studies. The missionaries who formed a central component of European colonialism around the world and the civil servants of the British Empire published extensive collections of folklore. Colonialism is hardly absent from histories of folkloristics. Disciplinary and predisciplinary work on folklore thus turns out to be even more important to histories of both "the West" and "the rest" than previously suggested.

While building on studies of folklore research in contexts that are explicitly colonial, we suggest that colonialism has shaped folkloristics from the time of its prehistory through the present, including times and places where colonial political relations were absent. We accordingly draw on a long time span, from the late fifteenth through the twentieth centuries, and include both predisciplinary precursors and scholars who wrote as and for folklorists. We bring together critical interventions into established genealogies in urging a transformed practice of folkloristics, which we refer to as *multi-genealogical*, as a mode of shaping the present and future of the discipline.

POSTCOLONIAL POSITIONALITIES

In his sophisticated account of the birth of modernity, postcolonial scholar Dipesh Chakrabarty's (2000) concern is with how modernity came to be seen as providing a universal measure of "man." Where, he asks, did this story originate, and how did it come to be seen as a means of comparing people across time and space? Chakrabarty argues that this supposedly universal framework is provincial in origin, springing from self-representations of elite, white males in seventeenth-century northern Europe. The trick, he argues, was how it got "deprovincialized," decontextualized from its point of origin and used in generating European projections of—in a word, "man"—to the rest of the world. Given its social, geographic, and historical underpinnings, modernity could only map in partial and distorted terms onto the people it recognized as "Others," dislocating them to varying degrees "to an imaginary waiting room of history" (8). Subjects situated at some distance from white, male, European (and later Euro-American) elite models could only endeavor to assimilate an ideological package that they could not shape or ever fully embody.

A very different reading of modernity and traditionality emerges in the genealogy presented by Dussel ([1992] 1995), Quijano (2000), and other decolonial scholars, including Mignolo (2000). Dussel and Mignolo urge us to see modernity as emerging not in northern Europe in the seventeenth century but in the Iberian Peninsula starting in 1492—with the expulsion of the Jews and Moors and the conquest and colonization of the Americas. They argue that modernity was not produced in Europe and then exported through a form of Orientalism (Said 1978) to lands that lay beyond "the West," but was hammered out through the violent extension of the Occident to the Americas. Dussel describes modernity as a world phenomenon that emerged simultaneously through Europe's constitution as a center and the location of the Americas, Africa, eastern Europe, and other areas as peripheries. European modernity thus "originates in a dialectal relation with non-Europe" ([1992] 1995:9). As such, modernity was produced in the very context of colonialism, and its emergence required racial Others for its inception and definition, not just its expansion. Here modernity was forged not simply in stable European centers but in movement, crafted in violent and unequal relations that were spatially dispersed and included nonwhite agency, a picture that resonates strongly with Paul Gilroy's (1993) conception of a Black Atlantic. Mignolo (2000) thus uses the term *modernity/coloniality*, suggesting that race and violence were connected to modernity from the start and continue to be deeply imbricated in it. The modernity/colonialism connection, he argues, is not severed when colonialism as a political system ends, as was the case in most areas of Latin America in the early nineteenth century; race and violence continue to be evident in how modernity is displayed as a social and political force. Aníbal Quijano (2000) and Mignolo (2000) thus stress the continuing legacy of race, colonialism, and violence in modernity, apart from formal political structures of colonialism, as "the coloniality of power," whence comes the title of this chapter.

One immediate implication of this map of the history of modernity is that the prehistory of folkloristics starts earlier and on a much broader geographic scale. Before Brits Camden and Aubrey began their work on forms of traditionality, Spanish missionaries were deeply engaged in inscribing Indigenous literatures in the Americas. Long before literacy became a means of constructing a great divide between premodern and modern English subjects, Spanish missionaries projected alphabetic writing as a border that separated civilized from uncivilized, rational from irrational. Projects of conquest included proto-ethnographers who crossed this constructed border and claimed the Americas for modernity—through the inscription of Indigenous historical and mythological narratives, along with accounts of what were considered to be superstitions, customs, and rituals—thereby helping to shape emergent projects of modernity.

The potential of this formulation for folklore is immense. The "colonial difference" is located in problematic oppositions between orality and writing, generating narratives in which alphabetic writing has been constantly privileged over oralism—even in those instances in which other forms of writing were clearly apparent (such as Incan and Mayan societies). These conceptions of an orality/literacy gap, of its status as a fundamental source of inequality, emerged in the course of practices of inscription that were very much part of colonial enterprises—informing the king of his new lands and subjects, missionization, surveillance, control, disciplining resistance and rebellious subjects, and justifying imperial and colonial ventures, as well as sometimes in resisting or complicating these projects. On the global scale of colonial difference, Eric Wolf (1982) suggested that people without writing were represented as people without history who were often judged to be quite low in human intelligence and civilization. Modernity, from the start, was fundamentally involved in projects in which "people with history could write the history of those without" (Mignolo 2000:3). Nevertheless, recent accounts of Indigenous participation in colonial inscription suggest that Indigenous elites were actively involved in creating colonial practices of representation—and thus shaping modernity (Hanks 2010).

Narratives of modernity did not always go uncontested. Dussel points to the role of Bartolomé de las Casas, the sixteenth-century bishop of Chiapas, in challenging the legitimacy of the conquest as bringing modernity to peoples enslaved by barbarous traditions. Dussel draws attention to de las Casas's realization that countering violent projects of modernity required challenging texts that purported to be inscriptions of barbarous words, beliefs, and customs. In de las Casas's words, "Ultimately we have written to make better known all these nations . . . whom some have defamed . . . by reporting that they were not rational enough to govern themselves in a humane and orderly fashion . . . I have compiled the data in this book to demonstrate the contrary truth" (quoted in Dussel [1992] 1995:70). De las Casas thus pointed out, nearly five centuries ago, that textual constructions of premodern Others played a key role in defining and legitimizing notions of modernity and their claims to rationality and universality, thus tracing intimate connections between poetics, power, and the politics of knowledge.

How might we use these competing accounts of the advent of modernity in rereading genealogies of folkloristics? An initial point of departure is provided by returning to Richard Dorson's (1968) genealogical charter for folkloristics, viewed here not in terms of its substantial role in establishing folkloristic boundary-work (see chapter 1) or projecting traditional communicability (chapter 2) but in how it provided a model for simultaneously including colonialism in disciplinary histories while denying its place as a constitutive force in folkloristics. It is useful not only insofar as it influenced Dorson's students, drawn from around the world, but also with respect to how critical engagements with it can reproduce its foundational parameters even as they challenge what Hayden White (1978) refers to as its mode of "emplotment"—narrative structures that shape how the story is told.

The British Folklorists opens as Dorson recalls how he spent the summer of 1948 in London exploring the history of British folkloristics. He continues this origin story of his own narrative as follows:

> During the years since that first summer, the power and eloquence of these giants of folklore were never long out of my mind, even when I was deeply immersed in my own American folklore. More and more I came to feel that familiarity with the brilliant history of folklore science in England was as indispensable for the American, and indeed for the European, Asian, or African student of folklore, as for the British. The birth and growth of the idea of folklore and the magnetism in that idea for many powerful minds in diverse callings formed a story as marvelous as any folktale. Here I have tried to tell that story. (1968:v)

In this passage, Dorson defined his book as a disciplinary meta-genealogy. Describing this history as "a firm thread" (441) that runs continuously from the publication of William Camden's *Britannia* in 1586 to "the fading of the British folklore movement ... as one of the collateral tragedies of the Great War" (440), Dorson constructs the study of folklore as an autonomous discipline, a bounded and delimited intellectual pursuit that is defined by its possession of a distinct object and set of methods, texts, and scholars. This genealogy provides him with a script with which to inscribe and circumscribe his mission to construct an autonomous discipline of folklore in the United States. No less than the Grimms a century earlier, Dorson provides a Eurocentric charter for a cosmopolitan discipline that is framed as the evolution of the theory and practice of folklore in England and its export "throughout the British Isles, the British Empire, and the world at large" (1).

Our motivation in starting with Dorson is not founded on the belief that he is still, in the new millennium, the fundamental point of reference for folklorists.[1] We rather wish to extend to folkloristics the sort of criticism that James Clifford (1988) afforded anthropology—analyzing how texts on folklore construct their object, assert their own authority, create disciplinary boundaries, and place traditionalism in relationship to other modern phenomena. In Hayden White's (1978) terms, the mode of emplotment of Dorson's narrative is that of the romance, in which a linear succession of heroic struggles results in a disciplinary victory; Dorson nevertheless moves to a tragic mode in projecting the postwar demise of English folkloristics. We are particularly interested in how Dorson's narrative renders colonialism both visible and invisible.

Dorson locates the emergence of folkloristics squarely with the work of John Aubrey in seventeenth-century England. He anoints Aubrey as folklore's forefather by virtue of the "sure instinct" with which he "recognized" (1968:5) an object that was lodged in the English countryside—"oral folklore" (6). Folklore is thus a naturally occurring object within the social world; discovering it required a particular form of "extraordinarily acute insight" (6) and a specific set of methodological practices for obtaining traditions "at first hand, from [Aubrey's] own immediate world" (8) and transporting them into the modern world, which is defined by literacy. As I suggested in chapter 1, Dorson's rhetoric creates a sense of disciplinary boundedness and continuity by constantly reiterating the purity of the folkloristic gaze that could discern the central disciplinary object, folklore, amid the contamination of modern technologies and scholarly intertextuality, embodying the affective posture of "ire and zeal" (11) that became the mark of Dorson's own disciplinary advocacy and scholarly authority (Bronner 1998).

The "Great Team" of folklorists in the nineteenth century provided an institutional basis through the establishment of the Folk-Lore Society. Recognition of a distinct object, a concern with methods, production of knowledge as a scholarly collector (versus being a "mere cataloguist" [294]), a sense of zeal, and concern "with the cause of folklore as an independent science" come to be complemented by active participation in folklore societies in creating a "fraternity of folklorists" (286) and excluding "the popularizer who wrote without regard for their principles and in complete disregard of the movement" (297).

Dorson defined folkloristics apart from race and particularly from colonialism, spatializing it as the exploration of rural areas of the British Isles: an engagement with subjects defined by lack of literacy skills, education, and modern technology and constituted as a pursuit befitting modern, elite subjects, "the walking tour." The work of Camden, Aubrey, and Bourne provided a model for the emergence of a national identity—"the self-discovery of England proceeded through the tour over improved roads" (1968:13). Aubrey's practice of walking provided an early example of the transformation of rural walking from a utilitarian activity undertaken by the poor and possibly criminal into a model of leisure, mobility, and cosmopolitanism—that is, of class difference. Just as walking becomes a quintessential embodiment of mobility and circulation (see Urry 2007), the study of what came to be known as folklore could similarly be both produced and rendered mobile, capable of ready decontextualization, by "the walking tour."

Note the intersections between Dorson's and Chakrabarty's genealogies, albeit in reverse. Chakrabarty constructs modernity as an ideological project, while Dorson describes it as a real, dynamic historical force embodied in literacy and technology. Similarly, Chakrabarty challenges the romantic and teleological character of modernist narratives like Dorson's. Nevertheless, modernity, in both accounts, was developed apart from traditionality or Otherness; the cultural forms associated with European peasants emerged independently of modernity, and they did not contaminate the male, white, elite ideology that modernity deprovincialized. Both modernity, for Chakrabarty, and folkloristics, for Dorson, emerged from whiteness and elite status, only becoming discourses of racial difference when whiteness was exported through nineteenth-century colonialism; modernity and traditionality got mixed up with race, coloniality, and violence at that point.[2] The emergence of a modern British subject and the recognition and entextualization of its (still white) opposite in the countryside is largely a cultural project, one that exists apart from the profound political-economic effects of the enclosures of the commons that were transforming the English landscape, displacing just the sort of people Dorson positions as Aubrey's interlocutors (Neeson 1993; Thompson 1963). The "improved roads" that Dorson cites were tied to the growing penetration of capitalist trade and agriculture into rural areas—and ironically often deteriorated by increasing traffic in carts and carriages (Copeland 1968). The expansion of English capital and technology during what is generally referred to as the industrial revolution was closely related to the possibility of imagining traditional Others in the countryside.

To be sure, contemporary genealogies often tell the story in rather less naturalistic, teleological, and heroic ways. Bauman and Briggs (2003), for example, characterize Aubrey's work as a crucial part of the production of modern subjects, spaces, and epistemologies through the creation of their cultural and political opposites; the "discovery" of the traditional Other was thus co-produced with modern science, politics, spatial dynamics, education, political economy, and language. These authors seek to demonstrate to practitioners in history, science studies, linguistics, and other areas that the history of folkloristics is a vital part of other genealogies—thereby attempting to secure a broader claim on scholarly landscapes. Nevertheless, their work reproduces crucial features of Dorson's narrative—Aubrey's texts are construed as representations of the English countryside and its occupants, and their history similarly begins in northern Europe in the seventeenth century.

Dussel's, Mignolo's, and Quijano's accounts of modernity open up the possibility of rereading this disciplinary prehistory. In both his *Essay Concerning Human Understanding* (1690 [1959]) and *Two Treatises of Government* ([1690] 1960), John Locke draws on his fascination with travel literature in according Asia and the Americas a crucial role. In the *Essay*, as Bauman and Briggs (2003) argue, Locke strips received understandings of language of such seemingly extraneous dimensions as rhetoric and poetics, arguing that language's core is referential (semantic), rational, transparent, and reliable. He suggests that "men" in Asia and America can reason quite adequately "who yet never heard of a syllogism" (IV.xvii.4). His baseline for constructing notions of language, mind, and rationality is provided by the site of nature, which he describes in the second *Treatise* as "the Woods and Forests, where irrational untaught Inhabitants keep right by following Nature" (I.vi.58), thereby constructing what human beings must be like when they have not been corrupted by performative uses of language—uses of speech in *creating* knowledge and social relations rather than confining speech simply to parsimonious and transparent reflections of what we already know. Colonial projections of racial Others thus provide Locke with a crucial mode of fashioning modern subjects.[3]

John Aubrey, like Locke a member of the Royal Society, similarly inhabited a textual world shaped by trade, conquest, and colonial projects that fundamentally informed his account of folklore.[4] Chapter 8 in his *Miscellanies* (1972) provides a cartography of "Magick." To be sure, Aubrey sometimes locates the site of linguistic anti-modernity in the English countryside. Nevertheless, it takes a great deal of work—and selective reading—to follow Dorson in suggesting that Aubrey's project consists simply of traveling to the English country, locating genuine artifacts of tradition, recording them, and transporting them to modern readers. The chapter opens with the statement "In Barbary are Wizards, who do smear their Hands with some black Ointment" as a mode of divination (83). Aubrey's source is not personal experience: "This Mr. W[yld] C[larke] a Merchant of London, who was Factor there several Years, protested to me, that he did see. He is a Person worthy of beliefe." Clarke was placed in "Santa Crux Barberie," now Ifni, on the Moroccan coast, through the global expansion of British trade; Aubrey drew upon circuits of science, knowledge, and capital (of which more later) to ask Clarke to gather information as well as botanical specimens.

From Morocco we travel back to England to witness "a Parallel Method" of divination using exposure of eggs to the sun. Aubrey then takes us to India, following the "wonderful Stories of the Bannians in India, viz. of their Predictions, Cures &c. of their Charming Crocodiles, and Serpents" (1972:83). Without seeming to take a breath, we travel back to England, where Aubrey reveals his observations of young women searching in a pasture on the Day of St. John the Baptist for coals under the root of a plantain "to put under their Heads that Night, and they should Dream who would be their Husbands" (83). Aubrey framed this description as having emerged "accidentally" while he "was walking in the Pasture behind Montague House." From there Aubrey moves to a general statement, "The Women have several Magical Secrets handed down to them by Tradition, for this purpose," before quoting Ben Johnson, Alexander Tralianus's *Of Curing Diseases by Spells, Charms, &c.*, John Dee's *Book of Spirits* by way of Casaubon, the English translation of a French historical encyclopedia (Louis Moréri's *Grand diccionnaire historique*), a work on magic by "Mr.——Schoot, A German," a manuscript by Elias Ashmole and a personal communication from him, Syrian Neoplatonist philosopher Iamblichus's *De Mysteriis de nomibis divinis*, quoted in Latin, a series of cures without any attribution, and cures provided by "an experienced Midwife," "a Yeoman in Surrey" (87), "Mr. Nicholas Mercator, Astronomer," "Mr. W. Lilly's Astrology" (88), "Mr. Sp.," and Thomas Gages's *A New Survey of the West-Indies* (89).

Thus, "the self-discovery of England" springs not simply from a "tour over improved roads" but from a heteroglossic (in Bakhtin's 1981 terms) project that constructs omens, dreams, apparitions, magic, festivals, oaths, and divination through a complex intertextual fabric drawn from classical antiquity, global trade, and European colonialism as well as the English countryside. The location of modernity's opposite, tradition, is not consistently mapped by a binary opposition between a rural, illiterate, female, traditional subject and an urban, highly educated, male modern one, but rather extends into the British aristocracy. Moreover, the sources that Aubrey cites do not all distance themselves from tradition. "Sir William Neal's Son, a very stout Gentleman," for example, nearly committed suicide from the pain of a toothache, only to be saved after bleeding his gums with a new nail (1972:87). "Gentlewomen" engage in divination, just as "Mr. Nicholas Mercator, Astronomer" not only provided information on a means of staunching bleeding but "told me that he had tried it with effect"; Aubrey reports that "Mr. Will. Nash a Chyrurgeon in Salisbury" used it to cure King James II (88). Although Aubrey sometimes distanced himself from "the old ignorant times" (289), it is not always easy to discern how he positioned his own voice. To his account of the healing power of a seventh son named Samuel Scott, Aubrey appends: "I am very well satisfied of the truth of this Relation, for I knew him very well, and his Mother was my Kinswoman" (79).

In short, it requires considerable textual erasure to construct Aubrey as a thoroughly modern subject who confidently journeys from the modern city along country roads and across a boundary defined by class and the city/countryside dichotomy to discover a pristine folkloric object, all the while remaining inside a sphere of racial homogeneity untouched by colonialism. He wrote about Irish folklore in the wake of Cromwell's violent suppression of the Irish Rebellion of 1641, massive land expropriation, and the growing but complex hegemony of the Anglo-Irish Protestant elite.[5] The England that Aubrey discovered was an empire shaped by diverse colonial projects and global expansion of capital and by textual imaginaries of Greece, Rome, biblical antiquity, North Africa, and Asia. Aubrey's fragmented subjects emerge through shifting, ambiguous, and seemingly ambivalent relations woven in multilingual, heteroglossic texts that are shot through with the coloniality of power. If Aubrey discovered the traditional object that would constitute what later became folkloristics, it was a traditional/colonial object.

Italian Giuseppe Cocchiara's encyclopedic *The History of Folklore in Europe* (1981), on the other hand, provides a genealogy that attends specifically to the fruits of colonialism in shaping the emergence of folkloristics. Contra Dorson's vision of an inwardly focused "self-discovery of England," Cocchiara argues that "the savage was a touchstone . . . [that] constitutes the beginning of the history of folklore" (28). He traces the importance of accounts by "missionaries, travelers, and historians of the American Indian" (15) and the impact of Orientalist literatures on such figures as Montaigne, Rousseau, Vico, and Herder. To his credit, Cocchiara mentions de las Casas and other debates regarding violence and justice in the treatment and representation of Native Americans, but his focus on texts and authors underplays the importance of processes of dissemination and reception and locations within broader political economies. In short, Cocchiara's *History* provides a fruitful point of departure for tying the emergence of folkloristics to complex intersections between modernity, traditionality, and colonialism. Nonetheless, his account of the way that "in Europe the discovery of America nourished a new humanism" (13) calls out for more attention to how constructions of modernity and traditionality were woven not only into textual visions of a pacific "noble savage" but into the racial violence of colonialism and the expansion of European capital as well as the enduring impact of these connections on disciplinary concepts and methods.

COLONIAL INSCRIPTIONS OF COLONIAL FOLKLORISTICS

When we examine genealogies of nineteenth-century folkloristics, we encounter the opposite problem—here colonialism is hardly erased, nor could it be. Nevertheless, colonialism often gets contained within particular spaces (particularly India), periods, and characters—British colonial officials and missionaries—thereby drawing attention away from how colonialism is connected with other spaces, subjects, and times, such as our own.

In Dorson's narrative, the evolutionists ("the savage folklorists"), the consolidators of folklore as a science ("the Great Team"), and the institutionalizers ("the Society folklorists") are carefully distinguished from the colonial folklorists. Dorson occasionally comments on the racist overtones that enter texts (1968:352). To his credit, Dorson points to "the Empire theory of applied folklore" that turned folkloristics into a vital part of colonial enterprises in India, Africa, and other parts of the empire (332). For Dorson, however, colonialism did not constitute folkloristics as a discipline or shape it in keeping with colonial epistemologies and practices; indeed, techniques of textual fidelity and textual annotation were "applied" in such a way, to quote Dorson quoting leading colonial collector Richard Carnac Temple, as "to strictly conform to the method adopted by the Folk-Lore Society of England" (337).[6] Rather than folklore collecting and publishing being part of the work of colonialism, Dorson conceives of the practice as a leisure-time activity for the odd colonial official, missionary, or family member. Dorson remarks of Temple, "One marvels how the 'hard-worked official,' as he described himself, writing in his spare hours remote from libraries, could have produced so well-informed a collection" (338).[7] The result is a "happy fusion of islands-and-empire folklore research" (345) in which, to extend the optimistic tone of Dorson's triumphalist narrative, "intellectual and administrative ends thus happily coincided, with *fortuitous* results for folklore collecting" (333; emphasis added).

Indeed, a common set of methodological concepts seemingly guided work in the English countryside and in the "splendid colonial laboratory of folklore" (Dorson 1968:440) provided by the "inexhaustible treasure houses of native traditions" (333). Speaking of William Crooke and Richard Carnac

Temple, Dorson writes, "By the time of the First World War, their untiring efforts and earnest purpose had firmly grounded the science of folklore in India, in keeping with the principles of the leading English folklorists, and helped make available a whole library of unwritten traditions" [1968:348]. The way that collectors "turned to the experts of The Folk-Lore Society for advice in processing their hard-won harvests from the field" (333) assured that colonialism would become a tool for extending the folkloristic canon rather than folkloristics being transformed in keeping with racial economies and colonial interests. Temple's status as president of the Folk-Lore Society does not seem to trouble Dorson's separation of the roles of "expert" and "colonial collector." Institutional contexts, including libraries, universities, professional societies, prisons, courtrooms, colonial administrative offices, military units, and the British East India Company, were deeply connected, in part by the production, circulation, and consumption of colonial folklore. Nevertheless, just as they are not allowed to infect the science of folklore, race and colonialism seemingly become irrelevant again as Dorson's narrative shifts to tracing how nineteenth-century collectors made "the most exciting discoveries" in Scotland, Wales, and Ireland—"their own Isles" (391). Britain was similarly deeply involved in the slave trade, deeply enmeshed in a "Black Atlantic" sphere that circulated slaves, goods, cultural forms, technologies, and epistemologies between Africa, Europe, and the Americas (Gilroy 1993).

Note how British colonialism in these areas and *"their own* Isles" (emphasis added), as well as long histories of anticolonial and working-class resistance, all seem to merge in a single English national identity, which somehow appeared long before the emergence of nationalism as a stable, obligatory, totalizing illusion (Anderson [1983] 1991). Dorson's account both connects and disconnects colonialism and folkloristics. Dorson uses a spatial vocabulary in separating England from the colonies and creating a single trajectory: knowledge about folkloristics emanated in the metropole and then "firmly grounded the science of folklore in India" (1968:348). Dorson's agricultural metaphor, folklore as "hard-won harvests from the field," naturalizes the establishment of folklore science in India, the extraction of knowledge, and its transport to the metropole for consumption. He seems to miss the implication that folklore and colonialism had become so entwined that the coming demise of the colonial venture helped undermine the expansion of British folkloristics.

We are, of course, now able to take advantage of a number of efforts to rethink colonial folkloristics in questioning colonial narratives of colonialism. Nicholas Dirks (2001), Johannes Fabian (2000), Michael McBratney

(2006), Gloria Raheja (1996), and others point to the embeddedness of the collecting enterprise in the administrative, military, missionary, domestic, and extractive everyday activities of colonialism, which paralleled the use of colonial accounts by Edward Tylor ([1871] 1889) and James Frazer, author of *The Golden Bough* ([1922] 1950), in consolidating the disciplinary status of evolutionary anthropology in Britain (see Stocking 1968). What has been less adequately documented is the role of folkloristics in producing commodified texts that provided an intimate, affective, and domestic space for colonialism in homes back in the metropole. Indian folklore, which came from diverse languages and social, religious, and philosophical contexts, was translated into English. It is easy to imagine that these folklores followed diverse genres and poetic structures, as well as different narrative and performative styles. It would be right to assume that they also had in the minds of the (Indian) performers and their audiences meanings and functions different from those received by their colonial rulers. If we take these factors into consideration, we will not hesitate to agree that this context—that of the colonial empire—was a highly complex situation that must have offered many challenges to the colonial collectors. A British collector might have been resident and ruler in the colony, but in the act of collection of folklore he or she confronted all the hurdles that any other collector faces—of language, method, and interpretation.

The works of the colonial collectors represented different kinds of efforts at resolving these issues, shaping the emergence of colonial folklore scholarship. Methods of recruiting contributors, who sometimes included servants in the colonial officers' own households and were accorded the roles of "assistant," "translator," "guide," and the like, were deeply woven into relations of race, power, capital, and military force that structured colonialism and its techniques of political control, resource extraction, population surveillance, and incarceration. When we place Indian "assistants," many of whom had levels of education equivalent to their employers', into the picture, the coloniality of accepted images of colonial folkloristics becomes evident. Naithani's (2010) study of British colonial collections brought forth the role of native associates. Pandit Ram Gharib Chaube—associate of the famous William Crooke—was a very special scholar in the context of colonialism. His method of folklore scholarship is not imaginable in any other context, and as such it reveals a great deal not only about him but also about Crooke. While in Crooke's employ, Chaube compiled a massive collection of Indian folktales (Naithani 2006) and played a key role in Crooke's published texts.

Mignolo emphasizes the importance of "critical border thinking" in colonialism and coloniality, perspectives that emerge along borders of modernity and traditionality, dominant and subaltern forms of knowledge, which "implies to think from both traditions and, at the same time, from neither of them" (2000:67). Indian scholars, assistants, translators, and writers, located within the colonial space of race but having received training in colonial forms of knowledge and inscription, engaged in complicated and creative forms of border thinking, which are evident in colonial folklore texts, even as their explicit traces are generally erased or reduced to a line in the acknowledgments.[8] Genealogies like Dorson's find no place for exploring the role of such border thinkers in the construction of folklore collections that were printed, discussed, and institutionalized in England, and critical counter-narratives regarding colonial collecting often reproduce these silences. Indeed, sustaining the illusion that colonial collecting simply extended metropolitan methods of inscription and control into new contexts requires that "the writing/inscribing practices of Indigenous collaborators are erased" (Clifford 1997:23).

The spread of the term *folklore* and its more specific categories, however, could not be arrested in this binary opposition. It spread among the colonized as concept and method. The colonized were asked for "folklore," asked to record it, and asked to translate it—and could therefore not remain unaware of the concept and object of "folklore." Word spread across the boundaries of the colonial empires that the colonized could be known through their folklore. The colonizing world formed images, and the colonized became aware of those images of themselves and often used the same images to create anticolonial and postcolonial identities (Naithani 2001:183–88), as Homi Bhabha (1994) suggests.[9]

Even when (post)colonial subjects were trained as folklorists, Naithani (2010) suggests, the imposition of Eurocentric categories and methods helped strip texts of their power to expose and challenge coloniality. Colonialism was apparent not only in the production of colonial folklore but in its reception as well. Within colonial empires, collections were published in European languages in Europe and were meant for European readers. In other words, infrastructures of knowledge and their products, like printed folklore, libraries, and archives, were to remain out of the reach of the colonized, even if officials may have performed their knowledge of folklore orally in order to address colonial subjects on what seemed to be their own terms (Raheja 1996). This issue has profound implications for the growth of the discipline. Having euphemistically dubbed colonial folklore collectors not as "colonial" but as "the overseas folklorists," Dorson discusses colonial folklore scholarship from other continents—Africa, Asia, Australia, Oceania, and the Far East—in about forty-five pages

(1968:332–78). In representing their work as extensions of British scientific folkloristics as applied in colonial encounters and then exported to the metropole, Dorson directed attention away from the role of colonial research on folkloristics and colonial folklorists' participation in societies and educational organizations. We suggest, on the contrary, that colonial practices of research, writing, and reading were forged in the production and the movement of knowledge, people, and objects between Europe and the colonies—and that they have shaped international folklore studies up to the present.

THE COLONIALITY OF FOLKLORISTICS AND THE DILEMMAS OF THE CONTEMPORARY

This exploration of British folkloristics suggests two things. First, race, violence, and colonialism, deeply inscribed into the traditional/colonial object from the time of folkloristics' prediscovery emergence in the seventeenth century, have remained central right through its efflorescence in the nineteenth and early twentieth centuries. Second, extant genealogies have (dis)connected, limited, and contained connections between folkloristics and colonialism in many ways. Nevertheless, as we suggested earlier, our concern is less with "correcting" disciplinary histories than with the implications of these patterns of representation and erasure for the present. Science studies suggest that rethinking historical genealogies provides a sine qua non for creating new ways of doing work in and on the present (Latour 1987; Anderson 2006). Rather than pretending to provide a comprehensive account, we engage here with work that seems to both reflect how coloniality shapes contemporary folkloristics as well as work that attempts to confront this legacy. The previous chapter's focus on the work of Américo Paredes provides a key example of traditionality/coloniality, including how he defined folklore through racial difference, power, and conflict and the way he was denied a more central role in shaping folkloristics. Here we provide three shorter examples.

Take 1: Postcolonial India

India provides an ideal site to challenge coloniality and create alternative genealogies. Infrastructures for folkloristics, including a number of doctoral programs and state support for research and public programming, are relatively strong. India and the diaspora have been the hotbed of postcolonial theory. Continuing with the nationalist fervor of the freedom struggle and Marxist influence, revising colonial history was a major item on the scholarly agendas of the 1960s and 1970s. In the 1980s, subaltern studies challenged nationalist-Marxist perspectives, transforming study of colonial India and freedom struggles. Contributions by Homi Bhabha (1994), Dipesh Chakrabarty (1989), and Gayatri Spivak (1988) are well acknowledged. As Chakrabarty (2000) urged, subaltern studies has become not simply a means of critically engaging accounts of Indian history that emerged from British colonial historians and nationalist elites but of mounting a challenge from the Indian subcontinent to the supposedly universal categories and subject positions that have organized dominant discourses. Edward Said (1978) stimulated a rethinking of colonial aspects of culture. Dirks (2001), Raheja (1996), and others brought folklore centrally into discussions of colonialism, and Veena Das (2007) powerfully revealed the importance of narrative to contemporary South Asian politics.

Nevertheless, a distinctive postcolonial folkloristics has yet to emerge. A fundamental tenet of subaltern studies, clearly signaled in Ranajit Guha's (1982) foundational essay, is Indian subaltern agency within colonial contexts. The importance of Indian folklorists working for colonial collectors, however, is largely missing. Moreover, although peasant insurrections receive substantial attention, how subaltern Indians used folklore in critically engaging colonialism has not become a focus of scholarly attention. In other words, the notion that folklore can constitute a positive historical force for the oppressed, as suggested, to name just a few examples, by Paredes (1958) for Mexican American folklore, John Roberts (1989) and Lawrence Levine (1977) for African American folklore, Cutcha Risling Baldy (2015) and Christopher Teuton et al. (2012) for Native American narrative, and James Scott (1985) for Indonesia, has not become central. British imposition of the categories and practices of European-derived folkloristics has been well documented, but how Indians reworked colonial structures in dialogue with precolonial forms remains largely unexplored (Naithani 2010). Much work on Indian folklore still embraces an anthropological paradigm rooted in nineteenth-century concerns with kinship, caste, and rural versus urban populations, and researchers seldom move beyond description. Even when researchers have embraced more contemporary approaches—say, performance-centered or gender perspectives—theory is often not conceived directly in relation to the context of research. There is a considerable amount of folklore research in India conducted by folklorists and anthropologists from Europe and the United States in which the terms of reference may be contemporary and situated in current debates, but the concepts and controversies are located in the academic contexts of Europe and North America and also find their areas of influence there. Debates about folklore that take place among Indian scholars show an awareness of the works of European and American scholars.

The political usage of folklore for constructing national pride and ethnic cultural identity receives state support in India. But a sensitive, truly postcolonial concern and engagement with expressive cultures got lost along the way, with some notable exceptions (Das 2007; Chatterjee and Mehta 2007), partly due to the epistemological agendas that structure folklore infrastructures. Although folklore collection, translation, and publication started in the 1860s and British colonial collectors themselves were instrumental in creating such institutions in Britain, scholarly loci of folklore research were not established in India until after independence in 1947. In the 1980s, the Ford Foundation funded some folklore research projects, and Indian folklorists participated with commitment in Udupi, Chennai, Shillong, and Jodhpur. From these the group in Chennai has coalesced into a National Folklore Support Centre and is doing commendable work of documentation and archiving. A few folklore departments located in regional universities, particularly Guwahati University in Assam and North-Eastern Hill University in Shillong, have brought forth a new generation of folklore scholars who will make a difference to Indian folkloristics in the near future. Yet, training in contemporary methods of collection and archiving requires much attention. At an overall level, folklore as a subject of study in higher education is in the outer margins of Indian academia.

Nevertheless, there is a growing body of recent work by scholars based outside of India that dialogically engages fascinating vernacular reflections on categories and identities associated with caste, gender, and class. Amanda Weidman (2006) uses postcolonial theory in scrutinizing the making, engendering, and technological transformations of voices that represent Indian pasts and presents. Kirin Narayan (Narayan and Sood 1997) places storytellers as both performers and critics of the social and religious worlds they occupy and critically engages her own positionality as an Indian American "halfie" scholar. Leela Prasad (2007) locates narration as a key means of managing complex and competing ethical positions. Frank Korom (2006) explores how west Bengali scroll painters critically engage the technologies, circuits, and forms of commodification that insert their work in global markets. Joyce Burkhalter Flueckiger (2006) enables us to see how a Muslim spiritual healer in south India moves across borderlines of gender, religion, and class in treating her Christian, Hindu, and Muslim patients. Finally, *Gender, Genre, and Power in South Asian Expressive Traditions*, edited by Arjun Appadurai, Frank J. Korom, and Margaret Mills (1991), and *South Asian*

Folklore: An Encyclopedia, edited by Margaret Mills, Peter Claus, and Sarah Diamond (2003), are important collections that reveal the complexity of current debates, engage a multiplicity of perspectives, and demonstrate careful attention to issues of inclusion and representation.

Although the displacement of colonial and postcolonial genealogies of folkloristics in India is occurring slowly and unevenly, two lines of research seem particularly significant. One is rethinking the role of Indian scholars who were cast in the position of assistants or translators to colonial British folklorists. For example, a lapse of nearly sixty years separated India's independence and the publication of Ram Gharib Chaube's work (Naithani 2002, 2006). Chaube's emergence as an active and conscious participant forms an ironic contrast to postcolonial folkloristics. Within the tight framework of the colonial intellectual world, Chaube's effort was to rise above it—subversively, reflecting colonial splits in Herderian projections of the unity of language, nation, and mind. Chaube knew Indian languages—including classical and colloquial dialects as well as Sanskrit and Hindi—Persian, and English. Yet, it was his historical compulsion to write in English, and he did this without a perceivable hitch. Furthermore, he wrote both as an outsider and an insider to the "traditional" tales. As a border thinker, his acts of translation show an awareness of colonial folkloristics and, simultaneously, a historical distance from it that is often missing from postcolonial Indian folkloristics.

Although Mignolo (2000:39) seems to glorify border thinking as a "multiplication of epistemic energies," Chaube perhaps best fits W.E.B. Du Bois's characterization of "double consciousness," in which racial Others must also see themselves through the denigrating lenses through which they are envisioned by members of the racial dominant. Double consciousness, according to Du Bois, results in "a painful self-consciousness, an almost morbid sense of personality and a moral hesitancy which is fatal to self-confidence" and "a peculiar wrenching of the soul, a peculiar sense of doubt and bewilderment" ([1903] 1990:146). Frantz Fanon ([1952] 1967) similarly described the splitting of the colonial subject as pathological and violent. Chaube died in his village of Gopalpur—a destitute driven to insanity by lack of recognition and support. His former employer, Crooke, did not write an obituary (Naithani 2002:211). Chaube's century-long anonymity and lack of influence on Indian folkloristics are more than his personal destiny. Denial of acknowledgment of Chaube's work in his lifetime transformed a personal tragedy into a postcolonial Indian folkloristics without a distinct identity. The continuing coloniality of folklore research has required erasure of the role of Chaube and other "assistants."

If Crooke had acknowledged Chaube's contribution, Dorson might have thought about British "overseas folklorists" from another perspective. Had Chaube's voice been heard in his lifetime, or even after independence, the nature of Indian folkloristics and international scholarship on Indian folklore could not have remained oblivious to the continuing effects of its own colonial past.[10]

Another important locus involves documentation of unexpected sites of circulation and performance of well-known Indian folkloric genres, which help counter the lingering effects of the coloniality of folkloristics in limiting both research agendas and their potential for reshaping public policies and political discourses. Muslim performers of Hindu epics provide a case in point. The Muslim Jogis (ascetics) of Alwar, Rajasthan, perform local, oral versions of the great Indian epics Ramayana and Mahabharata, and the stories of the Hindu god Shiva. They perform even in Hindu temples. They provide a record of the way conversion to Islam in medieval India took place, simultaneously revealing how local practices of Islam are under threat by current fundamentalist and hegemonic concepts of a universal Islam. For a folklorist, the content of these folk versions of the great epics are themselves a record of the perspectives from the margins. For example, the characters highlighted in these versions are those completely marginalized, and even missing, from the renowned epics. The style in which the protagonists are addressed and portrayed differs significantly from the official versions. Here we see a perspective on society and gods from the margins, where the narrators themselves are placed.

Most performers across India are classified as "lower caste," and in the narration of the genealogy of their caste (which often forms the opening texts of the performance) they address the issue and seek to establish their equality through a story of divine origin. The literature on colonialism shows the British preoccupation with reifying complex and shifting social and religious distinctions into rigid categories, including caste distinctions and a Hindu versus Muslim divide; the British then used these categories in a divide-and-conquer strategy that created the illusion of distinct, opposed, and mutually unintelligible populations who needed the British to unify them. As a number of scholars have suggested, folklore research by missionaries and colonial officials played a central role in this process. These Muslim performances of Indian epics, like the South Indian spiritual healer that Flueckiger (2006) discusses, provide one of the many contemporary sites in which dominant genealogies are critiqued and challenged, opening up critical spaces of dialogue. The colonial legacy of folkloristics rendered such phenomena largely invisible to folklorists, thereby thwarting practitioners' potential for making important interventions into tremendously consequential political debates; new work that identifies such sites is thus particularly significant.[11]

TAKE 2: GERMAN FOLKLORISTICS IN THE TWENTIETH CENTURY

When we speak of transformations, particularly positive ones, we must return to Germany. The significance of German scholarship goes beyond the pioneering roles of late eighteenth- and early to mid-nineteenth-century scholars to include the complex history of twentieth-century German folkloristics. Relevant to our discussion here is the *Auseinandersteęung* with the disciplinary history that folklorists undertook in 1960s and 1970s in response to the experience of National Socialism and German *Volkskunde*. Hannjost Lixfeld (1994) suggests that by aligning itself with Volkskunde, National Socialism sought to gain a scholarly legitimacy that could then advance the fascist agenda. (See also Bausinger 1994; Dow and Lixfeld 1986, 1994; Stein 1987.)

A broad postwar debate was enjoined among folklorists, even if it emerged slowly and encountered resistance (see Dow and Lixfeld 1994). Christoph Daxelmüller (1994:73) suggested, "There is no indication that German folklorists were directly guilty of exterminating Jewish life," but they were sympathetic to those who were responsible for genocide. Daxelmüller points out how German folklorists before Nazism had been uninterested in Jewish folklore and often encouraged jokes against Jews. After the war, Will-Erich Peuckert (1948:130–35) offered the theory of two Volkskunde in Nazi Germany: a populist version that collaborated with the fascists, and a scholarly Volkskunde that remained aloof to the politics of the state. This thesis, along with the notion that National Socialism morally corrupted an innocent discipline, was challenged in the 1960s and 1970s by Hermann Bausinger, Wolfgang Emmerich, and others. Bausinger states: "We must deal with the eventuality that National Socialism did not somehow introduce foreign ideas and did not just strengthen the peripheral elements but emphasized throughout the primary ideas within this scholarly discipline, and this makes a confrontation with National Socialist scholarship even more indispensable in Volkskunde than in other disciplines" (1994:11). Emmerich (1971) argued that Romantic Nationalism, folklore scholarship, and conservative political projects were tied together by a long history rather than a short-term twentieth-century misappropriation; he shows how Romantic Nationalism and German folkloristics contributed to conservative social and political perspectives and helped recruit the petty bourgeoisie for fascist politics. Bausinger and Emmerich thus locked horns with dimensions of violence and racism in folklore scholarship in a larger time frame than that of National Socialism.

The attacks on the extremity of the Nazi experience articulated during the 1960s produced several important effects. Folklorists felt it necessary to create a focused, critical, and wholesale engagement with their own history; most Volkskunde departments changed their names to *Kulturanthropologie*, European Ethnology, or *Empirische Kulturwissenschaft*. Scholars shifted away from traditional songs, stories, proverbs, and riddles and embraced social scientific perspectives on contemporary cultural phenomena and everyday life and critiques of folkloristics' epistemological and political foundations (see Bausinger [1961] 1990; Bendix 1997). Nevertheless, Dow's (Dow and Lixfield 1994) earlier enthusiastic and hopeful appreciation of these changes seems to have given way to disappointment by 2008: "The virtual rejection of a grand theory and the opening up of new research areas . . . have resulted in diffuseness in place of problem-oriented ideas, dispersion instead of a broadened concept of culture" (Dow 2008:59). He notes with concern that no new departments for the study of folklore have opened, including in the wake of German reunification.

The German experience of the twentieth century speaks importantly to issues of the coloniality of folkloristics. National Socialism appears to have drawn more on Volkskunde scholarship of the mid-nineteenth century and afterward than directly on Herder.[12] Nevertheless, romantic naturalization of a vision of a homogeneous national community made folklore scholarship and popular consumption of folklore texts exceedingly useful for National Socialism. We must not oversimplify Herder's work. He was deeply in dialogue with Enlightenment notions of modernity, and he acknowledged the influence of British philologists such as Thomas Blackwell, Robert Wood, and Robert Lowth, whose work sprang from a textual universe shaped by British colonialism and trade (Bauman and Briggs 2003). The effect of James Macpherson's textual imaginary of Scottish Highland bard Ossian is apparent in Herder's journey through time as much as space, as he pondered, a copy of Ossian at his side, amidst the waters "where long ago skalds and vikings with sword and song plied the seas" ([1877–1913] 1967:169). That Germany had no colonies at the time did not impede Herder from informing his vision of modernity, traditionality, and nationalism through works on Native Americans, Inuit, Tahitians, and Brazilian Indians or the Orientalism of his *The Spirit of Hebrew Poetry* ([1782] 1833). Indeed, Herder could no more have written his "Essay on the Origin of Language" ([1772] 1966) than Aubrey could have penned his *Miscellanies* without assimilating a textual universe that was tied in political-economic as well as cultural terms to colonialism and the expansion of European capital. Chapter 3 traced how Herder's vision of folklore as emanating outward from "the patriarch's hut" to the nation inscribed notions of whiteness and racial homogeneity, like patriarchy, into his construction of folklore and nationalism.

National Socialism thus did not take notions of traditionality and modernity that lacked racial referents and bend them to genocidal ends but rather transformed generally implicit dimensions of their indexical histories into nightmarish visions of embodied threats to a supposedly bounded and homogeneous cultural and racial group. Andre Gingrich (1998:119) similarly argues that colonial relations with Balkan Muslims shaped a "frontier Orientalism," remembered through such cultural forms as "folk tales, village chronicles, baroque pillars, Turkish museum collections, school textbooks, and rural toponyms" that has continued to produce ambivalent and contradictory reactions to Muslims during the past half century. We thus see as particularly significant the work of postwar German folklorists who addressed the underpinnings of difference and violence that had shaped Volkskunde and struggled to produce critical alternatives.

Take 3: Confronting Traditionality and Nationalism in Latin America

Néstor García Canclini ([1990] 1995) and Renato Ortiz (1985, 1992) have examined Latin American connections between folklore, nationalism, and state violence. García Canclini argues that "the dramatization of the patrimony is the effort to simulate that there is an origin, a founding substance, in relation with which we should act today" (110). Folklore becomes "the most secret basis of the social simulation that keeps us together as a group" (108), even as it naturalizes the boundaries between dominant and subaltern sectors by expelling the latter from modernity. Folklore is always subject to practices of preservation, restoration, and dissemination that enhance "patrimonial conservatism" as culture is transformed into part of the national landscape, becoming "natural like a gift" (111). Naturalizing folklore is particularly valuable when nationalism projects a social body as deeply connected to a natural body—the national territory and its natural resources (see Coronil 1997). Ortiz writes of Brazil that "popular culture is part of the construction of the Nation-State; it is the symbolic element that permits intellectuals to become conscious and express the peripheral situation in which their countries live" (1985:66–67, translation ours). Constructing folklore in such a way that Latin American nation-states seem to spring naturally from *el pueblo* (the people), Jesús Martín Barbero ([1987] 2003) suggests, cast elites as leading a pedagogical project required to free the premodern masses from barbarism.

Recent scholarship has provided new research foci and analytic interventions. Argentine folklorist Martha Blache (1998:27) challenged the notion that folklore involves an "authoritative norm or static and immutable force," positioning it as a continual reconfiguration of understandings of past and present.[13] In Venezuela, Yolanda Salas (1987) who, lamentably, died in 2007, traced distinct class trajectories of national hero Simón Bolívar: the Bolívar of the oppressors (the rich) and the Bolívar of the oppressed. Her work also examined how a leading tobacco company dominated public representations of folklore in Venezuela (2003) and how inmates reconfigured national narratives and symbolic practices. Jesús Chucho García (1992) analyzes the "folklorization" of Afro-Venezuelan culture and proposes its "de-folklorization," that is, its extraction from the sorts of constructions of tradition criticized by García Canclini and Ortiz.

Nevertheless, Latin America also presents a paradox. At the same time that some work performed in state, academic, and nongovernmental sectors conservatively reifies nationalist conceptions, other academic and public folklorists are actively exposing the role of coloniality, race, and violence in shaping these representations; the latter collaborate with communities of difference in reframing how folklore is defined and researched. In Argentina, for example, Fernando Fischman has used folkloristics as a tool for documenting Jewish memory and anti-Semitic violence (Fischman and Pelacoff 2015). Rather than creating a vibrant context for academic training, however, folkloristics is losing ground in most Latin American countries, and there are relatively few graduate programs. Dictatorships in Argentina and Chile and other conservative and repressive governments projected folklore as a common cultural heritage that constituted a sphere of consensus that required a pedagogical, patriarchal state that could supervise, teach, and speak for the people. In Argentina and Chile, folklorists were courted by repressive governments, while more left-leaning social sciences were institutionally and/or violently suppressed, leading many contemporary scholars to eschew the term *folklore* and locate work that could provide a basis for transforming the discipline into "cultural studies," "anthropology," or studies of "popular culture."[14] These difficulties spring from the foundational role of colonialism, difference, and violence in constituting folkloristics, whose regional predisciplinary history is rooted in entextualizing Indigenous peoples as a part of conquest and colonization.

TOWARD A MULTI-GENEALOGICAL PRACTICE OF FOLKLORISTICS

As suggested in chapter 3, Américo Paredes presented in the 1950s a systematic critique of the coloniality of folkloristics and offered a vision of how the field could become a key site for analyzing the ways that social identities and relations are produced and critiqued. John Roberts (1999) argued that folkloristics has fared poorly in the contemporary US academy because it celebrates bounded cultural niches while other disciplines explore how boundaries are formed through conflict, appropriation, and erasure. Scholars in women's, LGBT, ethnic, cultural, and American studies have focused on how researchers reproduce and extend social categories, borders, and relations. If folkloristics had followed Paredes, it would have been decades ahead, shaping understandings of diversity and the politics of culture rather than wondering why it often gets left out of the game. Folkloristics would be enjoying a stronger institutional and intellectual position.

Some disciplines have renewed their epistemological foundations, creating more inclusive infrastructures by redefining their objects of study. In the 1980s, as critics proclaimed the conquest of space by time through digital technologies and forms of transport (Castells 1996; Harvey 1989; Jameson 1991), geography seemed to be failing, and many departments closed or lost ground. Nevertheless, critical work by Lefebvre ([1974] 1991), Soja (1989), and others abandoned a conception of space as a preexisting object requiring expert cartographic knowledge to focus on situated social and political-economic practices for *producing* notions of space. Rather than a naturally occurring object, space became a problematic social product. Geography is now a thriving discipline. American studies has similarly shifted from documenting a common American historical and cultural legacy to studying difference associated with race, ethnicity, gender, and sexuality; challenging received notions of "American culture," the field critically examined its own genealogies (Lipsitz 2001). The study of race and ethnicity similarly shifted from mapping preestablished identity categories to examining how they are co-constructed with understandings of gender, sexuality, and disability (see, for example, Gutiérrez 1991; Omi and Winant 1994; Ralph 2014; Stoler 1995).

Anthropology's claims to a monopoly on scientific studies of culture through fieldwork in subaltern populations earned it the reputation of being a tool of colonialism and racial dominance. "Poetics and politics" critiques subjected ethnography to rhetorical and political scrutiny, reducing scientific claims of ethnographic authority to problematic narrative techniques for creating "the Other" (Clifford and Marcus 1986; Clifford 1988; Marcus and Fischer 1986). As ethnographers embraced a call to research elite actors at home (Nader 1972; Ortner 2003) and to critically scrutinize their own politics of knowledge production and entextualization, ethnography came to be viewed as a valuable but problematic enterprise; many ethnographers engage in critical, reflexive, and rhetorical scrutiny and experimentation even as they practice it. Linguistic anthropologists similarly transformed claims to have objective knowledge of linguistic structures into research on "language ideologies," viewing all representations of language—including their own—as politically interested, historically shaped, and materially consequential (Schieffelin, Woolard, and Kroskrity 1998; Kroskrity 2000). Medical anthropologists shifted from being cartographers of folk theories of subaltern healing practices to critical analysts of the production of medical epistemologies and technologies and notions of the body, health, disease, death, and race (see Cohen 1998; Farmer 1992; Menéndez and Di Pardo 1996; Scheper-Hughes and Lock 1987). As a result, anthropology has regained intellectual and institutional strength.

We see four relevant tendencies in folkloristics. One clings to reifications of the discipline's object of study, projecting its woes as resulting from the failure of many folklorists to zealously participate in boundary-work—thereby rejecting revisionist perspectives, poaching by nonscholars, cross-disciplinary promiscuity, and objects of study that are "not folklore."[15] A second casts the concept of folklore itself as a problem. Due to its imbrications with nationalist projects and nineteenth-century perspectives and its association with life-worlds irrelevant in a globalized and postmodern era, we should erase the term *folklore* and embrace designations that seem to have less baggage—and might accordingly lead to rosier institutional futures (Bendix 1988a; Kirshenblatt-Gimblett 1996).[16] This debate registers in some other areas of the world, such as Latin America, but it has no expression in the writings of Indian folklorists in India.

Nevertheless, reifying, extending, *or* rejecting foundational terms and presuppositions would all lead folklorists to miss the sort of opportunities that have renewed geography, American studies, and anthropology and deny the discipline the sort of new beginning that Paredes envisioned fifty years ago. Abolishing the term also promotes the idea that we can simply wipe away a problematic genealogy. It fosters what we would call *magical nominalism*, as if banning words (*folklore, tradition,* and *authenticity*) can ipso facto erase associated representational practices and institutional positionalities. Simply changing names could provide yet another excuse for not facing the coloniality of folkloristics. Terminological discomfort can rather prompt us to critically examine problematic genealogies.

A third response extends received notions of folklore to include new objects and routes of transmission; here the perspectives on folklore and media discussed in chapter 8 loom particularly large. Dundes (1980:17) argued that a fallacy of nineteenth-century definitions of folklore was how they were negatively tied to communicational technologies and social-change processes; he rather suggested that new technologies *produce* new varieties of folklore. Bausinger tied shifts in folklore to broad transformations of technologies and political economy ([1961] 1990) as their conditions of possibility. Bauman has examined how US notions of performance—and of politics and citizenship—were transformed by phonographic recording and other technologies (Bauman and Feaster 2005; Bauman 2010). Internet-based folklore and folk art, which Robert Glenn Howard (2008) locates in relation to what he refers to as the "vernacular web," are important areas of research (see Blank 2012). Scholars are now pushing the boundaries of folklore and performance beyond the human (Mechling 1989; Thompson 2010, 2018), urging folklorists to embrace "the animal turn" (Magliocco 2018). These paths are highly productive, but they will leave problematic foundational assumptions in place if they do not challenge the persistence of coloniality in the conceptual stock-in-trade of folkloristics.

In urging folklorists to address issues of coloniality, Paredes opened up a fourth possibility. He suggested that when folklorists erase issues of power, hegemony, conflict, and resistance from their work, they curtail its scholarly power by becoming complicit in the reification of existing social categories and hierarchies. In 1971, Paredes's young colleague Richard Bauman (1971) drew on these insights in suggesting that the creation of "differential identity" forms the core of the "social base of folklore" and should constitute its scholarly focus. He critiqued Dundes (1965) and Brunvand (1968) for defining folklore as shared cultural knowledge, arguing that folklore is not always a collective representation that belongs to everyone. It may be so, he suggested, but it may also be differentially distributed, differentially performed, and differentially understood (Bauman 1971:38). Bauman took the threshold that Paredes had opened up for folklore along the Mexican-US border and showed folklorists how to cross it.

Some features of his formulation limited its transformational possibilities. By suggesting that "folklore may be found in both symmetrical and asymmetrical relationships; members of particular groups or social categories may exchange folklore with each other, on the basis of shared identity, or with others, on the basis of differential identity" (1971:38), Bauman did leave space open for defining folklore in the usual fashion. Tying folklore to face-to-face performances, Bauman somewhat narrowed the scope of his intervention. Perhaps reflecting his experience as a journalist, Paredes (1958) stressed how legends and other forms articulated social boundaries as they circulated through newspapers, state discourses, and everyday interactions as well as oral performances. Paredes argued that studying difference is differentially structured—the folklorist's own positionality shapes how she or he portrays culture, requiring critical reflection. By extending Paredes's challenge to the field as a whole, Bauman's article offered a challenge that has not been fully answered.

To be sure, folklorists continue to build on these insights, conducting research that cuts to the heart of the issues raised by the coloniality of folkloristics. Barbara Kirshenblatt-Gimblett (1998a) explores how folklorists and scholars in adjacent fields have shaped and been shaped by the politics of artifact, display, and heritage in museums, world's fairs, tourist attractions, and festivals. She locates their emergence in charged loci for the production of difference, power, and notions of scale, demonstrating their continuing authority through the present. Regina Bendix (1997) provides a critical genealogy of folkloristics' foundational concept of authenticity, tracing how it has shaped the field and imagining the sorts of work that could be done in a post-authenticity folkloristics. Diarmuid Ó Giolláin (2000) challenges received conceptions of Irish folklore by tracing their imbrication in shifting and contested notions of modernity and traditionality as they traveled through the work of leading social scientists and nationalist projects in Estonia, Finland, Italy, Spain, Sweden, and Brazil. He knocks genealogies of European folkloristics off balance by viewing them through a Latin American lens drawn from the work of García Canclini ([1990] 1995), Martín Barbero ([1987] 2003), and Ortiz (1985, 1992). Colombian ethnomusicologist and folklorist Ana María Ochoa Gautier (1996) has explored the elevation of *vallenato* to the status of a Colombian national traditional music, the role of folklorists and the music industry in creating aural representations of modernity in Latin America (2006:803–25, 2014), the place of culture and policy in relationship to the politics of violence and state power in Colombia (2003), and the creation of archives of traditional cultural forms as a means of (re)constructing regional identities among internally displaced Colombians. José Limón's (1994) *Dancing with the Devil* provides a critical genealogy of folkloristics in Texas, including an analysis of the work of military folklorist John Gregory Bourke that demonstrates the similarities between Bourke's military and folklore pursuits, much like British colonial folkloristics in India. Limón's work also provides ethnographic analyses of folklore, music, food, and dancing that shake loose the study of Mexican American expressive culture from its legacy in the coloniality of folkloristics, tying it to vernacular reflections on social difference and power. Cristina Bacchilega (2007) traces how narratives framed as legends were delegitimized as possessing historical and legal significance and appropriated for use in producing an exotic legendary Hawai'i that could be consumed by tourists and other non-Hawai'ians. In India, in addition to the authors we cited above, scholars and activists such as Ganesh N. Devy have done pioneering work in bringing "tribal" and other marginalized voices into the public domain through activism and promotion of the study of "tribal" languages and folklore.[17]

These and other works provide critical genealogies that force us to rethink the baggage that comes with established concepts and methods, which we see as crucial for the present and future of the discipline. We build here on these efforts by identifying what we have argued is the constitutive contradiction of folkloristics—its emergence from within colonialism and its erasure of coloniality in genealogical narratives of its origin in white European self-portraits of cultural similarity. Nevertheless, our goal has not been to "correct" existing genealogies or to provide a master genealogical narrative for adoption by all practitioners. Our goal is rather to suggest that scholars embrace *a multi-genealogical practice*. In proposing this concept, we wish to advance five propositions for future research and analysis:

1. *Multi-genealogical practice and boundary-work.* We are sympathetic to Deleuze's and Guattari's ([1980] 1987) anti-genealogical spirit, to their call for destabilizing dominant genealogies, particularly the ones they refer to as "arboreal"—which rise vertically and in unilinear fashion from a single set of roots. Nevertheless, in sync with their "rhizomic" view of roots that extend horizontally and provide complicated, multiple, and heterogeneous foundations, we propose the notion of a multi-genealogical practice. By articulating multiple roots for key concepts and practices, scholars can expose their assumptions and expand possibilities for changing them, thereby opening up alternative meanings and potentialities and increasing the power and creativity of the analytical frameworks on which they rely. By locating genealogies beyond narrowly defined disciplinary histories, folklorists can draw productively on other frameworks and genealogies and show scholars, policy makers, and other constituencies that the implications of their work extend in important ways beyond the boundaries of the discipline.

2. *Multi-genealogical practice as a part of folklore scholarship in general.* Critical genealogies should not be confined to occasional historical and theoretical works but should be a part of the everyday practice of folkloristics. Even research on contemporary folklore should scrutinize the underpinnings of terms and practices it uses in locating and analyzing its objects. As such, rather than stable objects that stand on their own, genealogical tracings should form assemblages (Deleuze and Guattari [1980] 1987) that are put together in contingent and unstable ways in order to illuminate a particular project.

3. *Multi-genealogical practice and vernacular philology.* A multi-genealogical practice will draw greater attention to the politics of knowledge, to the critical issue of who is accorded rights to create genealogies and determine the uses to which they will be put. This proposition resonates with Richard Bauman's (2008:29–36) call to recognize the centrality of "vernacular philology" to the discipline, to the ways that scholarly investigations of cultural forms rely on genealogical inquiries undertaken by "the folk" and inscribed in both performances and commentary. Scholars generally claim a monopoly on genealogical inquiry, as enshrined in the foundational assertion so assiduously advanced by the Grimms that the folk only possess an unreflective ability to perform folklore—only scholars can discern patterns and trace genealogies. As a result, folklorists often either present vernacular genealogies only in order to discredit them, thereby legitimizing their own, or simply claim them as their own, resulting in forms of appropriation that amount to plagiarism. The approach we are advocating places genealogical collaboration at the heart of field and archival research, documents the dialogic unfolding of multiple genealogies, and acknowledges all contributions. This, we would argue, is the thrust of much of the recent scholarship that we have cited.

4. *Multi-genealogical practice and research on emerging cultural forms.* Opening up multiple genealogies will be of far more than "purely historical" significance. Many folklorists are now interested in how cultural forms are produced and circulate through new social media; Bausinger ([1961] 1990) and Bauman (2010) show that both the mediation and remediation of folklore by

new technologies is itself not new. Nevertheless, we are often in the position of using concepts and scholarly practices forged by previous technologies, social formations, and regimes of capital in exploring phenomena that travel to the beat of quite different drums (with apologies to Cher). Wiring multi-genealogical practice into research on emergent forms and social practices will help us challenge assumptions that dull the edge of available frameworks, thereby rendering existing tools more useful and enhancing our ability to create new ones.

5. *Multi-genealogical practice and the future of folkloristics.* Finally, discerning new pasts opens up possibilities for creating new futures. As Roberts (1999) pointed out, folklorists have often been less successful than practitioners of other disciplines in recognizing how new politics of culture challenge entrenched disciplinary perspectives, practices, and institutional structures. Both clinging to dominant genealogies and using existing frameworks in ways that render their genealogies invisible foreclose possibilities for leaving behind tragic narratives of grim futures for folkloristics and imagining how more promising disciplinary futures can be created. Rachel González-Martin (2017) poignantly reported how the lasting effects of what we could call the pervasiveness of whiteness and coloniality in the graduate training she received in folkloristics undermine minority scholars' place in "a discipline that remains uncertain of who we are and what we do" (21). In 2020, increased scrutiny of the pervasiveness of whiteness and racism in disciplinary infrastructures and broader recognition of antiracist struggles underline the importance of uprooting dominant genealogies and forging new ones that accord a central and transformative place to scholars from racialized minority groups if disciplines are to become more diverse, equitable, and inclusive.

As argued in chapter 1, folklorists crafted genealogies, like Dorson's, that made it seem as if the discipline arose through spontaneous generation, springing up naturally as Aubrey and others recognized the distinctive qualities of those autochthonous objects that came to be called folklore. Bauman and Briggs (2003) presented an alternative genealogy, one that places the study of folklore and language at the center of major social, philosophical, and political shifts associated with modernity, science, civil society, history, nationalism, and cosmopolitanism. In arguing that constructions of tradition helped constitute these dominant projects and imbue them with authority and positive affective and ethical auras, they point to ways that folklorists can contribute centrally to larger scholarly and public projects. At the height of the Cold War and surrounded by legal means of enforcing racial injustice, Américo Paredes, to use Walter Benjamin's (2003:391) oft-quoted words, offered us a means of "appropriating a memory as it flashes up in a moment of danger." For Paredes, defining Mexican American folklore through difference, conflict, and violence promised to fashion the discipline into a "heightened presence of mind," again in Benjamin's (1968:238) words, that could open up new understandings of the past, suggest scholarly and public strategies for engaging the present, and facilitate brighter disciplinary and more just political futures.

We have addressed other moments of danger, particularly those associated with colonialism in early modernity and nineteenth-century India, in suggesting how awareness of the coloniality of folklore can foster a heightened presence of mind capable of renewing the discipline. Our collaborative efforts here form a contribution to what we see as an emergent multi-genealogical practice that holds the potential for creating broader dialogues, connecting folklorists who stand in different relationships to legacies of colonialism, thereby sparking new debates about the discipline's stock-in-trade. In this way, folklorists can creatively transform analytic tools, conduct more prescient research on how traditionalities are currently produced for global markets, and displace the colonial legacy of the internationalization of (Eurocentric) folkloristics in favor of a collaborative and critical *global folkloristics*.

NOTES

1. In a presentation of this research at the American Folklore Society in 2007, Elliott Oring pointed out that few folklorists even read Dorson nowadays. If so, this neglect is most unfortunate, given Dorson's outsized role in infusing Eurocentrism and whiteness deeply within dominant genealogies of folkloristics.

2. Note, however, traditionality subsequently gets much more imbricated with modernity for Chakrabarty than modernity does with traditionality for Dorson.

3. See also Goldberg 1993.

4. As boosterish chronicler Thomas Sprat ([1667] 1958:155–56) emphasizes, the Royal Society devoted considerable efforts to compiling existing accounts of exotic lands and peoples using lists of questions to transform the experiences of "Seamen, Travellers, Tradesmen, and Merchants" into information that could be discussed in "weekly Assemblies" and distributed in their journal, *Philosophical Transactions*, as well as through individual publications and correspondence. (See Stagl 1995.)

5. On the city/countryside binary, see Williams 1973. On the place of folklore in Irish history, see Ó Giolláin 2000.

6. See McBratney's (2006) account of Temple's folklore collecting, how it shaped and was shaped by his other activities as a colonial officer, and his role as Folk-Lore Society president.

7. Dorson (1968:344) echoes William Crooke's self-projection in suggesting that "Crooke's achievement was the more remarkable since, like Temple, he had to snatch time 'in the intervals of the scanty leisure of a District Officer's life in India' at a far remove from libraries."

8. George Hunt similarly worked for Franz Boas for decades, helping to produce a massive collective of "Kwakiutl" texts. Although Boas is to be credited for including Hunt as coauthor, he erased the indexical traces of the coloniality of racial difference that shaped their creation. See Berman 1996:215–56; Bauman and Briggs 2003.

9. Luise White (2000) similarly provides fascinating narratives from twentieth-century British colonies in Africa, in which African narrators cast colonial functionaries as vampires. Narratives that represented colonialism as the source of epidemic diseases were also common in India (Arnold 1993).

10. To be sure, fascinating efforts are being undertaken in other parts of Asia, Africa, the Caribbean, countries of the former Soviet Union, and elsewhere to rethink genealogies of folkloristics and their impact on contemporary scholarship and the politics of culture. We do not attempt to examine them here in order to avoid foreshortening complex histories and scholarly projects.

11. This material is drawn from 2009 fieldwork by Naithani, conducted in collaboration with Sudheer Gupta; his film, *Three Generations of Jogi Omar Farookh* (Public Sector Broadcast Trust New Delhi), illustrates these issues.

12. We thank Matti Bunzl and Regina Bendix for an illuminating email exchange on this point.

13. See also Dupey 1988.

14. In Brazil, however, the study of folklore was sometimes connected with a more progressive politics of culture; the coup d'état of 1964 accordingly led to the abolition of a number of institutions of popular culture that included interest in folklore (see Ortiz 1985; Vilhena 1997; Ó Giolláin 2000:90–92).

15. See the differing positions taken on these issues in a 1998 special issue of the *Journal of American Folklore* entitled "Folklore: What's in a Name?" (vol. 111, no. 441).

16. See the 1998 special issue of the *Journal of American Folklore* and, for a critique, Dundes 2005.

17. See www.adivasiacademy.org.

Part II
Rethinking Psychoanalysis, Poetics, and Performance

5

Reconnecting Psychoanalysis with Poetics and Performance

MY GOAL IN THIS CHAPTER IS TO EXPLORE crucial but largely underappreciated connections between approaches centering on psychoanalysis and on poetics and performance. Beyond deepening dialogues between them, my goal is to breathe new life into both. Even as Alan Dundes championed psychoanalysis as a privileged framework for analyzing folklore, he frequently complained that "as far as mainstream folkloristics is concerned, it is as though Freud never lived" (1987a:ix). Here I attempt to provide a broader basis in psychoanalytic theory, including works that seem more deeply tied to the concerns that underlie research in the analysis of cultural forms. Similarly, the influence of performance-centered approaches was inescapable in the 1970s and 1980s. Even as their fundamental insights have been incorporated into folkloristics and other disciplines, a focus on poetics and performance seems to have slipped into the background, partly due to its assimilation within dominant approaches as well as critiques that called for more attention to gender, power, embodiment, and other issues (Limón and Young 1986; Sawin 2002) and also simply as other concerns and approaches gained prominence. Oddly, a broad conversation between psychoanalytic and performance-centered approaches has not emerged. Performance-centered scholars largely just turned their backs on psychoanalysis. For his part, Dundes frontally rejected poetics and performance: "I do not consider either so-called feminist theory or performance theory to be 'grand theory.'" He went on to suggest that neither is really theory at all: "As far as I'm concerned, they are simply pretentious ways of saying that we should study folklore as performed, and we should be more sensitive to the depiction of women in folkloristic texts and contexts" (2005:389). In short, my first goal is to rethink and reinvigorate both approaches by creating a new sort of dialogue.

In advancing this project, I emphasize Freud's *The Interpretation of Dreams* ([1900] 1965) and *The Joke and Its Relationship to the Unconscious* ([1905] 2002) which, Dundes suggests, "pointed out the enormous potential of psychoanalytic theory as a tool for deciphering the symbolic content of myths, folktales, legends, and other forms of folklore such as custom and belief" (1987a:viii–ix). These texts are, accordingly, crucial for "the application of psychoanalytic theory to folklore, [Dundes's] major intellectual goal as a folklorist" (x). In seeking to create a more intimate relationship between psychoanalysis and poetics and performance, I may be casting myself as one of the central figures in the Jewish jokes that Freud analyzes, the *schadchen*, or marriage broker, trying to coax mutually distrustful parties into an unlikely match. But my argument is really more subversive: I argue that psychoanalysis and interest in poetics and performance have been married from the start.

If many students of poetics and performance have been reluctant to incorporate psychoanalytic perspectives, I think the obstacle lies in part with how the major advocate for psychoanalysis in folkloristics represented this approach. Dundes (2005:391) identified psychoanalysis with "Freud's Oedipal theory." Elliott Oring (1998:63) suggested that Dundes espoused a "narrow psychoanalytic band of psychological study" that "seems artificially restricted."[1] Simon Bronner (2007:x–xi) argued, in contrast, that Dundes modified Freud's approach to the psychoanalytic study of folklore in order to render it less androcentric and universalistic and to excise its evolutionary underpinnings, incorporating work by other psychoanalysts. Dundes (1987a:xii) complained that later psychoanalysis sacrificed "the original Freud" to a fashionable revisionist process. Here I take a different approach in finding that poetics and performance played a central role in forming "the original Freud."

In arguing that psychoanalysis enables scholars to reveal meanings that structure cultural forms but that are inaccessible to performers and audiences, Dundes's analyses of symbols that underlie a wide range of genres confronted two orientations with deep roots in folkloristics. First, as Oring (1981:43–45) has suggested, insofar as psychoanalytic approaches focus on unearthing singular factors that deterministically structure cultural forms, they reduce the particularity and complexity of a joke, folk narrative, social identity, game, or worldview to a small set of sexual conflicts or types of corporeal eroticism (see also Oring 1998). The particularities of genres, forms, and performances can get eclipsed as they are fit into familiar explanatory endpoints. Dundes (1987a:x) defended himself against the charge of reductionism by arguing that the ultimate goal should be "to explain a hitherto enigmatic piece of data" (xii). Ultimately, he said, "one of the goals of social sciences is, or ought to be, to make the unconscious conscious" (xiii). Central among these is Dundes's binary opposition between conscious and unconscious and the resulting tendency to position the meaning of all cultural forms into a single unconscious basket, a move that shortcircuits the more complex and nuanced approaches of current psychoanalysis. Another limitation of Dundes's psychoanalytic folkloristics is that he largely relied on decontextualized examples. By documenting the complexity of cultural forms and the multiple ways they are embedded in naturalcultural life, ethnography provides a basis for countering the sorts of reductionism that can give psychoanalysis a bad name among folklorists and anthropologists.[2]

On the other hand, work in poetics and performance sometimes seems to cast performers as master composer/conductors who have a totalizing grasp of aesthetic elements and how they fit together. I argue here that psychoanalytic and performance-centered approaches can gain a great deal by looking closely at how cultural forms engender ways of thinking and feeling, listening and speaking, that operate on multiple levels and by resisting (as it were) the appeal of trying to explain everything with a single set of explanatory principles. *Dreams* and *The Joke* point the way to a new psychoanalytic approach, one that provides a means of circumventing these difficulties and helps scholars make important advances on major issues, such as subject formation, the status of aesthetics, and the reason why the formal dimensions of cultural forms play such a crucial role in shaping the worlds in which we live. Folklorists and anthropologists also have a lot to contribute to psychoanalysis by bringing poetics and performance into psychoanalytic texts in which they have not been considered. This chapter lays the analytic groundwork for rethinking psychoanalytic foundations, tracing the role of poetics and performance in shaping them, and extending a poetic psychoanalysis; chapter 6 uses deep ethnographic immersion in poetics and performance and with vernacular theorists in rethinking a key psychoanalytic text.

A legacy of nineteenth-century folkloristics is the idea that people have folklore but only professional folklorists can identify, describe, and analyze it. Jacob and Wilhelm Grimm suggested that the folk "are fortunately not consciously aware of their own quiet poetry" ([1816] 1981:4; see also Bauman and Briggs 2003). Recall that disciplinary boundary-work seeks to keep out not just other scholars but laypersons as well. If a psychoanalytic approach claims unique authority to identify "enigmatic" meanings and provide a definitive interpretation of them, then it will reproduce nineteenth-century understandings of folklore and sustain the race- and class-based global hierarchies that undergird the coloniality of folkloristics (see chapter 4). In the introduction, I described how my approach emerged through apprenticeships with people in New Mexico and Venezuela, mentors whose grasp of the complexities of naturalcultural worlds laid the basis for analytic perspectives that have taken me decades to appreciate. A psychoanalytic approach—or any approach that locates interpretation exclusively in a subterranean level accessible only to scholars—goes against the grain, in my view, of taking lay perspectives seriously as sources of analytic insight, not just data. Another problem with psychoanalytic theory as it is often deployed in folklore—in striking contrast to how it emerged in Freud's work and that of other practicing psychoanalysts—is that psychoanalysis is construed as a set of distal principles that are imported into an encounter with specific cultural forms.

POETICS, PERFORMANCE, AND THE EVERYDAY IN FREUD

Freud's argument in *The Joke* might seem to lend itself to the idea that folklore is fundamentally about repression. Freud invoked repression in analyzing the "tendentious joke," which puts itself "in the service" of a purpose, tendency, or intention ([1905] 2002:85). The difference between obscene, aggressive or hostile, cynical (critical, blasphemous), and skeptical genres and "innocuous jokes" is marked by "those sudden outbursts of laughter that make tendentious jokes so irresistible" (92) versus the agreeable feelings and slight smiles elicited by innocuous jokes. Such hearty laughter is tied to how "our culture's work of repression" deprives us of "primary possibilities of enjoyment" through internal censorship; thus, "tendentious jokes provide a means of reversing renunciation and of regaining what was lost" (96). Nevertheless, as Oring (2015) argued, the common reduction of Freud's argument simply to a characterization of jokes as modes of releasing repressed unconscious impulses overlooks both its scope and complexity and how Freud locates jokes in relationship to psyches, aesthetics, and social relations.

Freud is concerned with how jokes question social conventions, such as jokes centering on the schadchen and the *schnorrer* (Jewish beggar). Freud suggested that the latter gives voice to doubts about whether self-denial will be rewarded ([1905] 2002:105). In Jewish jokes, "the intended criticism of protest is directed against one's self, or, put more circumspectly, against a person in whom that self has a share, a collective person, that is, one's own people" (106). Oring suggested that there existed "some deep and personal relationship between Freud and his Jewish jokes," that they were tied to his economic struggles and ambivalence about his marriage and Jewish heritage (1984:4), and that they constitute "a set of defensive, even retaliatory, measures undertaken in the context of an oppressive environment," specifically "the oppression by the non-Jew, the *Goy*" (1992:119–20).

Sexual repression is not absent. Freud took us "back to fundamentals" in his analysis of obscene jokes, the desire to gaze on genitals being "one of the original components of our libido" ([1905] 2002:93). In a masculinized formulation, Freud argued that the need to use speech arises from a desire to engage a particular woman sexually, an attempt to stimulate a corresponding arousal in the woman, and "a defensive reaction" on the woman's part (94). Rather than examining a realm of decontextualized psychic processes, Freud explored how tendentious jokes require three classes of participants: the first is the teller, the second a "person who is taken as the object of the hostile or sexual aggression, and a third in whom the joke's intention of producing pleasure is fulfilled" (95). Thus far, Freud has only defined smut, the "bawdry" observed among country people or in lower-class taverns, uttered in the presence of the second participant, "a barmaid or the landlady." The obscene joke appears "only when we reach a higher social level" (94), requiring the *absence* of the second. Although Freud suggested that a shared background of class (and, one might add, gender and sexuality) is required for first and third participants, their roles emerge through their different relationships to the sense of revelation that the joke produces—enjoyed directly by the third and only at secondhand, that is, vicariously, by the first.

Poetics, along with the absence of the second, transforms smut into an obscene joke: "Only when we rise into more cultivated society do we find the addition of the formal requirements for jokes. The bawdry becomes witty, and is tolerated only if it is witty" ([1905] 2002:95). I use poetics here initially in the sense developed by Roman Jakobson (1960): a focus on formal features—expanded to include acoustic, visual, bodily, and material as well as textual elements—as objects of scrutiny, elaboration, and pleasure. Freud shared a concern with aesthetics that was important in nineteenth-century Germanic intellectual traditions (see Harries 1983), but his is not a disembodied, abstract, and internalized Kantian aesthetics—rather, it is one located in everyday life. We cannot overlook the problematic sexism, classism, and heteronormativity that positions "cultivated," heterosexual men as the creators, performers, and audiences for jokes and women as absent objects. Freud also suggested, however, that obscene jokes constitute sexual violence against an intransigent woman ([1905] 2002:94): her refusal to yield to verbal sexual assault, would—if she were physically present—dismantle the performance and interrupt the aggression.

Herein lies the power (as well as a key limitation) of *The Joke* for constituting a new psychoanalytic approach. One of the forms of repression that jokes release is how adults are required to suppress the pleasure of playing with language; Freud's extensive analysis of "the techniques of the joke" suggested that jokes enable us to explore phonetic, semantic, syntactic, and pragmatic dimensions of language and other semiotic modalities, reminding us that "words are malleable material, allowing all kinds of things to be done to them" ([1905] 2002:25). Published a decade before Ferdinand de Saussure's ([1916] 1959) *Course in General Linguistics, The Joke* contains a remarkably sophisticated philosophy of language, one that challenges referentialist views of language. "Given the part jokes play in our mental life" ([1905] 2002:1) and the insights they reveal, analyzing "the techniques of the joke" prompted Freud to fundamentally link psychoanalysis to poetics, again understood here as a reanalysis of units of form in their complex relationships to meaning and use. The poetics of the joke connect linguistic, psychic, interactional, and broader social dimensions in ways that evade any neat binaries of conscious/unconscious or poetic/everyday language.

This is a remarkable point of departure for rethinking psychoanalytic approaches. Rather than positing a gulf between psychoanalysis and folkloristics and then attempting to bridge it or positioning psychoanalysis as a universal "grand theory" that can be applied to folklore, *The Joke* presents us with a psychoanalytic framework that sprang precisely from reflections on poetics and performance. In what could be considered a precursor to the ethnography of speaking, Freud captured the dynamics of class, gender, and genre that emerge as a woman's presence sparks smut and her absence enables men to feel licensed to tell sexual jokes. Audience participation is central, as Freud read how hearty laughs and bemused smiles distinguish performances of tendentious and innocuous jokes. His attention to context is thus less a flatfooted description of cookie-cutter roles than one that presages Erving Goffman's (1981) concern with how roles are constituted as "participation structures" that are created in and shape interactions. Freud also pointed ahead to Jacques Derrida's ([1967] 1976) critique of the "metaphysics of presence": the absent second, the person denigrated by tendentious jokes, is as crucial for joke performances as the bodily presence of the joker and audience. The work of the joke in constituting subjects and (often) dimensions of class, gender, sexual, and ethnoracial difference lies in their iteration (Derrida 1988; Butler 1997), both in further performances and in relations to other denigrating discourses, such as smut and "the jokes made about Jews by outsiders [*Fremden*]," which "are mostly brutal comic anecdotes" (Freud [1905] 2002:106) (meaning anti-Semitic goys). The differences between the first and third are similarly constructed, not only in terms of the teller's skill but his (and I do mean *his*) focus on enabling the third to experience the moment that the joke releases words and other semiotic forms from their usual automatization and ties them to aggressive thoughts, long after this moment of revelation has passed for the teller. Finally, Freud placed tendentious jokes, albeit lodged in classism, sexism, and heteronormativity and cautiously avoiding overt challenges to anti-Semitism, within a broader economy of difference, inequality, and symbolic violence.

My goal, however, is not to argue that Freud is a proto-folklorist but rather to suggest how *The Joke* reveals ways that key concerns of poetics and performance and psychoanalysis *were co-produced*. As Oring (1984:6) suggests, components of his argument are not always well connected. Freud positioned libidinal sexual urges as prior to speech, and he sometimes separated "the content of the thought" from "its clothing as a joke" ([1905] 2002:87). Although jokes critically explore features of language, interaction, difference, and power, making these connections was reserved for rare individuals who possess "a special aptitude" that is "so frequently fulfilled in neurotic persons" (172). Here, unfortunately, Freud limited creativity to the *production* of new joke texts rather than performance, particularly how first, second, and third are constructed in telling jokes. Even if Freud limited the scope of his insights, he insisted that connections between psychic and poetic elements cannot be isolated analytically.

In *The Interpretation of Dreams*, on the other hand, Freud granted authorship, the power to use poetics to produce subjects, to all of us, characterizing it as a part of everyday (or every night) life. *Dreams* thus complements *The Joke* in forging a base for a psychoanalytic approach in which poetics, performance, and the psyche are linked from the start. In keeping with his anti-referentialist ideology of language, Freud drew attention to rhymes, puns, and other plays on words, analyzing how dreams separate sounds from referents in fashioning novel associations. Anticipating contemporary concerns with language and materiality (Keane 2007), Freud pointed out how words and names can be treated as objects in dreams, just as people and objects can be transformed into linguistic forms. In Peirce's ([1940] 1955) terms, Freud thus attended to how dreams explore indexical and iconic possibilities for unlocking the power of symbols, thereby transforming quotidian understandings of objects, events, and linguistic elements into novel meanings, perceptions, and arrangements.

Freud also opened up new ways to think beyond unproductive binaries of poetic versus ordinary language, everyday versus the extraordinary. Dreams are both mundane, revolving around everyday interactions, experiences, and concerns, and utterly alien. Poetic features of dreams rework everyday interactions and subjects. Dream narratives thus foster greater awareness of both the power and the indeterminacy of the ordinary—a point emphasized by Veena Das (2007). These insights reach deep into the roots of contemporary folkloristics. Trained in folkloristics, Jakobson (1960) and his fellow "Russian Formalists" explored how language becomes automatized, increasingly reduced instrumentally to the referential function. The Formalists suggested that literature disrupts the semiotic automatization of the everyday, opening up linguistic forms to scrutiny and change. Years before the Formalists launched their project, Freud suggested that dreams and jokes disrupt the power of received codes, linguistic and social, in the course of everyday life, charging these disturbances with condensed affects and meanings.

Dreams are infused with ambiguity: the way that dream elements are located vis-à-vis multiple pasts, presents, and futures and their symbolic significance and affective resonances are not immediately apparent ([1900] 1965:376–77). In *The Joke*, Freud mapped a genre; in *Dreams*, he studied how individual constructions of self and world are always embedded in emergent dialogues of genres. More than decontextualized signs pointing to abstract sexual conflicts, such elements are rooted in what we could call, following M. M. Bakhtin (1981), the heteroglossic character of dream narratives and their status as mixed genres that incorporate such forms as jokes, quotations, songs, proverbs, legends, and popular customs. Building on Richard Bauman's (2004) extension of Bakhtin, genres are not simply juxtaposed in dreams but blended in such a way that our reflexive understanding of their relationship to experience and to each other is heightened, unsettled, and potentially transformed.

Folklorists gravitate toward narratives that are well-structured wholes; an emphasis on poetics and performance deepens the search for "keys" or "frames" (Bauman 1977) that reveal cohesive formal patterns. Freud, like Das (2007), rather invites us to look for narrative *fragments*. The narratives that reveal dream-content are not fully formulated stories whose aesthetic properties can be appreciated per se; rather, they emerge as fragments whose meaning and power appear only in shifting relations with other texts. The condensation that shapes the transcription of dream-thoughts into dream content revolves around a process of "overdetermination" that highlights elements and infuses them with affect, creating "nodal points" through "a sort of manipulative process" ([1900] 1965:317–18) and emphasizing elements forming "an intermediate common entity" between "multiple fields" (330). This process links different times, conversations, images, stories, experiences, and relations. Poetic dimensions—including acoustic, visual, and other sensual aspects—are central to condensation and the way its charged elements are recontextualized. Freud extended this analysis in *The Joke* by exploring how "the joke lies only in the linguistic expression produced by the process of condensation" ([1905] 2002:20); condensation can take the form of "substitute-formation," creating an unusual and striking "composite word" (12) or using similarities of sound and/or meaning to create novel linguistic effects. There Freud showed how relations between poetic details, interactions, bodies, and spaces engender transcendent meanings through processes of condensation and displacement, the latter process revolving less around linguistic features than a change in the "train of thought" that produces a "displacement" as the "psychological emphasis" shifts "to a different theme from the one first broached" (41), such as when, for example, a shift from medical to sexist modes of referring to a woman's body forces us to rethink the meaning of a word (28). Returning to *Dreams*, rather than a simple, mechanical process of reducing preexisting material, the condensation that occurs as extensive "dream-thoughts" are "transcribed" into "dream-content" actively produces both memory and forgetting. Crucially, Freud referred to "the remarkable preference by the memory in dreams for indifferent, and consequently unnoticed, elements in waking experience" (1965 [1900]:53). This powerful production of meaning and memory emerges as the most mundane elements of everyday words and interactions get highlighted and connected with other words, persons, times, and events, thereby potentially becoming sources of insight. Condensation and displacement transform elements of the everyday as they become charged with affect and provide keys to a precarious, uncertain process of unlocking events, experiences, and relations. Simplistic binary oppositions between the everyday and the eventful, the ordinary and the poetic, the conscious and the unconscious fall away in this formulation.

RECONFIGURING POETICS AND PERFORMANCE THROUGH PSYCHOANALYSIS

The promise of psychoanalysis for analyses of poetics and performance—along with the narrative constitution of selves and social life—can thus be limited by failure to appreciate that poetics and performance form a fundamental part of psychoanalysis' DNA. Although this is not my concern here—nor am I adequately qualified to advance the following statement in more than cautious terms—I would suggest that psychoanalysts from Freud onward have been clinically trained to be particularly attentive to the psychoanalytic implications of features of poetics and performance. Finding the sort of prominent place for psychoanalysis that Dundes envisioned thus involves, I suggest, starting with their points of overlap rather than importing a theory that seems entirely alien to poetics and performance and whose application often strikes folklorists and anthropologists as potentially doing violence to the particular features of cultural forms. Now I would like to further develop this intimacy—still playing my role as the schadchen, or marriage broker—from the other side, by suggesting how valuable psychoanalysis can be in clarifying and deepening approaches to poetics and performance.

Bauman has referred to Roman Jakobson's (1960) classic essay, "Concluding Remarks: Linguistics and Poetics," as one "of the most prominent shaping influences" on performance approaches (2012b:97). Jakobson discerned six "constitutive factors in any speech event, in any act of verbal communication," which he refers to as addresser, addressee, message, context (here something of a euphemism for the referent, given his reservations about the latter term), code, and contact ("a physical channel and psychological connection between the addresser and addressee"). Jakobson then stipulated that each of the six factors is associated with a different "function," adding that "a set (*Einstellung*)" toward "the predominant function" primarily shapes "the verbal structure of a message" (1960:353). Jakobson, of course, was primarily interested in "the POETIC function of language," which he defined as "the set (*Einstellung*) toward the MESSAGE as such, focus on the message for its own sake," which he deemed the "dominant, determining function" of verbal art (356; emphasis in original). Jakobson immediately complicated the model by suggesting that the point is not that a single factor eclipses all others but that it shapes "a different hierarchical order of functions" (363). This conception of the poetic function is central to Bauman's original definition: "Performance thus calls forth special attention to and heightened awareness of the act of expression," of how performer and audience focus on "the way in which communication is carried out, above and beyond its referential content" (1977:11). Jakobson's formulation suggests that other functions do not disappear, nor are they entirely banished from consciousness. Rather, the "hierarchical order of functions" becomes dynamic—often shifting in the course of an act of communication—in such a way that less dominant functions are often imbued with new possibilities even as they recede from the center of attention.[3]

Freud can help us extend this analysis. In both Jakobson's and Bauman's formulations, relations between factors and functions seems to be a matter of artistic and interactional design, as crafted by the performer (but also affected by the audience). Jakobson's model seems to imply a somewhat mechanistic sense of this poetic design process through his emphasis on "the verbal structure of a message" as produced by a "*determining* function" (my emphasis). Bauman pointed us toward "heightened awareness" and the emergence of artistic and interactional control through the acquisition of competence. Freud would rather lead us to see poetics as pointing to ways that discourse and naturalcultural life are, like dreams and dream narratives, always if to varying degrees *out of control*. Rather than focusing on the spectacular moments in which the impressive potential of language, aesthetics, and interaction emerge in crystalline form, either in celebrated works of literature or performances by individuals regarded as the best verbal artists, Freud (1960) directed our attention in *The Psychopathology of Everyday Life* to everyday parapraxes (slips of the tongue and other verbal "mistakes") and interactional disruptions. He demonstrated that we can learn a great deal by looking at what seem to be clear manifestations of *in*competence, poetic patterns that emerge not by design and when our awareness is *not* heightened. In dialogue with what would later become a touchstone for medical philosophy through the work of Georges Canguilhem ([1966] 1989), Freud urged us to explore what seem to be abnormal cases as a means of going beyond accepted analytic conceptions: "I should prefer to stress the fact that here, as so often in biology, normal circumstances or those approaching the normal are less favourable subjects for investigation than pathological ones" (1960:273). Freud thus pointed to the ability of dreams, jokes, and slips of the tongue to disrupt the power of received codes, linguistic and social, charging these disturbances with condensed affects and meanings. Disability studies provides an even more radical opening, suggesting how attention to stigmatized bodies and minds calls us to attend to ways that notions of "normal," "abnormal," and "pathological" are continually made, reified, and destabilized (see Schmiesing 2014; Blank and Kitta 2015; Shuman 2016).

True, Freud's account of jokes did, as I suggested above, lodge their creative and disruptive possibilities too much in what he saw as the crafting of a joke rather than in its everyday work of performance. Even there, however, the disruptive role of the absent second—even as this denigrated figure makes the role of first and third both possible and precarious—is never fully contained. I think that Freud's account of dreams points us to a more fundamental way of rethinking Jakobson's "different hierarchical order of functions." Beyond criticisms that many writers have lodged against the analytic boundaries that Jakobson drew around notions of "message" and "act of verbal communication," I would emphasize how Freud's insights prompt us to dismantle the boundaries of "the speech event." *The Interpretation of Dreams* points to a dynamic way that recent conversations, objects, and observations intersect with distal interactions—especially, disturbing childhood and other experiences—and thus shape the role of poetics in everyday life. The meaning of any word or conversation is thus constantly in flux, potentially reconfigured at any point as new pasts and presents emerge and new futures are imagined. Dimensions of skill in verbal art, which Freud clearly appreciated in his work on jokes, do not enable performers to create aesthetic designs that control the meanings and effects of their words and actions, either for themselves or their interlocutors. Here we find a new opening for the influence of M. M. Bakhtin in thinking about how any "utterance" is shot through with other texts, discourses, and registers; Freud would push Bakhtin to think more carefully about why *particular* intertextual fragments emerge and how they reshape *particular* words, interactions, images, objects, and relations. As I suggest below, Freud's notion of condensation is particularly applicable here.

I've been fairly cautious so far in connecting psychoanalysis with poetics and performance, but now I want to take a larger risk. Three decades ago, Bauman and Briggs (1990) used the term *entextualization* to emphasize the importance of infusing discourse with particular sorts of patterning in order to shape its social life in specific sorts of ways. The term helped us get away from the sense that poetics is either an aesthetic layer that is added on the top of discourse or an immanent, intrinsic, stable feature of "the verbal structure of a message" (Jakobson 1960:353). We rather pointed to an active process of imbuing discourse with features that are metacommunicative, in Gregory Bateson's (1972) sense of the term, that provide roadmaps of how discourse is structured, how it is to be interpreted, and where it should subsequently travel and how. We argued that entextualization reflexively shapes how discourse will be perceived and interpreted (as a joke or a personal narrative, for example). Entextualization thus invites *decontextualization*, providing affordances for future discursive trajectories. Some, but not all, dimensions of entextualization are aesthetic, involving patterns that are infused with sensuous properties as associated with particular types of responses. What is at stake here is more than entextualization, if the "text" component of that term limits us to a narrow construal of the verbal; rather, this reflexive organization shapes the disposition of bodies, nonverbal dimensions of voices and soundscapes, gazes, objects, and the like in addition to the structuring of words. *Recontextualization* pointed to interdiscursivity, to how entextualization projects a stretch of discourse implicitly or explicitly as enacting various sorts of relations between discursive acts and thus different contexts, speakers, genres, registers, and the like. Bauman and I argued that entextualization renders discourse extractable, "making a stretch of linguistic production into a unit—a text—that can be lifted *out* of its interactional setting" (1990:73; emphasis added). Given that the task of this chapter involves forging relationships between psychoanalysis and work on poetics and performance, I want to take this point in a different direction: I want to trace how discourse gets *into* bodies and psyches.

Goffman's notion of "response cries" provides a particularly valuable point of departure. He defines them as "emissions from a source [that] inform us about the state of the source—a case of exuded expressions, not intentionally sent messages" (1981:100). "Oooh!" (uttered after experiencing a pleasant sensation), "brr!" and so forth cast those who hear them less as recipients of a message than as overhearers of something like a reflex emanating from within the speaker. This seemingly natural character disguises the status of response cries as conventional indexes that are inflected by the utterer's perception of who is likely to perceive them, sensitive to dimensions of gender, age, social status, kinship, and context. Thus, what seem to be direct emanations from a bounded subject that are oblivious to adjacent others performatively construct selves and naturalcultural relations in particular ways.

Here I would like to bring in psychoanalyst Melanie Klein ([1940] 1948). Klein pointed to the internal images of external objects that young children construct, dynamically internalizing them as new people and experiences are added. We slowly develop a mechanism for relating the worlds of internal and external objects. Argentine-born psychoanalyst Juan-David Nasio can help us build on Klein by the way he reworks Freud and Lacan. Nasio uses a metaphor to suggest how we build relations by internalizing the image of another person so as to "cover him or her over as ivy covers a stone wall" (2004:29). This process enables interpersonal relations to go beyond being external connections between two bodies to become ways that we infuse parts of our selves into other humans and such nonhumans as pets, just as elements of others become part of us, much as ivy attaches itself to particular "cracks and crevices" of a wall (31).

Alright, here's the analytic leap! I would like to extend Freud's argument regarding "overdetermination" beyond dreams. Entextualization heightens the semiotic power of the sensuous dimensions of signs and reorganizes acoustic, visual, tactile, gustatory, and olefactory dimensions in such a way as to provide "an intermediate common entity" with enhanced capacity to connect and disconnect "multiple fields" ([1917] 1957:330) of words, worlds, bodies, objects, times, and events. Here we can newly appreciate features that students of poetics and performance have highlighted, such as metacommunicative frames, parallelism, sound symbols, and techniques of verisimilitude,[4] as intermediate common entities that create links and/or gaps between multiple fields. Such features as the witch's evil laugh in a performance of a folktale or the creaking of the stairs in a ghost story similarly enter simultaneously into multiple spheres, connecting scary Kleinian internal objects, co-present bodies, performance spaces, and realms of the imagination. Like Goffman's response cries, entextualization structures discourse in such a way as to project how it comes from inside us and invites others to gain what is projected as privileged access to our internal states, thereby transforming relations between internal and external worlds. Like response cries, entextualization simultaneously reaches out to other beings as signs enter their bodies, including human and nonhuman ears, eyes, noses, hands, mouths, and skin. As entextualized signs enter other beings, their sensuous properties place our affects, desires, ideas, and imaginations inside of them. "Audience design," how discourse is patterned in keeping with what we expect to be our interlocutors' ways of perceiving, understanding, and reacting to our discourse, signals our perceptions of their internal objects and, simultaneously, our expectation that our discourse will become part of them and how it will do so. As V. N. Vološinov ([1929] 1973) brilliantly analyzed, reported speech (various ways of seeming to transmit the words of others) provides a range of tools for projecting entanglements of voices and subjects.

I do not wish to construct an analytic border between how entextualization unfolds in self and other. Lacan ([1966] 1977:181) suggested that we listen to and are affected by our own voices and physical movements; entextualization plays a crucial role here, shaping us as we listen to the way we incorporate and thus internalize the words, gestures, desires, feelings, and imaginations of others. Entextualization thus doubly shapes the sorts of psychic lives that signs will lead within us. To be sure, we also undertake this process through the referential function of language, as when I explicitly tell you that I am like this or am feeling that or ask you to think or feel about me in particular ways. Entextualization acts, however, in ways that are less subject to explicit scrutiny, acceptance, or rejection. It inscribes affects on the sensuous surfaces of words, sounds, gestures, facial expressions, and the like, but not in simple, mechanical, transparent ways. Entextualization claims space for what Julia Kristeva ([1974] 1984) refers to as "semiotic process," a concept that lies at the core of her project of linking linguistics, poetics, and psychoanalysis. Kristeva suggests that poetics draws on the materiality of signifiers in such a way as to enable subjects, meanings, and bodies to be dynamically configured as discourse unfolds; I return to her work in chapter 6.

Bringing poetics and performance into alignment with psychoanalysis also provides a way of transforming the former in response to some of the ways it has been criticized. In a trenchant feminist reflection on Bauman's (1977) *Verbal Art as Performance*, Patricia Sawin (2002) identified what she saw as an uneasy relationship between feministic folkloristics and Bauman's performance-centered approach. She tied their "incongruent" contours to a "lack of attention to the audience and to the emotional dimension of esthetic experience" (29). At root, as I read her, is the positing of a stable, bounded subject that seems to preexist the performance and whose competence it highlights. Replaying Bauman's classic definition of performance as entailing "the assumption of responsibility to an audience for a display of communicative competence" (1977:11), she counters that the gendered dimension of what is presented as a subject that is unmarked in terms of gender and sexuality is revealed by the way Bauman's definition identified the performer's role with behaviors that "were problematic for women: displaying competence and accountability, making one's actions subject to evaluation, calling attention to oneself" (2002:31).

Sawin's critique points to a critical need for further attention to the constitution of subjects in performance. I think that it might be most productive here to think less about what got left out than about how subjects do not just arrive—forms of competence in hand and/or head—at the scene of performance but how they are formed and fragmented in the process. Here the analytic requirements are demanding. Subjects are not only shaped by differential identities, to use Bauman's (1971) term and to invoke the legacy of Américo Paredes, but are partially but not deterministically preconfigured by the selves that they and others have previously enacted, are complex and heterogeneous, and shift even as performances unfold. As performance elements are extracted, internalized, and recontextualized, these selves continue to shift. In short, selves in performances are no more bounded or self-contained than utterances or "speech events." My reformulation similarly responds to criticisms that poetics and performance have not been sufficiently attentive to issues of bodies and embodiment. Entextualization, as reconfigured, provides powerful affordances for constructing and interpellating bodies and shaping their relations with other minds, bodies, materialities, nonhumans, and environments. Psychoanalysis pushes poetics and performance beyond its totalizing tendencies, looking less for cohesive patterns than for tensions, multiplicities, contradictions, fragments, and affects that operate on multiple registers.[5]

TOWARD A PSYCHOANALYTICALLY INFORMED ANALYSIS OF POETICS

Now I would like to reflect on how this framework for a psychoanalytically informed approach to poetics and performance might be useful in analyzing cultural forms. Here, I think, is some exciting news. My discussion of entextualization, Freud, Klein, and Goffman might lead readers to conclude that I imagine speakers as making up relations between poetics, psyches, and bodies out of whole cloth every time they open their mouths and ears or move their eyes, hands, and bodies. They don't! Rather, traditionalized cultural forms (see chapter 8), together with literary and media genres, provide elaborate, detailed, and flexible roadmaps for enacting the power of entextualization to project how worlds and words enter into the constitution of selves and others. Launching into a particular myth, folk song, personal narrative, lament, or proverb opens up astounding sets of resources for enacting this process without overdetermining its particular features or how they will be internalized. And folklore operates in this fashion along multiple dimensions, of which I would like to call attention to just two.

A first continuum is *distal versus proximal*. A personal narrative is about the performer, either as co-present or, for example, as the narrative unfolds on a blog or WhatsApp text and image. Here constructing the character explicitly goes hand-in-hand with entextualizing the manner in which this figure seems to emerge from and get reinserted into the performer. This does not mean that the entextualization process is necessarily fully (or even mainly) under the control of individual performers/characters. A wonderful example is presented by Ochs, Smith, and Taylor's (1996) analysis of a family dinner conversation in which a daughter's offhand remark about a classmate's school detention prompts her brother and parents to drag her reluctantly into telling a personal narrative about her own clash with school authorities. Given that the narrator's everyday identity and that emerging in the story are proximal, gaps that open up between the two highlight the power of poetics and performance to reveal the precarity of efforts to construct the self. By performing a myth or folktale, on the other hand, narrators can draw on elaborate and extensive scripts for constructing selves and naturalcultural relations that are designed to be maximally removed from the selves, places, and times they usually inhabit. Narrators may project their own subjectivities and positionalities as implicit reflections of the imaginary characters, events, and worlds they perform. Nevertheless, the distance between the two and the paucity of explicit, referential connections between them is what, according to many psychoanalytically inclined students of folk narrative, such as Alan Dundes (1987a, 1987b, 1991), Géza Róheim (1992), Francisco Vaz da Silva (2002), Maria Tatar (1992), and the much-maligned Bruno Bettelheim (1976), makes them powerful sources for psychological development.

This continuum overlaps with but is not identical to one that moves between *indexical and iconic connections* between recurrent symbolic content and the process of internalization. Charles S. Peirce ([1940] 1955) defined indexicality and iconicity as type sign modalities, alongside the symbolic. The latter involves relatively context-free relations between signs and objects, as existing in a code, which Ferdinand de Saussure ([1916] 1959) characterized as the arbitrary signifier-signified relations that lie at the core of language. Neither iconic or indexical modalities are arbitrary, and they are more based in phenomenal experience. Indexical relations are established in semiotic acts, either making connections to existing specific features of proximal or distal worlds or performatively bringing them into being (Silverstein 1976). Peirce emphasized the importance of existential connections between indexical signs and their objects, such that indexes denote "by virtue of being really affected by that Object" ([1940] 1955:102). Iconicity involves materiality and sensation, establishing relations of similarity between the material—acoustic, visual, olfactory, tactile, and so on—elements of sign and object. The performance of a joke or folk narrative can create powerful indexical connections by transforming the site of performance into the space of events, using gestures to point to features of an imaginary landscape as if they were right there before our eyes or, alternatively, revealing how the observed attributes of an actually existing landscape are in reality signs of natural/cultural/spiritual worlds that are no longer immediately perceptible (see Basso 1996). Performers' voices and bodies become the material for fashioning elaborate iconic works of art, producing sounds, gestures, facial expressions, and actions that seem to be those of the characters and actions they are depicting. These sign modalities are not mutually exclusive; Peirce suggested that photographs can function as indexical icons, positioning particular people, animals, and objects in time and space by virtue of the illusion that marks on photographic paper were inscribed at the very moment that they were copresent and iconically match their visual features. Entextualization supercharges iconicity and indexicality, turning them into powerful means of creating subject positions and subjectivities, imbuing them with affect, and enabling them to move between bodies, psyches, and environments. Specific genres and performances exploit the differential potential of these two modalities to different degrees and in different ways. Galit Hasan-Rokem (2014) beautifully analyzes how the bodies of women singing laments over their children's bodies iconically invoke the corporeal connections and separations of pregnancy, birth, maturation, and death and trace the relational indexicality through which mothers and their children's lives are co-produced.

In developing this framework, let me return to the proverb performance by one of my mentors, Córdovan wood-carver Silvianita López.[6] I was nineteen, conducting my first extended fieldwork in Córdova, and I had misbehaved. As I described in the introduction, I was living in a trailer near the Lópezes' house. One evening I accepted an invitation from peers to engage in a late-night bout of carousing. The next morning, Silvianita used a proverb performance to induce me to accept her advice: behave appropriately or risk expulsion from the community. Rather than stating her case directly, she employed a proverb text about horsebeans that bore no explicit relationship to my transgression and then used indexicality to suggest how I should internalize it. These indexical connections spanned multiple scales. Most immediately, I had inadvertently challenged her authority by suggesting that my high-school experience provided me with a sufficient basis for assessing the danger posed by the adolescents.

The proverb performance, particularly as validated by her husband George, restored her status as a knowledgeable elder and mine as a young newcomer who needed to learn, in her words, "how *a person* is *careful* . . . *a stranger* has to be *careful*" (her emphasis). At a broader scale, she placed my relationship to residents in relation to that of "los hippies," young whites who had taken up residence in Córdova. The youths whose behavior she criticized had used petty theft and hostile remarks to help displace these outsiders, who were buying up scarce plots of land on the tiny valley floor, bathing naked in the small stream that runs through the Quemado Valley, and condescending to residents, whom they considered ignorant and backward ("they're back in the '50s, man," one told me). At a broader scale still, like George's refusal to answer my initial questions about wood carving (see the introduction), the performance challenged the white domination of Spanish speakers and Native Americans that structured the racialized political economy of the region. The performance also indexically connected temporal scales, linking our conversation to a past identified with "the elders of bygone days" whose wisdom was encapsulated in the proverb, which is then positioned not as a relic of a disappearing premodern era but as a guide for collectively crafting more democratic futures. Think of the power of this short performance in X-raying the self that I was attempting to construct for myself, as knowledgeable and autonomous, which was suddenly replaced by the relational identity that Silvianita projected between the two of us. Given that I could not counter with another proverb performance, I was left with no option but to join George in affirming Silvianita's evaluation of her performance and its indexical power (and it's *true*, it's *certainly true*). Indeed, the performance became a turning point in my own development: I became the subject that she constructed.

Although, as I have suggested, folklore genres may operate primarily through either distal or proximal, iconic or indexical means, they do not occupy fixed positions in this regard. The remarkable myth performances by Santiago Rivera that I mentioned in the introduction included three renditions on separate occasions of the complex and sexist myth of the sun. During an annual festival, Santiago provided a full-scale, monologic version whose carefully crafted iconic voices of the mythological characters and gestural constructions of a mythic landscape brought a primordial world to life and invoked its ongoing but invisible power. Later, during a visit to his friend Manuel Torres, my Warao father and mentor, Santiago replayed only part of the myth; replaying scenes of rape and forced marriage conjured masculinized identities for the two co-performers, even as five wives were reduced to the status of overhearers. A third performance with Santiago's sons and sons-in-law centered on enabling them to internalize the role of deherotu, performer of myth. A single narrative thus moved from being maximally distal and iconic in the first instance, highly proximal and indexical in the second, and alternating complexly between the two poles in the third.[7]

I would like to provide an extended example that suggests how these dimensions can come together in a single performance by returning to the remarkable rendition of a Hopi I'isaw tale by Helen Sekaquaptewa that I initially discussed in chapter 2. I draw on a videotape prepared by Larry Evers and an article by Andrew Wiget (1987) that provides a translation and analysis.[8] Recall that the story involves an encounter between I'isaw, a figure generally (but, according to Risling Baldy 2015, incorrectly) translated as Coyote, and a flock of sparrows. The sparrows are busy winnowing seeds with plaque baskets. I'isaw observes their routine, which involves singing a song as they blow away the chaff and then flying up in the air before beginning a new round. Hoping "to enjoy a good snack," he proposes joining the wary sparrows in their activity.[9] At first, I'isaw pretends to learn how to winnow seeds and sing the song in order to prove that "I wouldn't do anything to hurt you" (Wiget 1987:302). His growing assimilation of the sparrow subject position leads him to attempt its complete internalization: he expresses his desire to fly upward in a circle with them. Seeming to accept his internalizaton of the sparrow subject position, each sparrow plucks feathers from one part of his or her body and places them on I'isaw. On the fourth time that he winnows, sings, and flies upward with them, the sparrows snatch away their own feathers, causing I'isaw to fall to his death. The narrative is thus richly iconic, entextualizing forms of self-formation in moving between a treacherous predator, his cautious would-be victims, and a figure whose desire to transform himself into an Other self leads to his own self-deception and destruction. The plot creates a distal, *tuuwutsi* (folktale) world, rendered a bit more proximal by placing the scene next to a village landmark.

Nevertheless, Ms. Sekaquaptewa uses her eyes, head, body, and gestures in such a way as to simultaneously indexically position herself and her grandchildren in this internalization process, creating a bodily transformation no less radical than I'isaw's becoming a sparrow. At first, she performs all of the roles herself, including singing the song. As I'isaw begins to sing along, however, so do her grandchildren, mimicking her gestures of shaking imaginary seeds and blowing away the chaff. (The camera and visitors seem to have produced signs of a sense of embarrassment that somewhat limited the grandchildren's participation.) Ms. Sekaquaptewa uses her hands, body, eyes, and face to extend this growing internalization of the sparrows' subjectivity by looking at each grandchild when the sparrows are conferring among themselves; she later reaches out and touches each grandchild, pretending to extract feathers. Her head movements suggest this increasing subjective identification as she first invites the children to look up at the flying sparrows but later positions them as collectively looking down toward the ground. Ms. Sekaquaptewa similarly looks at each grandchild in turn precisely when an internal state is crucially revealed, inviting them to try on each subjective state: I'isaw's initial trickery, the sparrows' wariness, I'isaw's request for help in self-transformation, the sparrows' pretended innocence as they dressed up I'isaw, and the birds' moment of vengeance and moral reprobation. The distal world of the tuuwutsi becomes proximal in the space of narration and the iconic entextualization of processes of self-construction feel indexically tangible as the participants become a multispecies, human-cum-sparrow-cum-I'isaw family. Watching the video extends these possibilities for participation. Recall from chapter 2 O'Neill's observation of how songs composed of what are often called nonsense syllables permit circulation across cultural and linguistic borders. Even viewers who know no Hopi can learn the song and gain at least some degree of entry into these sparrow/I'isaw/narrator/grandchildren subjectivities. As I watch over a hundred Berkeley undergraduates watch the video each year, I see how many—like Ms. Sekaquaptewa's grandchildren—a bit self-consciously begin to sing it and mimic the gestures.

Frantz Fanon's work invites speculation about a possible leap of scale that may underlie Ms. Sekaquaptewa's efforts to enable her grandchildren to explore the possibilities, limits, and costs of internalizing other subject positions. Fanon traces how the complex understandings of race and power embedded in "the oral tradition of the plantation Negroes" got displaced for children in the Antilles through "magazines [that] are put together by white men for little white men." Negative images of "the Wolf, the Devil, the Evil Spirit, the Bad Man, the Savage" contained in stories of Tarzan, Mickey Mouse, and comic books "are devoured by the local children" ([1952] 1967:146). Fanon traces the shock, the splitting of the subject that emerges when Antillean children internalize negative constructions of "the Negro" and "the Indian," then later come to see themselves through white eyes, realizing that their own bodies position them as the projected embodiment of sin, evil, savagery, and sexuality. Following Fanon, it is tempting to think that Ms. Sekaquaptewa's performance implicitly warns her grandchildren about the dangers of following teachers, mass media, and other sources in internalizing projections of white identities as normative, only to have their borrowed white feathers suddenly repossessed when a racializing comment transforms them into a negative stereotype of "the Indian." Such a possibility remains, however, at the level of conjecture.[10] Herein lies the beguiling magic of poetics and performance, particularly when entextualization draws attention to distal and iconic dimensions: it offers powerful affordances for constructing external and internal objects and imbuing them with charged affects without overdetermining forms of participation or foreclosing other possibilities.

To be sure, these two continua, distal and proximal, iconic and indexical, provide only a very preliminary starting point for transforming the admittedly dense and abstract framework I developed above into a program for guiding fieldwork, analysis, and comparison. Recent scholarship that focuses on the body, affect, the senses, violence, gender and sexuality, disability, and multispecies and environmental relations opens up a multitude of possibilities. To try to chart them here would be to turn what must be a collective enterprise involving a range of emerging mentors—including students, scholars, and practitioners, humans and nonhumans—into a pretentious individual assertion of authority, an ambitious form of intellectual colonialism that would reproduce precisely the politics of knowledge that I seek to challenge. And, as we have learned from so many scholars, positionality matters: we are moving beyond the point where a single white, heterosexual, North American man can convince anyone but himself that he can single-handedly chart new horizons. I can thus only hope that this discussion will help break down barriers between seemingly incompatible fields and perspectives and open up new futures.

CONCLUSION

Even as Dundes was portraying his advocacy of psychoanalysis in folkloristics as a quixotic task of tilting at windmills, psychoanalysis was becoming a powerful force in such fields as literary criticism, performance studies, anthropology, history, feminist studies, queer studies, and racial and ethnic studies. I would thus suggest that the more difficult task here is trying to figure out why psychoanalysis has *not* been a more visible presence in folkloristics. In the end, asking whether folklorists should use psychoanalysis might seem less crucial than asking what sort of psychoanalytic framework might be most valuable, how it can advance research, and what folklorists and anthropologists can contribute to psychoanalysis. I have advanced this project here by seeing how psychoanalysis can help us think through some thorny issues that have similarly plagued an arena that did have its dominant day, the study of poetics and performance. I think that extending the dialogue between these approaches would be of great value for psychoanalysis and poetics and performance.

In the end, my goal has not been to sell psychoanalysis or market a new and improved poetics and performance. I have rather used this discussion in wrestling with questions that my mentors have raised over the decades. Why is experience often so intensively heightened in performance? Why are cultural forms so powerful in shaping selves, relations, and politics? Why do performances open up the imagination so impressively, why are they so memorable, and why—particularly in the case of political performances of intolerance—can they so powerfully help facilitate some futures and demonize others? Think about Old Man Hawkins: how could stories construct him as a dangerous menace, leading to social isolation, when the circulation of his own stories found him a privileged place as a locus of knowledge, entertainment, and peaches? I suggested that certain elements, drawn from poetic, referential, acoustic, bodily, musical, material, and other dimensions, enter simultaneously in multiple processes of constituting subjects. Freud's concept of condensation provides a valuable resource for exploring this process. His notion was primarily lexical in focus, seeing how particular words could reshape meanings attached to others, even as he was acutely aware of the acoustic materiality of signs and dimensions of materiality and embodiment. By recasting condensation in terms of entextualization and vice versa, I have suggested that poetics and performance play a crucial role in this process of reconfiguring subjects, affects, and relations.

I clearly do not want to suggest that poetics is a sign of mental pathology. Similarly, I would agree with Bauman and others that the metacommunicative dimensions of entextualization can enhance reflexivity. I have suggested, however, that this reflexivity may not add up to a totalizing sense of conscious awareness, either of the discursive act in question or of processes of constructing selves and worlds. Jacques Lacan's ([1966] 1977) notion of the imaginary helps us understand why the reflexivity associated with entextualization does not constitute the sort of transparent, one-to-one correspondences of signs and their objects envisioned by John Locke ([1690] 1959). Lacan starts with what he terms "the mirror effect," the moment when infants of around six months of age recognize their image in a mirror as themselves. When they move their hands, so does the image. Nevertheless, mirrors distort, turning three dimensions into two and reversing laterality. Recognizing that we have selves that are not extensions of our parents thus involves dealing with the power of reflexivity and with its limits. Entextualization enables us to grasp features of distal and proximal worlds and provides us with powerful models for how we can internalize them. The forms of reflexivity that it affords, however, are always selective and interpretive. As Lacan suggests, it crucially depends on an Other who is listening and looking, touching, smelling, and tasting, one that exists both inside and outside of us. I recall Santiago Rivera's performance of "my myth," that of the emergence of white (and Black) people, which he used to project a non-Indigenous self for me that might reject racist expropriation, thereby inviting me to join an Indigenous anticolonial struggle. My Córdovan mentors similarly constantly used performances to X-ray racial domination and to challenge me to examine my own subject formation, particularly my race, class, and gender privilege.

A major problem, in my estimation, is that folklorists have generally incorporated the sorts of foundational psychoanalytic concepts that Frantz Fanon so forcefully challenged. I would not follow Dundes (1987a:23–26) in framing this issue as cultural relativism versus universalism. Fanon's point was not just that psychoanalytic constructions of "the family" were universalistic but that "the family is a miniature of the nation" ([1952] 1967:142): broader racial inequalities thus get inscribed in families in ways that socialize

Black children to internalize the very negative stereotypes that stigmatize them. Accordingly, a new synthesis thus requires, in my view, building on Fanon's and other reformulations of psychoanalysis and simultaneously using his work—along with that of Américo Paredes—to challenge similarly universalized notions of poetics, performance, performer, audience, language, and the body. Fanon's work suggests that entextualization is grounded in political economy, including colonialism and racial and other inequalities, and that it can provide a powerful means of producing, reproducing, and reifying them.

As I noted in the introduction, I designed part 2 of this book to put together two different takes on poetics and psychoanalysis. I argued that entextualization matters, that it constitutes an exceedingly important site for constructing, internalizing, and externalizing psychic worlds: poetics and performance thus provide key affordances. Nevertheless, this argument presents me with a dilemma. Does this not apply to scholarly writing as well? Conventional forms of writing invite conventional responses, even if the content waves a referential banner that pretends to call for new ways of thinking. I tried to disrupt this kind of academic entextualization by experimenting with the genre of the scholarly introduction. Since then, however, I have largely fallen back on conventional scholarly rhetorics. Now I'm ready for another experiment.

Here is my plea. As you read the following chapter, please be open to my effort to create a new form of entextualization, one that develops iconic and indexical features designed to facilitate different modes of interaction between poetics, performance, and psychoanalysis. Trust me: my motive is not to wow you with my creativity. This effort rather grew out of frustration and a sense of failure. I had long struggled to create a dialogue between several of my mentors: Sigmund Freud and women who used laments to mourn their children who died in a mysterious epidemic in Delta Amacuro in 2007–2008. For several years, I tried conventional academic rhetorics—using Freud as a theorist to help *me* (note the self-positioning here) make sense of *their* (Delta interlocutors') laments, narratives, and conversations. I had satisfied reviewers that the effort was successful, but I myself became less and less convinced. Freud had become a dead theoretician, not a mentor whose voice lived within me. The mothers and grandmothers were losing their status as mentors whose powerful insights into life, death, natureculture, and the psychic and political power of poetics and performance had helped Norbelys Gómez, Tirso Gómez, Conrado Moraleda, Enrique Moraleda, Clara Mantini-Briggs, and me diagnose the epidemic and fight for justice in health. I was inadvertently turning these women into mere producers of cultural forms that seemed to invite me to become a distanced and authoritative interpreter. I dragged a psychoanalyst and lamenting mothers out of their chosen forms of entextualization and into a homogeneous social scientific register that I dominated, simply bringing along the usual ethnographic traces of their words. But my own self could not settle for a rigid, hierarchicalized schema that muted these voices—I was still working through the trauma I had experienced when, myself a grieving parent, I was assigned the task of accompanying parents' failed efforts to save their children's lives and to join them in working through the pain and anger that followed.

Suddenly, I wondered what might emerge if I threw out all previous drafts in favor of addressing Freud in the form of a letter, an epistolary genre whose literary features lie precisely in connections and disconnections between a self and an other. Suddenly a writing process that had grown oppressive and frustrating became a tremendous source of pleasure. I stopped trying to dominate and demote my mentors in favor of exploring what they might have to say to one another, and to you and me. This genre gave me more room to engage with the registers used by the Delta women and Freud, to let them exert more power over the entextualization process, even if I admittedly retained control. If chapter 5, with its big words and many ideas, has created some distance between us, please join me as I return to a more personal, vulnerable form of writing, thinking, and feeling.

NOTES

1. Limón and Young (1986) similarly suggest the need to develop a psychoanalytic folkloristics that departs from Dundes's formulation; they stress the need for ethnographic engagement. Such problems are apparent in varying degrees in the work of Carvalho Neto (1972), Holbek (1987), and Vaz da Silva (2002). Rather than surveying the broad range of psychoanalytic perspectives on folklore and psychoanalytic interpretations by folklorists here, I focus more closely on particular issues.

2. See Mechling 2001 for an excellent example of a psychoanalytic analysis of ethnographic materials.

3. I do not rehearse here the many critiques that have been offered of the limitations of Jakobson's model, including its analytic isolation of the "speech event."

4. Dennis Tedlock (1983, chapter 5) used this term to describe a range of devices that narrators invoke to make the imaginary realms created through storytelling seem real. These include such features as using a local landmark in a folk tale, producing sounds for events taking place in the story (bang!), picking up a nearby object and inserting it into the story, and using gestures and movements of the head and eyes to make it seem as if the narrator is actually in the space depicted by the story.

5. I thank psychoanalyst Maureen Katz, MD, for pressing me on this point.

6. For a more extended analysis, see *Competence in Performance* (Briggs 1998).

7. See Briggs 2000 for an extended analysis of the three performances.

8. See Hymes 1992 for a rhetorical analysis of the narrative.

9. Please note that I have deleted the specific typographical features that Wiget uses in his transcription.

10. This point brings to mind Dell Hymes's (1981) analysis of the Clackamas Chinook myth of "Seal (and) Her Younger Brother Lived There," where a mother refuses to listen to her daughter's warnings about the strange behavior of her uncle's "wife," who turns out to be a murderer. Hymes (307) suggested that the story might provide a warning about the daughter's need to rely on her own observations and verbal knowledge in the face of racialized violence and cultural destruction.

6

Dear Dr. Freud

DEAR DR. FREUD,

I hope you don't mind my writing you. People might think it strange that I address myself to a dead person, casting the living as overhearers. Yet my letter is precisely about that subject, so this mode of address seems uncannily appropriate. And I think that this type of intimacy, which I hope does not seem inappropriate to you, will allow me more freedom to explore connections between two quite different sites that have opened up issues of grief and mourning for me. One is your essay "Mourning and Melancholia" and the psychoanalytic literature it inspired.[1] Another lies in laments I heard in the midst of a mysterious and frightening epidemic in the Delta Amacuro rainforest of Venezuela in 2008 and how they shaped Indigenous leaders' efforts to diagnose the disease and demand action. Your essay helped me think through poetic and acoustic features of the laments, the demands they made on listeners, and what they can tell us about the work of mourning and anthropology. I think that you and other psychoanalysts might discover new lines of thinking in how these parents, some of whom lost nearly all their children to an undiagnosed illness, displayed collective and critical ways of producing knowledge and placing it in circulation.

My goal is to reflect on my engagement with "Mourning and Melancholia" and the particular forms of mourning I encountered, not to position myself as critiquing psychoanalysis or anthropology. A letter will, I think, provide a more open space to explore insights that got lost in translation, literally. This format might help me respond more directly to what I perceive as the remarkably and productively tentative, even hesitant, tone you adopted in the essay, starting with your "warning against any over-estimation of the value of our conclusion," sustained in recurrent expressions like "I think" and "is not at all easy to explain." You opened up a space of indeterminacy by suggesting that mourning is both analytically perplexing and "is taken as a matter of course by us"; accordingly, you never seem to resolve the question of how we move between clinging to and reimagining "the object" and reality-testing. I want to further open up this space of indeterminacy and draw attention to its productivity.

Like many readers, I was captured by your expression "the work of mourning" and your sense that mourning is not pathological, so that "we look upon any interference with it as useless or even harmful." Your emphasis on the contradictory character of mourning engaged me deeply. On the one hand, the work of mourning involves hyper-cathexis, recovering and reinternalizing the image of the dead person and imbuing it with such intense psychic energy "through the medium of a hallucinatory wish-psychosis" that "the existence of the lost object is psychically prolonged," creating a fantasy world in which we allow ourselves to believe that the person never really died or will return. Nevertheless, "reality-testing" requires that "each single one of the memories and situations of expectancy which demonstrate the libido's attachment to the lost object is met by the verdict of reality that the object no longer exists," leading to a struggle "so intense that a turning away from reality takes place." Crucially, you pointed out that this juxtaposition engenders both the "extraordinarily painful" character of mourning and the emergence of a "compromise" between the two processes. I think that listening to laments will deepen our understanding here by drawing attention to some acoustic, bodily, and material dimensions of this contradiction.

Other readers have distanced themselves from how they see you as projecting the temporality of mourning. My colleague at Berkeley Judith Butler suggested that your essay "implied a certain interchangeability of objects as a sign of hopefulness, as if the prospect of entering life anew made use of a kind of promiscuity of libidinal aim." She thought that a linearity informs your distinction between mourning and melancholia, which would equate mourning with forgetting. Butler argued that you later changed your mind, admitting in "The Ego and the Id" that reincorporation of the lost attachment "was essential to the task of mourning." And the French psychoanalyst Jean Laplanche contended that "the Freudian theory of mourning" involves a unilinear process of stripping away memories. Julia Kristeva extended your thinking about the pervasiveness and persistence of melancholia, depicting it less as pathology than as a painful but productive force. Anne Cheng, Angela Garcia, and other writers have reflected on the complex ways that melancholia gets woven into the fabric of racial inequalities and vice versa, a point I want to discuss with you shortly.

I agree that casting mourning in linear and functionalist terms as a process that reestablishes a psychic status quo would be problematic. By suggesting that "when the work of mourning is completed the ego becomes free and uninhibited again," you do invite such readings, but recently I have come to doubt that your text points us squarely in this direction. During six delightful months in Germany, I spent a great deal of time with "Trauer und Melancholie" in German. That exercise, admittedly long overdue, convinced me that this projection of a unilinear temporality in your essay partially emerges through problems of translation. The translation of the crucial paragraph in which you characterize the contradictory nature of mourning suggests that the "orders" of the "respect for reality" "cannot be at once obeyed." The next sentence of the translation suggests that these "orders" "are carried out bit by bit, at great expense of time and cathectic energy."

Nevertheless, my reading of the German text suggests to me that these projections of a single, universal, unilinear temporality are absent. You continue: "Er wird nun im einzelnen unter großem Aufwand von Zeit und Besetzungsenergie durchgeführt und unterdes die Existenz des verlorenen Objekts psychisch fortgesetzt," which is translated, problematically I think, in the *Standard Edition* as "They are carried out bit by bit, at great expense of time and cathectic energy, and in the meantime the existence of the lost object is psychically prolonged." You point to the need to link a "great expense of time and cathectic energy" to the specificities of individuals and situations. The next sentence, "Jede einzelne der Erinnerungen und Erwartungen" ("Each single one of the memories and expectations"), lodges the call for considering specificities (*einzelne* reappears) precisely in multiple temporalities, both pasts ("memories") and anticipated futures; mourning seems to multiply the complexity of interactions between pasts, presents, and futures. The English translation of the next sentence suggests that this work "is carried out piecemeal," again seemingly suggesting a gradualist temporality, if less explicitly. Your German text rather repeats the word *einzel* (*Einzel-durchführung*), pointing once again to specificities in particular acts of carrying out the "orders" of reality-testing. This sense of open-endedness and indeterminacy prompts you to a stunning admission: "Why this compromise ... should be so extraordinarily painful is not at all easy to explain in terms of economics." The temporalities that unfold in the German text enabled me to find new ways of thinking about mourning, temporality, psychoanalysis, and anthropology.

I have always been perplexed, however, by the absence of an element that is prominent in *Jokes and Their Relationship to the Unconscious* and *The Interpretation of Dreams*. The anthropologist Vincent Crapanzano suggested that you regard language as a referential apparatus. This statement certainly rings true for "Mourning and Melancholia," but in these other two works you pointed to how people engage the formal properties of language reflexively. Oddly, you left poetics out of "Mourning and Melancholia," and I missed your reflections on the role of poetics in shaping the struggle between reattachment to the "existence of the lost object" and "the testing of reality." So I invite you to take a journey with me to Delta Amacuro, to meet people who not only lodge the work of mourning in poetics but also reflect deeply on this process. There I think that you will find an eerie resonance with your call to attend to the specificities of struggles and compromises, of hyper-cathexis and reality-testing.

ON THE THRESHOLD IN MUAINA

The morning of July 28, 2008, in Muaina (see figure 6.1) afforded one of those scenes that is both unimaginable and whose horror you know intimately, one where your feet seem to propel you inexorably into the middle of a disquieting space—and yet are susceptible to the urge to turn and run (see figure 6.1). The doorway, flooded with sunshine, led to a darkened interior that would confront us with our first direct encounter with death. Not just any death, but a body claimed by an epidemic of a "mysterious disease"—just one of numerous strange fatalities—in this small settlement where the rainforest meets the Caribbean in eastern Venezuela. Having recruited us for the investigation they were organizing, Conrado and Enrique Moraleda had invited Clara Mantini-Briggs, Norbelys Gómez, Tirso Gómez, and me to a *meeting*, a sober gathering in which measured voices would provide clues that might add up to a diagnosis. But this is what we saw:

First our eyes were directed to the right side of the house, where a wisidatu (a particular type of healer) with graying hair and a kind face was treating a young man in a hammock. His song, which called on hebu (pathogens treated by the wisidatu) to leave the body, was drowned out by the voices of five women and one adolescent who became visible as we took another step forward along the dock. Standing directly opposite the doorway, we also saw a young man lying in a coffin, bringing visual and auditory senses into disconcerting alignment. One of the faces, transformed into a mask of grief and fatigue by more than a day of mourning, belonged to Florencia Macotera (see figure 6.2), the mother of Mamerto Pizarro, the third Muaina resident to die from the unknown disease (see figure 6.3). Beside her Mamerto's grandmother, two of his aunts, a sister, and a brother rocked back and forth as they collectively composed and performed laments. The exhaustion that would have ordinarily weakened their

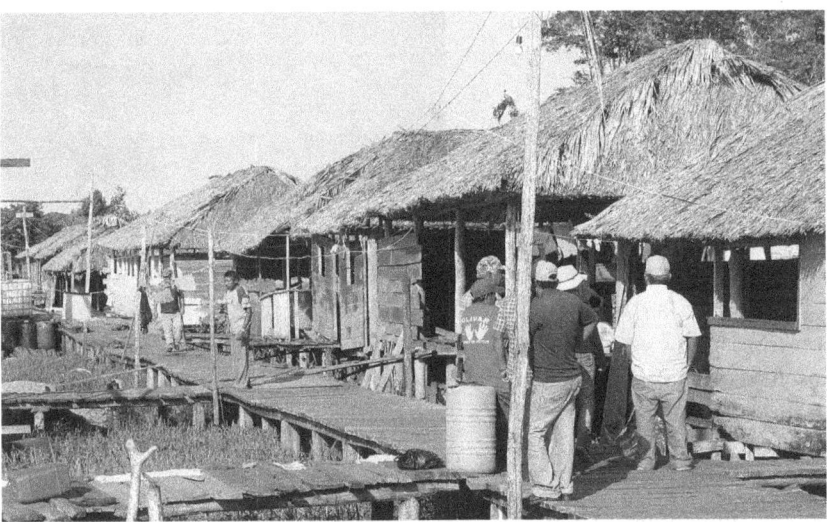

Figure 6.1. Muaina

voices by this time had been overpowered by the realization that they would soon take Mamerto to the cemetery.

In retrospect, witnessing that scene seems both accidental and overdetermined. My relationship to the Delta and its residents had been long and intense. I began working there in 1986, learned the language (Warao), and studied healing, narratives, Indigenous legal practices, gender relations, and the racialization of citizenship. Given the precariousness of health conditions, I witnessed numerous wakes and documented several; after a couple of years had passed and people wanted to hear my recordings, I sat with women for extended periods, transcribing their words and discussing performances. Clara, a Venezuelan public health physician, began working for Delta Amacuro's Regional Health Service (RHS) in April 1992, just months before a cholera epidemic killed some 500 Indigenous residents. She served as the assistant epidemiologist and the state director of health education. After collaborating with Indigenous communities to establish nursing stations and prevention programs, we researched the underpinnings, bureaucratic as much as epidemiological, of such extensive death from a preventable and treatable bacterial infection.

After years of working elsewhere in Venezuela, it was the book that documented this epidemic, *Stories in the Time of Cholera*, that brought Clara and me back in 2008. Collaborating with Norbelys and Tirso Gómez and residents of several communities, we were using income derived from royalties and prizes to explore new models for health programs. We had documented how President Hugo Chávez's socialist revolution had brought doctors, mainly Cubans, to live in many low-income urban neighborhoods in Venezuela. Nevertheless, other than the creation of two larger facilities, the revolution had brought few changes to Delta health conditions. More than a quarter of children still died, mostly as infants from treatable diarrheal and respiratory infections. Then an epidemic started in Mukoboina, a community of about seventy-five residents, in July 2007; by January, eight children had died. Then children started dying in neighboring communities. When strange symptoms appeared, parents took their children to healers and the local doctor, but neither could save them. Patients were referred to metropolitan hospitals, but all died.

As the president of the Health Committee, Conrado Moraleda observed the patients in the local clinic; parents and leaders pressed him to demand that public health officials take firmer steps to diagnose the disease and stop the epidemic. Cuban and Venezuelan epidemiologists visited, but they could not sort it out. Conrado appealed to the regional legislature, but the public meeting that resulted infuriated health officials. When a third wave of deaths began in June 2008 and the regional government seemed to have given up, Conrado and Enrique decided to form their own team to investigate the epidemic and take the results directly to officials and journalists in Caracas, the national capital. Having stumbled onto the epidemic,

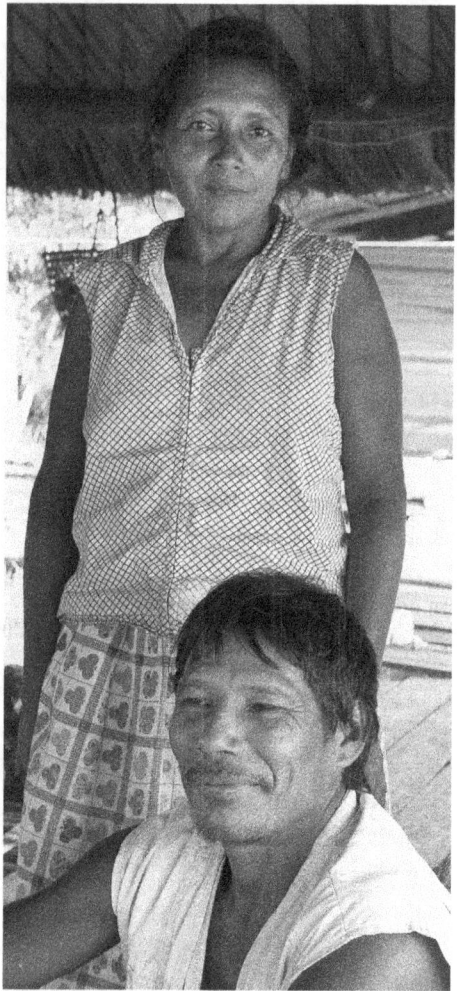

Figure 6.2. Florencia Macotera and Indalesio Pizarro

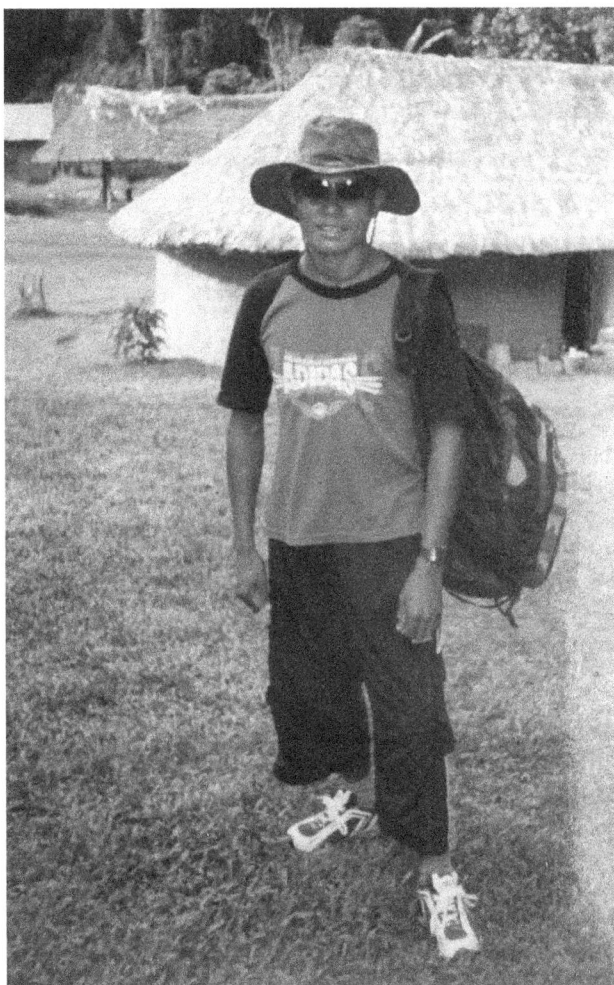

Figure 6.3.
Mamerto Pizarro
at the Indigenous
University
of Venezuela
(photographer
unknown)

we were looking for the resident physician to ask what he knew about the strange cases when Conrado buttonholed us as we ascended the clinic's stairs. "You have to help us! You, Dr. Clara, must work as a physician, and you, Dokomuru" (my Warao name), "you have to work with us in finding out what is killing the children." I was positioned as an anthropologist, but my training as a healer, my ability to translate between diagnostic languages, and my photographic training were also relevant. The investigation began in Muaina.

I think you would be fascinated to see how the features of the work of mourning you analyzed—its contradictory dimensions, the tremendous

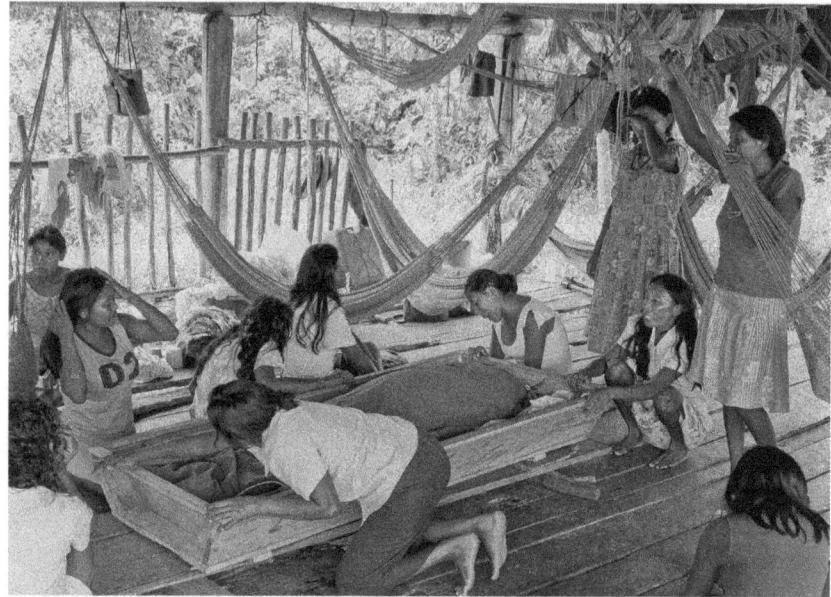

Figure 6.4. Singing laments for Elbia Torres Rivas, Barranquita

investment of psychic energy, and the depth of the pain—were highlighted by lamenters' words and voices (see figure 6.4). Each explored the specificity of the process of resurrecting *Erinnerungen*, memories, investing them with tremendous poetic, musical, and psychic energy. Mamerto's brother Melvi reflected on how they played together as children, traveled with their parents to their mother's natal community to garden and, shortly before Mamerto died, worked together constructing houses. His grandmother remembered that he sometimes slept at her house and brought her fish. Mamerto's mother reflected with pride on his studies at the Indigenous University of Venezuela.

Infusing our consideration of mourning with attention to poetic detail can provide insight into complex issues of temporality. In "Mourning and Melancholia," you used the power of German's noun morphology to build evocative phrases around complex nouns, as when you joined *Kompromißleistung* (accomplishment of a compromise), *Einzeldurchführung* (particular acts of implementation), and *Realitätsgebotes* (dictates of reality). Although Warao grammar can rival German in the complexity of nominal constructions, the poetic action in laments lies in the verbs: in the laments for Mamerto, mourners wove complex temporalities deeply into poetic images. Lamenters attached the present-tense marker *–ya* and the durative aspect form –*ha* to verb stems, sometimes both in the same word, to make images of the deceased seem as if they were unfolding at that moment and would continue indefinitely into the future. Performers created tiny imagist poems that placed listeners in the middle of actions, as if we were currently sharing these experiences with the performers. At the same time, a struggle ensued within each voice through verb endings marked as past and punctual, particularly –*(n)ae*; here reality-testing took each image and burst it apart.

This short passage from Melvi's lament suggests how finely the two temporalities were woven together.

1. *Mano, oko daobasa serebuya makina eku,*
   My brother, we were making boards together in the sawmill,
2. *ama ihi mamoae diana.*
   now you have left me.
3. *Ihi yakerakore aniaokawitu karamuyaba hatanae,*
   When you were well you used to get up right at dawn,
4. *planta aida esohoyaba gasoi hatanae tatukamo,*
   you were filling the large generator with diesel,
5. *oko yaotaya yoriwere dao sepeyaba,*
   we were working alongside one another planing the wood,
6. *ihi mate yakerakore, wabanahakore.*
   while you were still well, before you died.
7. *Ama ihi momi wabae.*
   Now you died apart from me.

In lines 1 and 3–6 we stand alongside Melvi as he is watching Mamerto get up at dawn and fill the generator and as the two brothers are milling lumber (see figure 6.5). Melvi uses grammatical features that suspend time, placing Melvi, Mamerto, and listeners in the middle of these scenes. Lines 2 and 7 contrastively place these memories and expectations in a past that has been sealed off from presents and futures. These features thus created the sort of struggle between multiple temporalities—lingering pasts, anticipated futures, and a harsh reality of temporal rupture—that you depicted. There is nothing either gradual or linear here. The presents that each performer constructed were not bounded points in a linear trajectory but sites in which shifting, violent, and unavoidable juxtapositions of multiple temporalities emerged. Struggles and compromises also became apparent in how these words were sung. In previous work I have referred to lines 1 and 3–6 as "textual phrases"; the focus is more textual than musical, consisting of bursts of words that invite listeners—including other lamenters—to con-

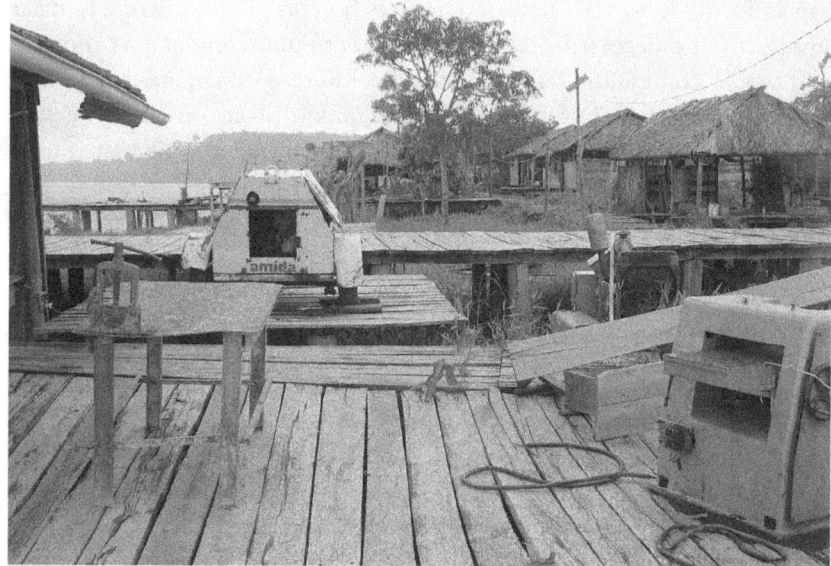

Figure 6.5. The contractors' sawmill at Muaina

centrate on their semantic content and poetic contours. Refrains, on the other hand, are associated with reality-testing; here narrative elaboration gives way to bald statements about the finality of death. These moments of reality-testing provided resting spaces in which lamenters listened to other performers.

The performance thus made this struggle explicit from moment to moment through both poetics and the musical materiality of voices. Putting poetics and acoustics into the equation could enable us contribute to how psychoanalysts have extended your discussion of mourning. I think Melanie Klein added a great deal to our language for talking about mourning. She suggested that young children build internal images of external objects (particularly of their mother and father), thereby possessing them inside their bodies as internal objects. This world of internalized objects is not static but changes continually through the incorporation of new people and experiences, real and fantasized. Klein echoed your insightful comments on the terrible pain of mourning, arguing that it is produced by losing the person in the real world, which induces distrust of the external world in general and a shattering of this carefully constructed internal world. Klein suggested that the work of mourning requires mourners "to rebuild with anguish the inner world, which is felt to be in danger of deteriorating and collapsing." Although Klein referred to "the slow process of testing reality in the work of mourning," seemingly subscribing to a gradualist view, she emphasized the conflicting emotions that emerge in juxtaposing "passing states of elation . . . due to the feeling of possessing the perfect love object (idealized) inside" with intense sorrow, distress, and hatred. Klein thus productively left room for iterability, arguing that grief moves in waves, much as we saw in the laments. Klein's formulation captures how each mourner began to rebuild her or his internal world, which initially fell apart after the death of Mamerto's younger brother, Dalvi. The poetics of lament are crucial here in suggesting how mourners repeatedly took images from a shattered external world and imbued them with wholeness, immediacy, and a sense of the real, as Jacques Lacan might put it. If the crucial process, following Klein, is reconstituting the mechanism by which internal and external objects are co-constructed, then the poetics and acoustic/bodily materialities of laments provide an impressive cultural form that simultaneously models how this process can be accomplished and demonstrates its precarity.

I think you might appreciate the work of Juan-David Nasio, an Argentine-born student of Lacan. Nasio followed you in tracing how love progressively dominates our internal world by taking in the image of someone we love in such a way as to "cover him or her over as ivy covers a stone wall." I would add that in grief we seem to painfully retrace how our love for a person has attached itself "in very particular places of the wall, in its cracks and crevices," revealing how deeply and minutely our lives became intertwined. The lament verses were like vines that extended simultaneously into the performer and into Mamerto, tracing how these experiences linked them psychically, thereby resulting in intense pain and disorientation when they suddenly seemed to have been severed. Psychoanalytic accounts of mourning and these laments similarly point to how we lose parts of ourselves as we lose another. In analyzing the element of the imaginary, Nasio complements the ivy metaphor by describing how internalizing the loved person in the unconscious enables us to see reflections of other internalized objects, including images of ourselves, not like "the smooth surface of a lens, but as a mirror broken up into small, mobile fragments of glass on which confused images of the other and of myself are reflected." Poetic and musical features of laments suggest how memories are fragmented, as in the ivy and mirror metaphors, but also linked by virtue of their inclusion within a poetic and musical structure.

Laplanche productively charted the complexity of temporality in his evocation of Penelope in Homer's *Odyssey*. She famously embodied her mourning for Odysseus by weaving a shroud for his father, frustrating her suitors for three years:

> "Young men, my suitors, now my lord is dead,
> let me finish my weaving before I marry . . ."
> So every day she wove on the great loom—but every night by torchlight she unwove it.

Laplanche used this metaphor to disagree with your account: "Penelope does not cut the threads, as in the Freudian theory of mourning; she patiently unpicks them, to be able to compose them again in a different way." Laplanche suggests that this work requires time, is repetitive and, thinking about Lacan's account of how prohibiting the use of the names of the dead constitutes a linguistic reserve, he argued that "it sets aside a reserve." My rereading of temporality in your essay suggests that Laplanche provides us with a rich metaphor less for challenging your account than for extending it.

ACOUSTICS AND AFFECTS IN THE COLLECTIVE WORK OF MOURNING

Reworking these issues through the lens of poetics, Kristeva suggested that mourning and melancholia can result in a dramatic disruption of meaning. She argued that when the "symbolic" (semantically based) process falls short, the "semiotic" process, which does not center on referential meaning, gains ground: "Melody, rhythm, semantic polyvalency, the so-called poetic form, which decomposes and recomposes signs," are crucial. Kristeva further opened up space for poetics and acoustics in taking up the relationship between beauty and mourning you discussed in "On Transience." "When we have been able to go through our melancholia to the point of becoming interested in the life of signs, beauty may also grab hold of us to bear witness for someone who grandly discovered the royal way through which humanity transcends the grief of being apart: the way of speech given to suffering, including screams, music, silence, and laughter." The anthropologist Renato Rosado similarly explored connections between poetics and grief through poems he composed after the tragic death of his wife, Michelle Zimbalist Rosaldo.

An essay by the sociologist Erving Goffman, "Response Cries," seems particularly revealing here. He suggested that such utterances as "Ouch" or "Whoops," exclaimed suddenly after some kind of mishap, signal a temporary loss of control. Providing what appear to be natural, involuntary indexes of the emotional and/or physical state of the person who uttered them, they seem to provide listeners, even strangers, access to our internal states. Nevertheless, "response cries" are conventional signals whose expression is shaped by our perception of those around us: children learn to emit different response cries when they drop something in the presence of peers, grandparents, or teachers. Goffman's formulation captures how such expressions seem to convey transparently what is happening within individual bodies and simultaneously to engage social relations, asking overhearers to interpret signs of internal distress as constructing both utterers and overhearers as particular types of social beings.

Despite his genius, Goffman was given to anecdotal examples. Attending to acoustic features of the laments for Mamerto can open up Goffman's concept and help us see how acoustics forms part of the work of mourning. In laments, pain adopts the acoustic features of crying, of moans and wails, yet at the same time it is stylized. Warao lamenters use "creaky voice," low pitch, high volume, and a special, affectively charged timbre, the suppression of the "singer's formant" between 1.8 and 3.8 kHz. These features are not read as consciously stylized, as in storytelling, but as involuntary, transparent embodiments of internal, affective states. This construction of acoustics/affect relations is said to generate their compelling effects on listeners: "What they're crying is entirely true; they couldn't cry lies." Goffman located response cries in words; thinking about lamentation would point to the centrality of acoustics. I found previously that if women use the same poetic structure but do not invest their words with these acoustic features, particularly the special timbre, they elicit a different response in listeners—they can be accused of faking it.

Goffman's work might lead us to imagine this projection of internal states as emerging accidentally. Kristeva, given the depth of her explorations of psychoanalysis, language, and poetics, unsurprisingly has much to teach us about how we are constantly providing iconic, in Charles S. Peirce's terms, constructions of internal processes. Her distinction between semiotic and symbolic processes opens up a space for rethinking Goffman's response cries. The subject does not enter into the semiotic process with a clearly defined identity shaped prior to and independent of the discourse; it is rather emergent through semiotic features. Poetics enters into both semiotic and symbolic processes; through the semiotic, poetic dimensions intersect with acoustic ones in providing extensive modes of constituting and voicing selves. I think, Dr. Freud, that given how referential content, poetics, grammar, bodies, music, and other acoustic dimensions come together in laments, they provide one of the contexts in which semiotic and symbolic processes come closest to merging. This, I think, constitutes part of the tremendous affective and social power of laments, and it suggests why they have interested anthropologists concerned with the relationship between acoustics and embodiment.

Reflecting on the work of mourning vis-à-vis these laments provides us with a new way of thinking through what has been framed as the problem of the limits of language in relationship to mourning. Eric Santner takes Paul de Man to task for "turning death into a purely linguistic operation," which leads de Man to preclude "the possibility of distinguishing one victim from any other." Bringing in specificities of historical circumstances, deaths, and acts of mourning, of bodies and materialities, of affects, of the social and psychic productivity of mourning seems to position it beyond the limits of language. But thinking about these laments suggests that the problem might rather lie in the adoption of a limited, referentialist view of language, in its reduction to Kristeva's symbolic process. Taking lamentation for a model of language in mourning would leave such binaries behind by linking symbolic to semiotic dimensions, to the specificities and materialities of bodies, acoustics, and poetics.

I think that we can bring Goffman's and Kristeva's analyses together productively, albeit keeping their differing approaches in mind. Although Goffman seemed to view response cries as pointing to broader dimensions of speech and social interaction, he framed them as accidental, unusual features. Reflecting on spirit possession, Vincent Crapanzano suggested that such outbursts can be therapeutic when their expression is structured. Elaborately and multiply patterned, laments are prolonged performances of response cries that provide seemingly unmediated reflections of internal states and yet simultaneously model how listeners should hear them and what they should feel. Kristeva characterized semiotic process as a ubiquitous dimension of everyday speech, and her concept pointed in the direction of broader acoustic, poetic, and musical patterns. Goffman suggested that the projection of internal states is social and interactional, always more than an internal splitting of the self. In talking about laments, listeners feel that these acoustic features create similar bodily and psychic responses *within them*, saying that they "cry along behind" lamenters; we could say, in Nasio's terms, that they, like fellow performers, are reflecting on the particular vines that extended between them and the deceased.

Here I hope you will find a powerful similarity between lamentation and psychoanalysis. Lacan defined psychoanalysis as practices of listening. He was struck by "the subject's relation to his own speech, in which the important factor is rather masked by the purely acoustic fact that he cannot speak without hearing himself" and by "the fact that he cannot listen to himself without being divided as far as the behaviour of the consciousness is concerned." In analysis, patients learn to listen to their own speech, including its silences and the multiple voices that constitute it, just as the analyst's role revolves around practices of listening. The locus of performativity and the possibilities for transforming the subject lie in listening as much as in speaking, in an interactive setting in which psychoanalysts are listening too. The lamentation process similarly requires performers to listen closely to their own voices—as echoed in the words and acoustic features of the voices of their fellow performers.

What I am suggesting, Dr. Freud, is that the effects of lamentation in splitting subjects and doubling processes of listening impact overhearers powerfully as well, pointing to crucial collective as well as individual and intrapsychic dimensions of the work of mourning. Mamerto's relatives performed laments *collectively*. One person took the lead at any given moment, contributing themes that were then taken up by others. The remaining lamenters did not voice the same words or sing at precisely the same time or with identical pitch or voice quality; rather, other singers transposed these lines, reflecting their own relationship with Mamerto and the most affectively charged aspects of their experiences. In musical terms, this relationship is called *polyphony*. Voices were coordinated in terms of pitch, volume, affective intensity, and timbre, as well as content, but these features never precisely coincided: voices never gave up their individuality. Composing, transposing, performing, and listening thus emerged together, with the emphasis shifting from one process to another from moment to moment.

In these laments, the orientation toward overhearers in the construction of internal states, which Goffman elucidated, extended beyond fellow performers. In Muaina, houses largely lack walls; accordingly, other residents were thrust into the acoustic space of mourning. Even if Mamerto was not their relative, the pain was inescapably *inside* everyone as their eardrums vibrated with the frequency of the affects generated by Florencia Macotera and other lamenters. As Nadia Seremetakis argued for Greek laments, listening engages a broader sensorium and interpellates the body. As my colleague Charles Hirschkind suggested for Islamic sermons on cassettes, listening requires listeners to locate themselves in affective and ethical soundscapes. Those in earshot could not avoid being interpellated by the sensory, ethical, affective, and bodily demands of the laments for Mamerto.

Accepting Enrique's invitation to the meeting (see figure 6.6) thus entailed becoming an overhearer of the lamentation. By the time Florencia crossed the dock from her house to take her turn in the white plastic narrator's chair, we had been listening all morning to how she moved between reinternalizing powerful images of her two sons to announcing the finality of their deaths. Florencia walked slowly, as if in a trance. All eyes shifted

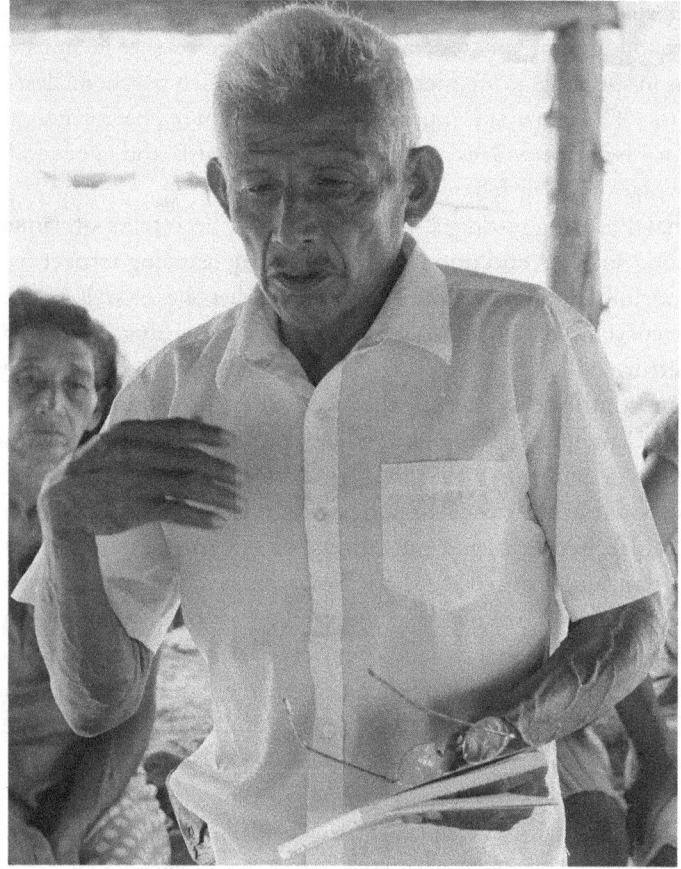

Figure 6.6. Enrique Moraleda

from the previous witness, who wrapped up swiftly; everyone stepped aside. Florencia was wearing a white blouse and a light green skirt. Her hair, hanging haphazardly in front and back, and her look of exhaustion inscribed mourning on her body. The force and passion of the ritual wailing did not diminish but seemed to move toward a crescendo as she began. Her three-year-old daughter hovered around her, listening intently while alternately wrapping around herself the dress that she was carrying, and twirling it (see figure 6.7).

Florencia focused her lament on Mamerto, but she wove in verses that evoked the prior death of her younger son. The effect was to heighten the iterative qualities and the affective surplus of fear, frustration, and determination she experienced as Dalvi's symptoms seemed to leap from his dead body into that of her oldest child. In the narrative she told at the

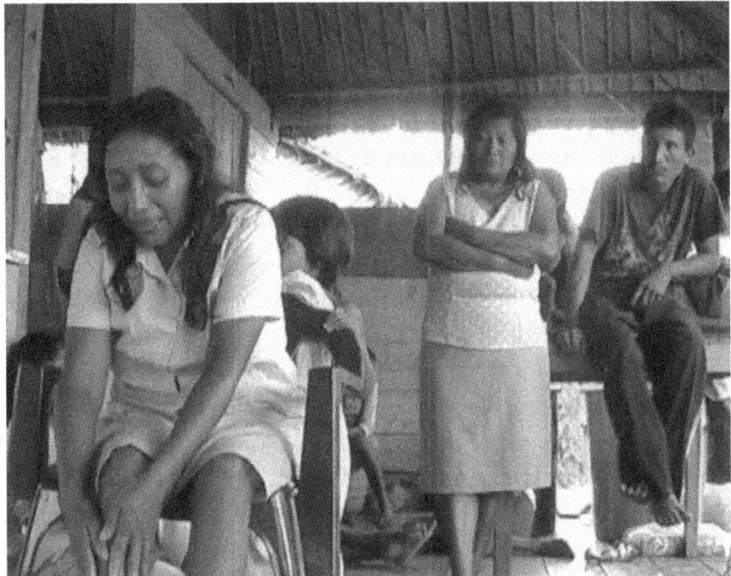

Figure 6.7. Florencia Macotera telling the story of Dalvi's death at Muaina meeting

meeting, Florencia recounted how Dalvi first grew feverish at the wake of a cousin, Muaina's first fatality in the epidemic. She weaves the story of the progression of Dalvi's symptoms into that of efforts by the local nurse and healers to diagnose and treat him. Given your training as a physician and your interest in poetics, Dr. Freud, you might not be surprised to learn that the narrative climax seemed to mirror the increasing severity of symptoms, particularly strange neurological manifestations. Arriving in a larger community where both doctors and more experienced healers were available, Dalvi seemed to be fighting cartoon villains regularly beamed into Muaina via DirecTV satellite dishes; as death drew near he declared, "Mama, the monsters have killed me, they have taken my heart." His voice began to fade: "Mama, I am leaving without you now, I'm going now. My dead cousin Eduardito has come to get me, he's with me, I'm going now, we're going now." Note how Dalvi's reported words seem to provide Florencia with lines for the lament that she would soon be singing. Attempting to hang onto Dalvi, Florencia pleaded, "Don't die yet son, wait a little longer for me." Moved, he comforted her, "Okay, I'll stay, I won't die. I'm not going to die, Mama." But she could see that his eyes were closed, his body growing cold, his voice fading away. "Mama, Mama, I won't die, I won't die, I won't die, Mama, for you I won't die. My body will grow cold, but I won't die. I'm going to come for you, Mama, wait for me, Mama. When I die, don't cry for me, don't cry for me." "And then," concluded Florencia, "he grew silent. My son Dalvi died." At that moment Florencia shifted quickly to recounting how Mamerto's symptoms began even as the family was returning from Dalvi's burial. Before she could finish telling of Mamerto's death, the grief became too intense, and she suddenly rose up, retraced her steps across the dock, and transformed her words back into lamentation.

The rich detail in Florencia's testimony helped us in the diagnostic process. The dying words of a nine-year-old boy, moving between fantastic battles with cartoon villains and a remarkably sensitive and articulate attempt to shield his mother from mourning, signaled to us that the disease might have a crucial neurological dimension. Florencia's emphasis on the emergence of identical symptoms—fever, headache, a feeling of itching in the feet that turned to numbness, then paralysis, and then ascended upward, along with hydrophobia—provided us with a major clue. Given your training as a neurologist, Dr. Freud, I bet you have already figured out that *rabies* was behind the epidemic. As she was leaving, Clara asked Florencia if either son had been bitten by an animal. When Florencia replied that both had received bat bites about a month before they developed symptoms, meaning that they had been bitten nocturnally by vampire bats, a hypothesis regarding the means of transmission emerged.

Listening sideways to Florencia's lamentation shaped how we subsequently heard her narrative, producing an involuntary doubling. The affective intensity of her narration, simultaneously etched onto her body, was doubled by the superimposition of the remembered acoustic features of her lament. Her narrative was overlaid yet again by the acoustics of the laments still emerging next door. Even the less charged words of other witnesses, such as those by Muaina's nurse and other residents, were shot through with the acoustic features of the laments in ways that we would never be able to disentangle, even as we transposed them into written documents for transport to distal sites.

TOWARD A POLITICS OF SPECIFICITY

Given your stress on specificities in the work of mourning, I would have liked to see you analyze particular cases, as you do elsewhere. You rely on two general figures, "the mourner" and "the love object" (*Liebesobjekt*). I miss here the personal introspection that provided such poignant moments in some of your other work. Matthew von Unwerth suggests that beyond

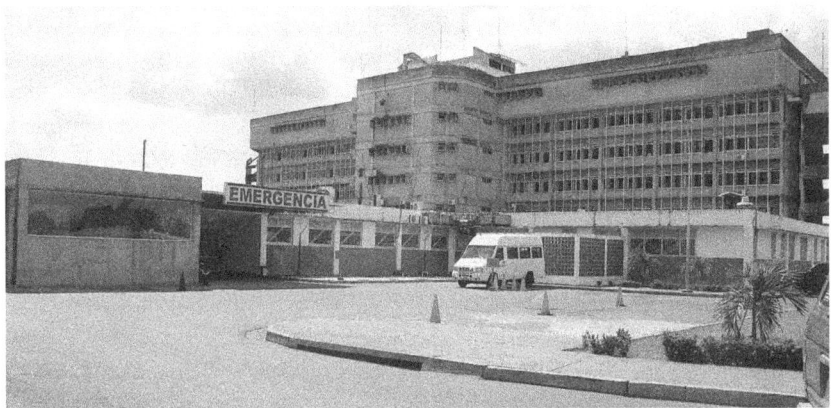

Figure 6.8. The Uyapar Hospital in Puerto Ordaz

psychoanalytic disputes that resulted in the loss of friendships, "reflection of the current affairs of a world gone mad" during World War I sparked a return "to a problem that had long been the subject of Freud's interest—the fate of pain and loss in human memory." Because I am an anthropologist rather than a psychoanalyst, please allow me to return to the encounter with Mamerto's mourners in reflecting on the importance of whose pasts are remembered, whose futures lost, and which realities tested. Subsequent conversations with Mamerto's parents and his brother Melvi taught me much about the nature of the reality-testing that had taken place.

Mamerto was wheeled into the intensive care unit on the fifth floor of the Uyapar Hospital in Puerto Ordaz, a city in neighboring Bolivar State (see figure 6.8). There a guard escorted Mamerto's father and wife through a strangely vacant waiting room. They noticed a large clock with red digital numbers of the same sort that seemed to proliferate in every corridor. The date and hour portions were strangely blank; to the right of flashing dots it read ":82," as if time had been erased or was out of whack. The guard's gesture forced them onto the landing, a space of about two-by-four meters in which around fifteen people were standing, sitting on the floor, or leaning against a mound of coolers, thermoses, pillows, and satchels. Two dozen more people were distributed in the stairwell leading to the fourth floor. Rather than welcoming Elbia Torres and her father-in-law as two more worried relatives of poor patients in a public hospital, people stared at them as if they were foreign objects. A boy of about eight pointed to them, looked up at his mother, and said, "Look, Mama, Indians!" This detail brought me back to the psychiatrist Frantz Fanon's reflection on a boy's remark, "Look, a Negro!" Fanon wrote: "My body was given back to me sprawled out, distorted, recolored, clad in mourning." After a sleepless night in a rural clinic, each step of the journey—a boat trip at dawn, anxious hours in the Tucupita Hospital, and two long ambulance rides—seemed to dislodge Mamerto's wife and father progressively from all that was safe and familiar. Being unwelcomed into this disorderly space in a modern, orderly hospital was just too much.

Retreating to the next landing, which had fewer occupants, Elbia sat in a corner and slept while Indalesio remained vigilant. At 5:00 a.m., a nurse appeared, leading people to jump up and push toward the entrance. She called out, "Indalesio Pizarro." Following her, a physician standing in the middle of the corridor told Indalesio matter-of-factly, "Your son is dead." Indalesio recrossed the waiting area slowly; the digital clock still read ":82." Awakening Elbia on the landing below, he seemed to mirror the doctor's curt, unfeeling words: "My son is dead." "What are we going to do?" she asked. "We have to wait."

Did Florencia's and Indalesio's reality-testing begin then, and were the multiple forms of symbolic violence that organized space in the stairwell part of that reality? Seeing Mamerto hooked up in the ICU, Indalesio sensed that death was near: "Everything fell on top of him. The machines failed him there—everything failed him." Did reality-testing begin then? Did the succession of medical technologies—and the clock's capacity to disjoint time—constitute the reality that was shaping this testing? Did it begin when Florencia first declared that Mamerto's symptoms were "just the same as his younger brother's"? Dalvi felt sick during the wake conducted for his cousin, Eduardito, whose symptoms had appeared as he returned from the funeral of a cousin in another community. And the deaths in Muaina were not the first: thirty-four children and young adults had already died. Did reality-testing begin when "Warao Radio," as regional word-of-mouth transmission is called, brought stories of the first death to Muaina? Or did reality-testing begin when two of the couple's children died as infants? In the eyes of health officials, losing just under 30 percent of one's children (prior to Dalvi's and Mamerto's deaths) was considered "normal."

But Mamerto did not die as a child, his death was not a "normal" death, and his life had been infused with important specificities. Enrique had particular reasons for launching the investigation next to Mamerto's body. Muaina, you see, was established by one of the most charismatic and creative Indigenous leaders in Venezuela, Enrique and Conrado's brother Librado, who was one of my closest friends. A socialist long before Chávez became president, Librado founded Muaina as a model socialist community. Paulo Freire would have loved it: Librado, an educator, created a critical pedagogy that juxtaposed Indigenous knowledge production with access to Spanish, literacy, and "Western" forms of knowledge. Librado also helped create the Indigenous University of Venezuela, hoping to train a new set of national leaders who could challenge anti-Indigenous racism. Facing terminal cancer, Librado sensed a potential leader in Mamerto and enrolled him in the university. Mamerto quickly distinguished himself by his intelligence, dedication, and vision; within three years he had written two short book manuscripts and translated portions of the Bolivarian Constitution into Warao. With Mamerto's death, reality-testing thus jumped scale: as Indalesio and Florencia were mourning their firstborn son, Muaina was lamenting the death of its socialist dream yet again. Enrique and Conrado were mourning the demise of their brother's dream anew.

CIRCULATION: ON THE POLITICS OF INDEXICALITY AND ERASURE

Our recruitment was doubled that day in Muaina, Dr. Freud; having been asked to join Conrado and Enrique's investigation, we were called to participate in the work of mourning for Mamerto. Both tasks involved practices of listening, but they were not focused solely on these genres or on the contexts of their performance. I have pointed to the importance of circulation, to how words, acoustics, and affects moved between performers, overhearers, and narrators. Processes of circulation were modeled multiply through poetic and acoustic features of lamentation narratives and frequent references to how news of the epidemic had been moving for more than a year and was circulating at that moment. Crucially, this modeling of past and present circulations was transformed into projected futures and distal contexts from the moment we arrived: lamenters charged the team to "take our words to Chávez!" Carrying out this charge required that the team, consisting of Clara, Conrado, Enrique, Norbelys, Tirso, and me, document the epidemic and take our findings to national officials and journalists in Caracas. In the remarks with which he opened the meeting, Enrique anticipated the verbal and visual materialities that would be required to make this jump in scale by asking Muaina residents for permission to record and photograph the proceedings, providing "a base, a support, a force to enable us to convey this painful situation that is taking place." He similarly told us after the fact what agreeing to join the investigation had entailed: collectively taking a report to Caracas.

The boldness and the potential political effects of this circulatory project struck us immediately. The projection of an Indigenous/non-Indigenous chasm that sorts human beings into two vastly unequal categories lies at the heart of everyday practices in Delta Amacuro's state government, including its Ministry of Popular Power in Health branch. The stereotype of "the Warao," despite 500 years of evidence to the contrary, suggests that "they" lack political agency and cannot rise above immediate material interests. One way that the racial status quo—and the viability of this feeble but enduring racial construction—is maintained is through the unstated rule that people classified as Indigenous can only report problems and demand actions in private meetings with state officials in Tucupita, but they can never take their petitions to Caracas. Worse yet, reporting an epidemic of an infectious disease would challenge the RHS's monopoly over the circulation of epidemiological discourse—backed, the RHS often asserted, by law. Starting in September 2007, the RHS had struggled to keep news of the strange disease from circulating; epidemiological reports were carefully guarded internal, rather than public, documents. No wonder officials became enraged when Conrado, after closed-door meetings failed to prompt effective action, went public about the epidemic in February 2008. Unless sympathetic national officials overrode the angry reactions of regional subordinates, we were in for trouble.

Making the work of mourning mobile raises complex issues. The sociologist John Urry has suggested that casting such phenomena as walking, bicycles, cars, and airplanes as immanent embodiments of mobility required broad transformations of bodies, landscapes, the built environment, and social relations; he reminds us that the same processes produce *im*mobilities. Mobilizing scientific and medical objects entails specific requirements. The science studies scholar Bruno Latour has argued that scientific facts and concepts are often projected as "immutable mobiles"—as capable of traveling anywhere without changing their significance. Given that these should rely on a single body of "gold standard" evidence and common diagnostic categories, a doctor's pronouncement "This is rabies" should mean the same thing in Delta Amacuro as in the United States (where people die periodically of bat-transmitted rabies, too). Geoffrey Bowker and Susan Leigh Star have suggested that rendering diagnostic categories and statistics mobile requires two things. Particular assemblages of practices, epistemologies, and technologies emerge at each site they are (re)produced. For example, reducing some 500 cholera deaths in Delta Amacuro in 1992–1993 to the official count of 13 involved inadequate health infrastructures, a "case definition" that rejected clinical in favor of laboratory evidence, limited laboratory testing facilities, racial profiling, and political pressure. Nevertheless, epidemiological discourse would be unlikely

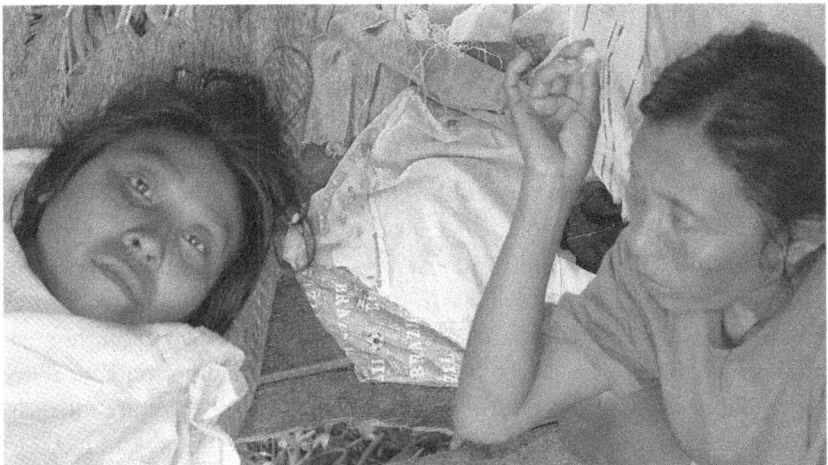

Figure 6.9. Elbia Torres Rivas, an hour before death, with her mother, Anita Rivas

to travel if these complex assemblages remained attached to statistics and diagnostic categories. Accordingly, Bowker and Star suggest, indexical histories must be erased for categories and statistics to become mobile.

Herein lies a fundamental contradiction the six of us faced in carrying out the parents' charge to carry their words to Chávez. Neither the laments sung over Mamerto's body nor the narratives unfolding in the adjacent house were likely to travel beyond the rainforest or to interpellate epidemiologists, health officials, or journalists—none of whom could speak Warao or would accept these genres as conveying scientifically valid knowledge. We were asked to construct a classic epidemiological formulation, "N people died from X disease over Y period in Z area," one that would have the mobility to reach national officials. Suddenly, we were not medical anthropologists who exposed *other* people's indexical histories or critically engaged *their* erasures. We documented thirty-seven deaths in fourteen localities in meetings that created a complex knowledge-production process, one that drew on political oratory, Indigenous medicine, dispute mediation, personal narratives, epidemiology, and clinical medicine. The long days of our investigation were punctuated by daily visits to Elbia Torres, Mamerto's wife, whose symptoms began while returning to Muaina from the urban hospital (see figure 6.9). Recognizing that her symptoms were identical, knowing that all patients had died, and remembering acutely the symbolic violence that she and Mamerto's father had experienced in the Uyapar Hospital, she decided to die in her parents' home. The indexical history we built thus included Clara's detailed examinations, Norbelys's provision of palliative care, and the photographs that the family asked me to take of her illness, wake, and funeral.

In preparing a report, we made painful decisions about what to erase. We had spent time listening to discussions of bad medicine (which anthropologists often refer to as "sorcery"). Nevertheless, Enrique stated: "After deep reflection, I reluctantly propose that all references to 'witchcraft' be erased from the final report—they shall remain with us." No one spoke; we understood all too well. Any allusion to bad medicine would render our efforts, to use the anthropologist Arjun Appadurai's phrase, incarcerated by culture: our report would be dismissed as reflecting superstition, not science. Nevertheless, the cost of creating mobility would be too high if we severed indexical links to bodies, laments, and narratives. Despite the risks, we made the journey. All of us supporters of the revolution, we framed our work as bolstering government efforts to confront health inequities and overcome discrimination against Indigenous Venezuelans. Nevertheless, Caracas officials initially refused to accept our report, denying its mobility. "You should have stayed in Delta Amacuro and delivered it to officials there," they insisted, thereby reinscribing the racialization of space and speech. "We told them over and over again," Conrado countered, "and they didn't listen." A three-hour standoff ensued in the ministry's lobby. The team held its ground. The situation attracted the attention of national health reporters and of Simon Romero of *The New York Times*. When the photographer for *El Nacional* appeared, Enrique handed out several of my photographs. Enrique held up a photograph of Anita Rivas watching her daughter die, Tirso a portrait of Elbia's grandfather, and Norbelys one of Arsenio Torres performing a lament over his daughter's corpse (see figure 6.10). In recirculating their account of the epidemic, they wanted to keep the images and laments attached to the account that the team had transported to Caracas, thereby preventing them from becoming abstract words and numbers or further "proof" of Indigenous stereotypes.

CONCLUSION: PSYCHOANALYSIS, ANTHROPOLOGY, AND THE WORK OF MOURNING

When asked why they had come to Caracas, Conrado, Enrique, Norbelys, and Tirso repeatedly pointed to the regional government's failure to respond adequately to the deaths. When the photojournalist's camera seemed to pose the same question, they took out photographs of a dying Elbia Torres, her family's grief, her father's lament. The *El Nacional* photograph would take viewers back to the contested act of witnessing these deaths in the ministry's

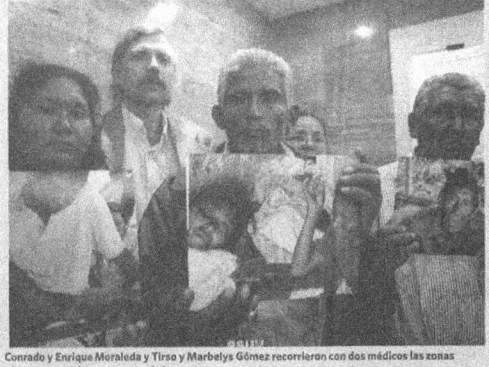

Figure 6.10. *El Nacional* photograph of team with pictures of Elbia Torres Rivas and her family

lobby. The psychoanalyst Jed Sekoff's reflections on a family photograph that includes a dead child seem particularly illuminating: "Looking at a photograph places us at the edge of a certain time . . . The dead are somehow conjured into life. And yet again, this very magic makes their death all the more certain; our loss stares us in the face." In addition to multiple edges, the *El Nacional* photograph pictures several uncertain times: one of the encounter in the ministry, another of a life slipping into death, and a third moment in which Arsenio, Elbia's father, attempted to acoustically conjure a death into a life. If photographs are indexical icons, as Peirce argued, tying images not just to what they reflect but to the moment of their creation, both reflections and points of origin get multiplied here in complex, unstable, and productive ways, especially when, to return to Nasio's metaphor, the mirror has been "broken up into small, mobile fragments of glass."

Butler suggested that in the face of pronounced inequalities, "certain lives are not considered lives at all, they cannot be humanized," adding that "if a life is not grievable, it is not quite a life." In opening the Muaina meeting, Enrique projected how racialization differentially values lives and deaths: "If this community was a *criollo* [non-Indigenous] community, or of the upper class, I have no doubt that health authorities would have already taken charge of the situation. It seems as if the lives of us Warao . . . aren't worth anything to the criollo world." The photograph multiplied claims to the grievability of Elbia's life, refracted through images of mourning and the trip to Caracas. In the *El Nacional* article, Enrique interpellates the body politic through the figure of Chávez: "We invite the President to come to our funerals," thereby ambiguously including deaths past and future.

This photograph and its interpellation of readers into the work of mourning might signal the end of our story, telling us wherein lies the work of mourning. But the issues you raised, Dr. Freud, suggest that the photograph might rather deepen our engagement with questions of grievability than effect their closure. You wrote that what distinguishes melancholia from mourning is "a lowering of the self-regarding feelings," suggesting that sometimes "it is all the more reasonable to suppose that the patient cannot consciously perceive what he has lost." Can mourning and melancholia be neatly separated in the wake of Mamerto's death? The literary scholar Anne Cheng has suggested that melancholia structures racialized inequalities in such a way that it "conditions life for the disenfranchised and, indeed, constitutes their identity and shapes their subjectivity." A decade before your essay appeared, W.E.B. Du Bois traced how racism complicated grieving for his infant son: "All that day and all that night there sat an awful gladness in my heart,—nay, blame me not if I see the world thus darkly through the Veil,—and my soul whispers ever to me, saying, 'not dead, not dead, but escaped; not bound, but free.'" Fanon famously stressed the individual and collective depersonalization that structures the violence and social death produced by colonialism. Enrique frequently disrupted epidemiologists' ahistorical interpretations of the deaths by citing 500 years of colonial violence in the Delta following Columbus's arrival in 1498. In such a situation, is it possible to speak of "normal grief" or to distinguish it neatly from melancholia?

I am also left with questions about the anthropologist lurking in the background of the photograph. How am I participating in the work of mourning? If the laments and their circulation can inform psychoanalytic understandings of mourning, what might they contribute to anthropology?

Ethnography, as classically framed, involved imagining a research object, usually an ethnos ("the X"), a journey to what was defined as the space of a culture, and a trip home, data in hand. Although this formulation has been widely critiqued, one of its central elements—interviewing—remains central. Interviews help anthropologists create and control the discursive events they use in producing knowledge and asserting rights to circulate their interlocutors' words and images. Despite limits imposed by institutional review boards, once consent is granted, anthropologists largely shape what becomes mobile and how it travels.

Which is why the epidemic provides such an interesting and troubling site to reflect on anthropology. I had not gone to the Delta to do research, and I did not conduct interviews. Nevertheless, I was asked to participate in the investigation that Conrado and Enrique organized because I am an anthropologist, and I was constantly told what it means to do the work of anthropology. As I have suggested, the meeting juxtaposed modes of knowledge production associated with political discourse, dispute mediation, alternative healing, testimonies, epidemiology, and media documentation, which all got overlaid with the poetics and acoustics of lamentation. I was not granted control over the circulation of words and images; I was rather interpellated by lamenters and leaders into a circulatory process, placed both behind the camera and in front of it. The way I contributed anthropologically to the investigation of the epidemic and the trip to Caracas was shaped from the start by how my participation was constructed as part of the work of mourning.

Juxtaposing your essay and the laments has led me to think of *anthropology as the work of mourning*. I am not trying to universalize a single model of the work of mourning—your call to attend to specificities is crucial. Nor would I want to privilege these lamentations as a sort of *ur*-mourning or archetypal mourning; I think that there is much to be learned from the narratives, home altars, Facebook pages, grief groups, and other forms of the work of mourning that are woven into everyday life and death in the United States, not to mention the home funeral movement that nostalgically resituates corpses, wakes, and funerals in family homes. Nor am I suggesting that anthropologists should be fixated on physical death; Du Bois, Fanon, Das, Pandolfo, and others have clearly suggested that we should think just as seriously about social death. Indeed, my interest here focuses more on work than on mourning per se.

Framing anthropology as the work of mourning evokes the work that anthropologists do in making images collaboratively and placing them in circulation, and it unsettles the usually unstated techniques we use to infuse images with particular sorts of affects. It can also help us think more complexly about how our work responds to and participates in efforts to make and understand worlds, including ways that humans and nonhumans cohabit with viruses and bats. Anthropologists might read this statement as suggesting that all anthropology must be engaged, activist, or community-based, but I think that framing anthropology as the work of mourning would challenge this interpretation in two ways. First, I have not presented the particular contours of how I was interpellated in the epidemic as providing some sort of general model for anthropology; I have rather focused on how attending to the poetics and acoustics of laments can extend the ways that anthropological research and writing are imbricated in the specificities of worldings, an issue that Kathleen Stewart has recently addressed. Second, "Mourning and Melancholia" demonstrated how attending to the specificities of memories and expectations, hyper-cathexis and reality-testing requires reflecting on persistent and productive conceptual puzzles. The work I was called to perform has required a collective process of rethinking knowledge production, poetics, cross-species relations, epidemiology, and circulation, and this work is by no means finished. Reframing anthropology as the work of mourning would thus require surrendering the engaged versus conceptual binary as a means of classifying anthropologists and projects.

Perhaps paraphrasing Karl Marx's famous statement in the *Eighteenth Brumaire of Louis Bonaparte* might help me clarify what I mean by anthropology as the work of mourning: anthropologists make their own stories, but they do not make them just as they please; they do not make them under circumstances entirely chosen by themselves. Crossing the threshold in Muaina called me to make knowledge anthropologically under circumstances that I had not chosen but that I did have a role in shaping. I was asked to make images, to build on Klein, as a part of collective efforts to (re)create mechanisms for building and connecting internal and external worlds that had been shattered through the colonial violence quintessentially embodied in thirty-eight gruesome deaths. I was asked to participate in creating pasts that would challenge the social death that preceded Mamerto's physical demise and in projecting futures that imagined the end of colonialism's violent grip on the Delta. The precarity of these futures was painfully evident in the chilly reception we received in the ministry lobby's marbled interior and the government's steadfast refusal to confirm the rabies diagnosis or to provide an alternative. The lability of futures and the affects attached to them were underlined subsequently when the roles that Enrique projected were reversed: it was Chávez who died and the six of us who witnessed his funeral. As I finish this letter in February 2014, the Bolivarian revolution seems to be seized in a precarious work of mourning as President Nicolás Maduro's efforts to sustain Chávez's image are tested by realities shaped by his corporeal and political absence.

Nevertheless, the power and the precarity of making pasts and futures, images and realities were signaled from the start in each verse of the laments sung for Mamerto. The rhythms and acoustics, polyphonies and affects of the laments, the way they turned listeners into overhearers but made demands on them nonetheless are what I want to capture in recasting anthropology as the work of mourning. Rethinking this notion through a dialogue between psychoanalysts and lamenters has suggested to me how anthropology as the work of mourning captures connections between the precarity of anthropologists' constant movements between image making and reality-testing and the precarity of the worlds they engage, of anthropology's specificities, struggles, and compromises.

You might conclude that I am trying to get psychoanalysis on the cheap by writing a letter to a deceased analyst, one whom I cannot pay. Here, I think, you would be wrong. I have done my work of mourning, and some psychoanalysis as well. But that's another story, equally unfinished and uncertain.

Your friend,
Charles

NOTE

1. Given that this text is a letter, I do not include citations in the text. A list of sources follows, tied to entries in the reference list. All citations within the same paragraph of the letter are grouped in the same line in the list of sources. My text revolves around retranslations of a number of key terms and phrases. When the translations are my own, I have included the German. Quotations not accompanied by the German are taken from the translation in the *Standard Edition*; an editor's note suggests that it was based on Joan Riviere's translation of 1925 but "has been very largely rewritten" by James Strachey and his collaborators (Freud [1917] 1957:239). The translations from Warao and Spanish are my own.

SOURCES

"warning against any over-estimation" (Freud [1917] 1957:243); "is not at all easy to explain" (245); "is taken as a matter of course" (245)

"we look upon any interference" (Freud [1917] 1957:244); "through the medium of a hallucinatory wish-psychosis" (244); "the existence of the lost object" (245); "reality-testing" (244); "each single one of the memories and situations of expectancy" (255); "so intense that a turning away from reality takes place" (244); "extraordinarily painful" (245); "compromise" (245)

"implied a certain interchangeability" (Butler 2004:21); "was essential to the task of mourning" (20–21); "the Freudian theory of mourning" (Laplanche [1992] 1999:251–52); Kristeva (1987) 1989; Cheng 2000; Garcia 2010.

"when the work of mourning is completed" (Freud [1917] 1957:245); "respect for reality" (244); "orders" (245); "cannot be at once obeyed" (245); "are carried out bit by bit" (245)

"Er wird nun im einzelnen unter großem Aufwand" (Freud [1915] 1946:430); "They are carried out bit by bit" (Freud [1917] 1957:245); "Jede einzelne der Erinnerungen und Erwartungen" (Freud [1915] 1946:430); "is carried out piecemeal" (Freud [1917] 1957:245); "Why this compromise" (245)

Freud (1905) 1960, (1900) 1965; Crapanzano 1981

Briggs and Mantini-Briggs 2003 on the cholera epidemic; Briggs and Mantini-Briggs 2009 on health programs and the Bolivarian revolution; Villalba et al. 2013 provide child mortality statistics

"Kompromißleistung" (Freud [1915] 1946:430); "Einzeldurchführung" (430); "Realitätsgebotes" (430). Osborn 1967 presents a useful analysis of Warao verbal morphology. With respect to the analysis of Melvi's lament, line 6 uses a different form, -*kore*, which similarly places the utterances in the middle of an unfolding time before illness and death gripped Mamerto. On the textual and musical structure of laments in Delta Amacuro, see Briggs 1992, 1993c.

"to rebuild with anguish the inner world" (Klein [1940] 1948:321); "the slow process of testing reality" (321); "passing states of elation" (322–23)

"cover him or her over as ivy covers a stone wall" (Nasio 2004:29); "in very particular places of the wall" (31); "the smooth surface of a lens" (34)

Robert Fitzgerald (Homer 1963:22) provides the translation of Penelope's lines. "Penelope does not cut the threads" (Laplanche [1992] 1999:251); "it sets aside a reserve" (252)

"Melody, rhythm, semantic polyvalency, the so-called poetic form" (Kristeva [1987] 1989:14); Freud (1915) 1957; "When we have been able to go through our melancholia" (Kristeva [1987] 1989:99–100); Rosaldo 2014

"On Transience" (Freud [1916] 1957)

Goffman 1981

Kristeva (1974) 1984; Peirce 1932. Some sources on affect, acoustics, and embodiment in lamentation: Feld (1982) 2012, 1990; Nenola-Kallio 1982; Seremetakis 1991; Urban 1988; Wilce 1998; Briggs 1992, 1993c; Hasan-Rokem 2014

"turning death into a purely linguistic operation" (Santner 1990:29); "the possibility of distinguishing one victim from any other" (29)

Crapanzano 1973

"the subject's relation to his own speech" (Lacan [1966] 1977:181); "the fact that he cannot listen" (181)

Seremetakis 1991; Hirschkind 2006

"reflection of the current affairs of a world gone mad" (Unwerth 2005:5); "to a problem that had long been the subject of his interest" (10)

"My body was given back" (Fanon [1952] 1967:113); see also Pandolfo 2018

Urry 2007; Latour 1987; Bowker and Star 1999

Appadurai 1988

"Looking at a photograph" (Sekoff 1999:110); Peirce (1932:142); "broken up into small, mobile fragments of glass" (Nasio 2004:34)

"certain lives are not considered lives at all" (Butler 2004:34); "if a life is not grievable" (34); "We invite the President to come to our funerals" (Weffer Cifuentes 2008)

"a lowering of the self-regarding feelings" (Freud [1917] 1957:244); "it is all the more reasonable to suppose" (245); "conditions life for the disenfranchised" (Cheng 2000:24); "All that day and all that night" (Du Bois [1903] 1990:154); Fanon (1961) 1963 on the violence of colonialism

Briggs 1986 on interviews

Hagerty 2011 on the home funeral movement

Stewart 2012 on how attending to the poetics and acoustics of laments can extend the ways that anthropological research and writing are imbricated in the specificities of worldings

Marx (1852) 1935

Part III
A New Poetics of Health, Multispecies Relations, and Environments

7

Toward a New Folkloristics of Health

THE STUDY OF FOLK MEDICINE HAS DEEP ROOTS in folkloristics. Both Richard Dorson's (1968) genealogy of the field and critical counter-genealogies (such as Bauman and Briggs 2003) locate John Aubrey's seventeenth-century cartography of traditional subjects and cultural forms as formative of what would become the field of folkloristics. Nevertheless, two less orthodox points here. First, folk medicine was central to Aubrey's notion of antiquities. The chapter "Magick" in *Miscellanies* (Aubrey 1972) traverses the English countryside and locations around the world as it describes curative practices, who used them, and the ills they were designed to ameliorate. Second, as Richard Bauman and I have suggested (2003), joining Boyle, Locke, Newton, and other members of the Royal Society in fashioning modern subjects, Aubrey helped create a binary opposition that separated modern from traditional. He subordinated the latter subjects, suggesting that "old customs, and old wives fables are grosse things" (1972:132) that constitute "Encroachments of Ignorance on Mankind" (xxxi). Nevertheless, Aubrey did not consistently position folk medicine as belonging exclusively to unlettered rural subjects. His survey included reports of traditional cures used by aristocratic men and women, such as when "a Chyrurgeon in Salisbury" used a new nail to bleed the gums of King James II in order to treat toothache (88). In short, at this formative moment folk medicine was central to what would become the study of folklore, and it stood on the border between what were projected as traditional and modern social spheres.

Jumping ahead three centuries prompts another pair of observations. First, folk medicine is flourishing, both in its everyday uses as well as in ethnobotany, complementary and alternative medicine, and drug development. Second, the *study* of folk medicine has nevertheless been relegated to a relatively marginal scholarly space, viewed by folklorists in general as a medical specialty that is of interest only to a small cadre of scholars. There were no folk medicine specialists among Richard Dorson's "young Turks" (1972:45), nor did *Toward New Perspectives in Folklore* seem to require a new statement on folk medicine (Paredes and Bauman [1971] 1972). The study of folk medicine is seldom celebrated as an endeavor that offers galvanizing new concepts or theories that become necessary reading for all folklorists.

I develop my argument in four sections. The first reviews an old trajectory in the study of folk medicine and suggests how contemporary manifestations engage actively in transdisciplinary dialogues. The second section points out dimensions of contemporary scholarship on health and medicine in anthropology, sociology, and science-technology-society studies that folklorists might find productive. I then explore some conceptual and methodological blind spots of other disciplines that correspond closely to areas in which folkloristics is particularly strong. The final section proposes a framework for retooling research on health and medicine, configuring this arena as a crucial location for tackling problems that lie at the forefront of folkloristic research.

Folklorists are specialists in documenting the social lives of stories, objects, and other cultural forms and tracking how they circulate and are transformed as they move through time and place. Unfortunately, folkloristic work on medicine has been limited by disciplinary compartmentalization; though traditional curative practices bring together a range of cultural forms, the scholarly literature generally leaves objects to folk art specialists, stories to narrative specialists, and medical beliefs and practices to folk medicine specialists. A more integrated approach would build on existing strengths. Further, folklorists have long cultivated the ability to locate social worlds defined by their opposition to "modern" knowledge, whether the relationship is one of exclusion, rejection, or parodic recirculation. Traditionalization, a major focus of the next chapter, was generally analyzed apart from the production of bodies, knowledge, and objects that get defined as new, thereby deflecting folklorists' gazes from closely related phenomena and precluding other scholars from appreciating folklorists' contributions to larger scholarly agendas (Bauman and Briggs 2003). Fortunately, recent work on museums, tourism, intangible cultural heritage, and the global circulation of traditional cultural forms is placing the co-production of traditionalities and modernities at the center of folkloristic agendas.[1] Because the study of folk medicine and ethnomedicine was designed to fill the holes left by cartographies of "modern medicine," it offers a useful vantage point from which folklorists can contribute to critical perspectives on the construction of new modernities.

Folklorists are now making important contributions to contemporary debates about health and medicine, and their work has received attention beyond the social sciences and humanities. Nevertheless, research on health and illness has not achieved visibility as a site for forging new perspectives with discipline-wide import. Here I suggest ways that the folkloristic study of health and disease can be reconfigured and repositioned in order to contribute significantly to transforming the discipline.

THE EMERGENCE OF RELATIONAL PERSPECTIVES ON HEALTH IN FOLKLORISTICS

Wayland Hand (1980) claimed a distinctive body of knowledge and practice for folkloristics: folk medicine. Bonnie O'Connor and David Hufford note that he placed this field, in keeping with contemporaneous understandings of the social and cultural location of "the folk," "in a sort of lower midsection between official, scientific medicine at the hierarchical pinnacle and 'primitive' medicine on the bottom stratum" (2001:13). At the same time, Hand claimed folkloristic authority over a domain that he carved out of biomedical authority: "Better than the doctor," he said, "the folklorist is able to see the interplay of these religious and magical forces" that constitute the domain of folk medicine (1980:xxvi). His efforts to identify a distinct object, claim it for folklorists, and defend its boundaries against other potential claimants were nonetheless juxtaposed with his interest in constituting folk medicine as an interdisciplinary arena to which biologists, biochemists, ethnobotanists, ethnopsychologists, ethnologists, travelers, cultural historians, and anthropologists could also contribute (Hand 1976).

Hand pointed to moments of what is often called medical pluralism, in which different epistemologies and practices intersect, only to separate dimensions that were cast as folk from those distinguished as modern and then order the two hierarchically: "In sickness, more so than in any other vicissitude of life, people will throw all caution to the wind, as it were, and resort to trials and actions that they would not even consider under ordinary circumstances. It is on these human proclivities and on this crisis and despair that quacks and charlatans thrive" (1980:xxv). Although Hand construed objects and epistemologies associated with folk medicine as distinct, their social distribution did not correlate perfectly with distinct classes or social groups: "Superstition is not the preserve of the unlettered only, but is a state of mind or way of looking at things that may befall even the most sophisticated members of society" (1961:xix). The following sentence in this passage extends the separation between folk medicine and rationality, suggesting that modern subjects leave their modernity behind when they resort to folk medicine: "Professional people of all kinds, no less than tradesmen, are prone to many of the same popular conceits and mental errors to which, for want of formal education, members of the humbler classes have fallen heir" (xix–xx).

Don Yoder carved folk medicine out of an arena that, for him, included three other spheres—scientific, primitive, and popular. Although he considered "primitive medicine" autochthonous, existing independently of modern medicine, folk medicine was fundamentally *relational*, even if this relationship was hierarchically ordered: folk medicine, he said, "shares the ground with and exists in tension with the higher forms of medicine" (1972:192). Nevertheless, Yoder undercuts this relational view by referencing a residual definition of folk medicine: he quotes Hanns Otto Münsterer's belief that folk medicine consists of "whatever ideas of combating and preventing disease [that] exist among the people *apart from* the formal system of scientific medicine" (193; my emphasis). As O'Connor and Hufford (2001) suggest, the location of folk medicine as a middle category between "primitive" and modern medicine, and the projection of biomedicine as gradually displacing its two supposed rivals, were stances deeply rooted in nineteenth-century cultural evolutionism. Still insisting on distinguishing educated classes from the popular and the folk levels, Yoder seems both to deny and affirm this evolutionary trajectory: "In the twentieth century, in fact, there would seem to have been an increase in irrational-medical attitudes and practices, particularly on the popular level of middle-class and mass levels of culture" (1972:210).

A generation later, Hufford and O'Connor have extended the notion that folk medicine exists in close interaction and competition with both official medicine and unofficial modalities, going on to expand this dynamic and relational perspective in several important ways. First, Hufford extracts folk medicine from the old oral/literate binary in suggesting that "most of the traditions studied as folk medicine use print to some extent" (1997:549). Although O'Connor and Hufford (2001) note that folk medicine relies more on oral transmission, and biomedicine more on print, they observe that word-of-mouth dissemination now intersects with use of a range of media. I would add that YouTube, videos placed on alternative medicine websites, and social media are now very much part of the mix. (In chapter 9 I analyze how deeply folklore and media interact with biomedicine and public health.) Second, Hufford argues that folk arenas are systematic and embrace "an entire set of attitudes, values, and beliefs that constitute a philosophy of life" (1997:547). O'Connor and Hufford (2001) add that the illusion of randomness and fragmentation in folk medicine is largely due to problematic assumptions and a lack of adequate research. Third, Hufford suggests that the very categories of folk and official are themselves shifting and continually constructed "in the local context" (1997:546); as a result, folk medicine is heterogeneous and shifting, continually constituted in practice as people pick up and combine elements, including those associated with modern medicine. He traces "the constant flow of influences among the health systems within a society" that not only bridges these systems, but also shapes their individual logics (548). O'Connor (1995) argues that nonofficial forms of care are based on generative principles, thus enabling them to formulate modes of addressing new situations in ways that are consistent with their own logics. Kimberly Lau's (2000) study of new age healing and work by Michael Owen Jones and his colleagues (2001) on *botánicas* used by immigrants in the Los Angeles area both provide striking cases in point. Here work by folklorists intersects in important ways with that of Argentine-Mexican medical anthropologist Eduardo Menéndez (1981, 2009), whose relational perspective I highlight below.

Recent folkloristic work on epidemics has extended this dialogue into clinical medicine and public health discussions. Diane Goldstein (2004) indicated that HIV/AIDS legends did not simply reflect but rather informed popular (mis)understandings of the disease and its transmission, taking existing forms of othering and repositioning them on a landscape of fear that promoted scapegoating HIV-positive individuals and "high-risk" groups. Her work demonstrates how narratives and folk beliefs structure perceptions of risk, thereby shaping the success or failure of prevention efforts (2001). Clara Mantini-Briggs and I traced narratives told about the cholera epidemic that began in Peru in 1991; documenting stories about the people who were infected and died, we spoke with hundreds of residents of a rainforest area in Venezuela and nearby cities, as well as with individuals employed by the national health bureaucracy, the World Health Organization in Geneva, and other sites. We suggested that narratives fundamentally shape both how epidemic diseases are treated and the way that race and disease are juxtaposed in epidemiology and policy (Briggs and Mantini-Briggs 2003; see also Rosenberg 1992; Treichler 1999; Wald 2008).

Folklorists have been successful in bringing their work beyond departments of folklore and scholarly publication venues into biomedical spaces. Goldstein's HIV/AIDS work gained national recognition in Canada from biomedical researchers and policy makers. Hufford and O'Connor have developed careers within medical school settings. Hufford (1982) juxtaposed folkloristic and biomedical perspectives in using an "experience-centered" approach in establishing commensurability between the experience of sleep disorders and traditions such as the Old Hag. Extensive work within biomedical settings enabled Hufford and O'Connor to chart how complexly folk and official logics and forms of treatment get interwoven, even in high-tech clinical settings. These shifting boundaries are formed, in part, by the incorporation of folk medicine into biomedical orthodoxies, which do not necessarily challenge the subordination of the former. O'Connor (1995) explores how patients incorporate contrastive therapeutic modes in developing their own plans for seeking care and participating in diagnosis and treatment. Extensive experience with patients and providers enabled O'Connor and Hufford to suggest that such connections are formed less between abstract and totalized systems than they are developed by individuals as part of personal medical systems (2001:32), thus combining what are often seen as incompatible and competing modalities (Brady 2001; Hufford 1988). Andrea Kitta (2012) brings a folkloristic perspective to the task of unraveling what has become a major challenge to biomedical perspectives and public health programs: the anti-vaccination movement in the United States. The success of these scholars' efforts to bring folkloristic perspectives to biomedical researchers is evident in their publications in biomedical journals (e.g., Jenni and O'Connor 2005). Hufford, O'Connor, and other folklorists have played roles in the Office of Alternative Medicine and the National Center for Complementary and Alternative Medicine; the latter, established in 1998, is one of the twenty-seven institutes and centers that make up the US National Institutes of Health. Recent publications suggest that work on health is gaining prominence in folkloristics (see, for example, Blank and Kitta 2015).

In spite of this impressive trajectory, research on folk medicine is seldom celebrated as offering galvanizing new concepts or theories that become necessary reading for all folklorists. Thus, I think it is time to ask why folkloristic work on health and medicine has not taken a more central place on disciplinary stages.

THE VIEW FROM ANTHROPOLOGY AND SOCIOLOGY

At the same time, studies of health and disease have mushroomed in anthropology and sociology. A strong initial focus of the field of medical anthropology was ethnomedicine, cultural and individual variability in perceptions of health, illness, the body, and treatment (see Foster and Anderson 1978; Nichter 1992). Anthropologist and physician Arthur Kleinman (1980) argued for a distinction between disease, defined through biomedical categories, and illness, seen through the experience of patients and their relatives. He suggested that anthropologists could contribute to health research by exploring the explanatory models that different parties build in the course of illness events, pointing out discrepancies between models constructed by patients and practitioners. Mark Nichter (2008) recently suggested that work in ethnomedicine is of continuing relevance for the field of global health.

Many anthropologists now focus on sites such as laboratories, testing centers, clinical settings, and biotechnology and pharmaceutical corporations where "scientific breakthroughs" emerge. Researchers have emphasized how new techniques and technologies are transforming fundamental definitions of life, death, the body, citizenship, and the state. Margaret Lock (2002) suggested that the demand for cadaveric organs for transplant operations has fostered new definitions of death, just as Lawrence Cohen ([2001] 2002) and Nancy Scheper-Hughes (1996) argue that a global traffic in organs from live donors has promoted neoliberal understandings of bodies as fragmented, modular sites of private ownership that permit their commodification and sale as spare parts. Scholars have charted the geographic, social, and institutional dispersal of biomedical knowledge production by tracing links between laboratories, marketers, clinicians, and patient populations around the world through clinical trials (Petryna 2009) and between researchers, pharmaceutical corporations, patients, and lay organizations in promoting research on and treatment for particular diseases (Rapp, Heath, and Taussig 2001). Michael Montoya (2011) explored how racializing blood samples for diabetes research as "Mexican" involves myriad details of scientific practice that often contradict scientific skepticism about genetics and race. Taking a topic close to the heart of folk medicine scholars, Cori Hayden (2003) traced the role of pharmaceutical corporations and international regulations in shaping what counts as Indigenous knowledge of medicinal plants, who gets to claim it, how it is commodified, and who sees the profits; it was thus an STS-oriented anthropologist who reshaped discussions of biopiracy.

The great visibility of STS has helped relocate the sociology of health and medicine. STS scholars have emphasized the sites, textual and social networks, infrastructures, technologies, organisms, and modes of representation required to produce scientific subjects and objects, enable them to circulate, and imbue them with authority. Few students seem to be able to get a PhD in the social sciences or humanities today without reading Bruno Latour. Just as work on medicalization (Zola 1972; Conrad 1992) drew attention to how social phenomena get placed within medical frames,

Adele Clarke et al. (2003) point to a contemporary shift in medical subjects and objects from medicalization to biomedicalization; they suggest that "the 'bio' in biomedicalization" points to "the transformations of both the human and nonhuman made possible by such technoscientific innovations as molecular biology, biotechnologies, genomization, transplant medicine, and new medical technologies" (162). Steven Epstein's (1996) earlier work examined how gay activists shaped research, treatment, and public discourse in the HIV/AIDS epidemic; more recently he tracked how a "difference and inclusion" paradigm has placed new biological essentialisms at the center of identities and struggles associated with LGBT, African American, Latinx, and women's social movements (2007).

Work in medical anthropology, STS, and the sociology of medicine reflects three key principles that have produced a fundamental reorientation and increased visibility. First, research foci (bodies, diseases, technologies, drugs, etc.) and scientific knowledge about them are not taken as preexisting objects. Like anthropological understandings of culture (Clifford 1988) and the way critical geographers approach space (Lefebvre [1974] 1991), attention is focused on the practices, epistemologies, technologies, and social/textual networks that bring these objects into being and imbue them with value, enabling scholars to document and produce different ways of understanding them. Second, scholars are interested in similarities and differences between how they and others—including scientists, clinicians, and patients—create knowledge; they accordingly explore how scholars and their interlocutors encounter one another, collaborate, and compete in the same spaces (Riles 2004; Strathern 2000). Finally, there is a tendency—by no means universal—to reject totalizing, reified categories ("biomedicine," "the state," or "the public") and binary oppositions—such as experts versus laypersons—in favor of formulations that make provisional claims based on concepts generated in close association with the phenomena they describe (Rabinow 2003; Stewart 2008).

This reorientation has transformed the study of medicine in anthropology and sociology: what were often considered marginal and technical subfields have become some of the most visible sectors of these disciplines—with substantial cross-disciplinary clout. Although it would be difficult to pinpoint a single factor that has brought research on health and medicine into greater prominence in anthropology and sociology than in folkloristics, I would like to point out a crucial difference. Critical medical anthropology (Scheper-Hughes and Lock 1987; Singer and Baer 1995; Castro and Singer 2004), STS, Latin American social medicine and critical epidemiology (Breilh 2003; Menéndez 2009), and other perspectives have led many anthropologists and sociologists to scrutinize biomedical authority and to investigate how biomedical and other scientific knowledge is made and how it is practiced. Folklorists have focused less on deconstructing dominant perspectives with regard to hegemonic medical epistemologies and practices.

A parallel to Dell Hymes's promotion of a dialogue between folkloristic and sociolinguistic perspectives is useful here. Hymes (1971) did not juxtapose existing approaches to folklore with an established field of linguistics; rather, he asked folklorists to join efforts to transform the study of language into the ethnographic study of the social and cultural constitution of language, and to use the ethnography of speaking to rethink folkloristics. Perhaps folklorists need to spend less time asking their biomedical colleagues to make room for them and their perspectives and focus more on using their tools to assess biomedicine's claims to dominate the politics of knowledge about health and disease.

BLIND ALLEYS

However, I am not suggesting that folklorists should ape their colleagues in anthropology, sociology, and STS. Indeed, I point out in this section how existing work in those areas reflects four crucial blind spots that have, in turn, generated some blind alleys. My goal is not to convince folklorists simply to address these blind spots, but rather to prompt reflection on how we can create a foundation that avoids the sorts of assumptions that give rise to myopia, thereby helping to open up new perspectives and reformulate old approaches.

First, fascinating work on new definitions of life, reproduction, death, the body, disease, and so forth sometimes lends itself to formulations that verge on new universalisms. Generalizing on the basis of research in leading laboratories, teaching hospitals, or biotechnology and pharmaceutical corporations can raise problems of scale and representativeness when the technologies, tests, drugs, and forms of treatment encountered there are projected as having transformed minds, bodies, and healing practices *everywhere*. At the same time that folklorists should be competing for the social scientist slot in labs, clinics, and national public health offices, there is a great deal of room for investigating the "old" epistemologies, practices, and political economies and inequalities that shape where "new" objects, technologies, and practices go (and don't go), and that also shape their effects. João Biehl (2005) has argued that in Brazil the pharmaceuticalization of public health simultaneously promotes the notion that medical justice means access to drugs and creates zones of "social abandonment" that deepen old inequities of race and class. Paul Farmer (2003) has argued eloquently that not only are fancy new diagnostics and forms of treatment still largely inaccessible to most people on the planet, but that "old" infectious diseases such as cholera, tuberculosis, and malaria—all preventable and treatable—still kill millions each year. This is not, of course, just a "third world" issue, given striking disparities of access to medical care in countries like the United States and the many middle-class whites who reject biomedical epistemologies and organizations. (Recently, I overheard the middle-class daughter of a geriatric patient in a US facility tell her mother, "When they give you a medication it fixes one problem and creates five more—I just don't trust doctors!") As this book goes to the printer, the "rollout" of COVID-19 vaccines could not provide a more poignant case in point: profound inequalities regarding which countries can afford to buy vaccines and have public healthcare systems in place that can transport and administer them will intersect with "vaccine hesitancy" on the part of those with access who say that they will not choose to be vaccinated—in ways that will, it seems, affect planetary viral futures.

Second, I am struck by the extent to which scholars in anthropology, sociology, and other fields often read narratives in flat-footed ways, as if a narrative elicited by a stranger who just showed up to conduct an interview provides a transparent window into the social world of the person who tells it and/or the phenomena he or she portrays. I think much recent work in the social sciences reproduces this failure to document and analyze the social lives of narratives. Examining narratives told by clinicians and epidemiologists provided Mantini-Briggs and me with a way to see how institutional strategies for deflecting blame for hundreds of preventable cholera deaths relied on converting problematic narratives of cultural difference into scientific truths (Briggs and Mantini-Briggs 2003). Looking ethnographically at these stories and how they circulated enabled us to X-ray epidemiological practices and public health policies. Work by folklorists on rumor, legend, gossip, and personal narrative has contributed to a more robust understanding of the role of narratives in constructing health- and disease-related beliefs and practices (e.g., Fine and Turner 2001; Goldstein 2004). Examining how the social lives of narratives shape health beliefs, practices, and policies is a crucial arena in which folklorists can push the envelope, and anthropologists such as Veena Das (2007) and historians like Luise White (2000) open up new approaches to health and narrative.

Third, Latour (1999) analyzes "circulating reference," the array of social networks, modes of classification, and techniques of visual representation needed to create scientific knowledge and make it mobile. Even in Latour's classic account of moving knowledge from the Amazonian rainforest to a scientific publication, however, the ethnographic impulse brings in a restrictive range of actors—people defined as "scientists." And Donna Haraway (1996) points out how race and gender inequities can be reproduced in who gets included in such accounts. What sorts of narratives, lexical items (forms of folk speech), and ways of using eyes, ears, bodies, lips, facial expressions, and the like might inform—or potentially contradict or complicate—the seemingly stable processes of narrative transfer that Latour documents? What counter-narratives emerge along the way? If a folklorist had made the journey from forest to laboratory, we might be able to answer these questions. As I noted in chapter 2, pathbreaking work by Geoffrey C. Bowker and Susan Leigh Star (1999) shows how biomedical knowledge (as quintessentially embodied in diagnostic categories and statistics) requires processes of contextualization vis-à-vis the technologies, political hierarchies and vulnerabilities, and epistemologies evident in each site it inhabits—as well as the erasure of these specific histories in order to render it mobile. Bowker and Star conducted their inquiry through archival records; by looking ethnographically at the broad range of bodily practices, narratives, and other cultural forms that inform the production, transformation, transmission, and reception of medical knowledge in specific locations, ethnographers could deepen our understanding of how some cultural forms get erased and how hierarchical configurations of the politics of knowledge get naturalized.

Fourth, I mentioned above the importance of Menéndez's relational perspective (2005, 2009). He draws attention to how clinical practices rely on what he refers to as *autoatención*, the labor performed by nonprofessionals outside clinical sites. Families—and particularly women—undertake daily work regarding nutrition, hygiene, health education, medication, and accident prevention. When signs of distress appear, family members, coworkers, friends, and neighbors provide initial forms of diagnosis and treatment and help determine whether a problem warrants a specialist's attention, what type of and which practitioner to consult, when and how to initiate contact, and how much household income should be used. They then help transport the person in distress, provide crucial diagnostic information, give social and emotional support, decide how to implement possibly competing treatment regimes, obtain needed medicines and other materials, determine whether to seek further treatment, and help with treatment regimes. Although biomedical professionals depend on this labor, they generally construct diagnosis and treatment as consisting only of those aspects they themselves provide or prescribe. Most nonprofessional labor is thereby hidden from view, and the elements that are recognized overtly are examined with respect to their possible deviation from biomedical epistemologies and practices—cast as forms of ignorance, resistance, and noncompliance that threaten the health of the patient and the success of professional treatment. Scholars similarly point to the concept of self-medication as a residual category used by professionals to pathologize the everyday medical work performed by laypersons (and pharmacists) (Nichter and Kamat 1998; Das and Das 2006). Menéndez (2005) emphasizes how health and healing require both a multiplicity of *saberes médicos*, of different types of medical (and not simply biomedical) knowledge, as well as the erasure of those varieties that do not conform to what he refers to as the hegemonic medical model (Menéndez and Di Pardo 1996). This work intersects with the research on ethnomedicine and folk medicine I outlined above, but Menéndez shows how lay practices relationally constitute biomedical knowledge and practice and vice versa.

ORIENTING PRACTICES AND GUIDING PRINCIPLES

What is needed, I think, is a new means for folklorists to define their sites of inquiry and to conceptualize their modes of intervention and analysis in such a way that existing categories, identities, and boundaries are not simply reproduced in methodological strategies and analytical principles. Folklorists should rather become key players in documenting and analyzing how such demarcations are produced and become consequential. In developing these practices and principles, I draw on some of the issues and strategies that have proven productive in other areas of folkloristics and beyond in suggesting how they could inform work on health and disease.

Orienting Practices to Deepen Ethnographic Inquiry

None of us can simply turn off our own commonsense categories and presuppositions and erase our positionalities in order to embrace an ethnographic openness that magically illuminates what generally gets left out or cast as subordinate. Similarly, celebrating marginalized or erased sites, subjects, bodies, objects, and forms of knowledge dodges the less romantic but crucial analytic work of determining how hierarchies get made and silences enforced; Amy Shuman's (1993) warnings against romantic celebrations of "the vernacular" are particularly valuable here (see also Goldstein and Shuman 2016). I thus think it just as important to "study up," in Laura

Nader's (1972) terms—to document elite actors and dominant social sectors and organizations as well as those that these subjects relegate to subordinate spheres. The following framework, organized around four types of practices that play crucial roles in constructing what is visible, what is pushed to the margins, and what is erased, can help us foster what Walter Benjamin (1968) referred to as "presence of mind," assisting in critically engaging implicit assumptions, boundaries, silences, and hierarchies.[2]

1. Siting practices. In general, commonsense notions of location are used in initiating and defining research. Research that focuses on clinics, hospitals, homes, laboratories, NGOs, and the like often rests on preanalytical notions of places. Critical geography suggests, however, that categories of space and place are produced through spatializing practices, modes of symbolic construction that shape materialities, access, value, and more (Lefebvre [1974] 1991).[3] Commonsense notions of healing spaces are reproduced in the spatializing practices that construct clinical spaces; patients' homes and doctors' offices are defined in opposition to one another, just as examination and reception areas are ideologically as well as spatially separated. What is needed here is a two-step process. First, Menéndez's (2009) critical approach would require not just documenting all of the spaces in which the phenomena in question are situated, but also tracking how spatial categories, boundaries, and forms of mobility and immobility are made. Tracing encounters among diverse types of medical knowledge in relationship to what is defined as a respiratory infection would require attention to everything from perceiving signs of illness in the home, workplace, and/or other sites to initiating telephone calls, text messages, and other social media contacts and searching the internet and social media and responding to advertisements to considering visits to medicine cabinets, pharmacies, health-food stores, doctors' offices, and alternative healers (who might be family members). As respiratory infections become key loci of biosecurity concerns and public anxieties in the wake of pandemics of influenza and COVID-19 (see chapter 9), case definitions and reporting requirements imposed by state and international health/security organizations become relevant. Rather than forming distal and unrelated spaces, news stories, CDC press conferences, and political pronouncements can become intimate components of conversations and actions that take place within domestic spaces and vice versa. As Menéndez argues, sites and relations between them should be determined ethnographically as the investigation unfolds, not defined before it begins. Second, the medical spatializing practices used by all parties should be documented, particularly with regard to how they organize spaces hierarchically on the basis of presumed medical knowledge, defining such places as homes, for instance, to be spaces of compliance, ignorance, or efforts to defy what is perceived as "deep state" control. In other words, just as we need to look beyond the received boundaries to see how they get made, we need to document the often discrepant spatializing practices of all parties, including the role of rumors, illness narratives, and news stories in shaping and embodying them.

2. *Subjectifying practices.* Researchers from Erving Goffman (1961) to phenomenologically oriented medical anthropologists (Csordas 1994; Kleinman 1988) have focused on how bodies are constructed, inhabited, and experienced as healthy or diseased. In terms of folkloristically informed work on medicine and the body, Katharine Young (1997) has been particularly attentive to how bodies and subjectivities emerge in encounters such as gynecological exams and autopsies. A wealth of research in various disciplines demonstrates two countervailing processes. One involves the co-production of subject positions, subjects, and subjectivities through highly unequal encounters that are relationally constituted. The other side of the coin, however, is their reification in what are often viewed as opposing subject positions that are independently constituted. Note the parallel here to Hayden White's (1978) account of how historians construct visions of the past and then create texts that seem to be transparent reflections of what actually happened. For example, the vast literature on doctor-patient communication is based on a foundational assumption that there are two distinct positionalities (or perhaps three, when patients are accompanied by parents or other relatives), thereby excluding consideration of other subjects (receptionists, nurses, laboratory analysts, etc.) and how information moves between contexts and modes of representation (Cicourel 1992). The positions of doctor and patient are further reified in transcriptions (often abbreviated as D: and P:).

As with siting practices, the trick here is to start without a set of categories in mind and then examine the complex similarities, differences, and relations in observed subjectivities; in addition, one should note how essentialized subjectivities are constructed and how people are recruited to play these roles. Finally, folklorists should remain attentive to how race, ethnicity, gender, sexuality, social class, disability, and citizenship/migration are both constituted and constituting. Howard Waitzkin (1991) famously analyzed how large-scale race and class inequities get produced and embodied in clinical spaces, even as protocols for "doctor-patient interaction" and the individualistic, mechanistic, and technologistic underpinnings of biomedicine (Menéndez and Di Pardo 1996) transform them into "structures of feeling" that are felt but generally not explicitly formulated (Williams 1977). Epidemics and pandemics become sites for mass-producing subjectivities as much as medicines and vaccines. Hundreds of deaths from cholera in Venezuela's Delta Amacuro State, to which I referred in the introduction, were the product of racialized state policies that denied potable water, sewage facilities, and adequate healthcare coverage to rainforest residents. In order to deflect the political fallout, however, public health officials circulated narratives that racialized affected communities as incarcerated by an Indigenous culture that rejects doctors and hygiene in favor of belief in "shamans" and "spirits" (see Briggs and Mantini-Briggs 2003).

3. Practices of embodiment and objectification. Investigations of bodylore (Young 1993) and studies of the body in the social sciences in general point to the way that bodies, like subjectivities, are constantly made and challenged through medical encounters, technologies, and media representations. Studies of the social life of things (Appadurai 1986), museumification (Kirshenblatt-Gimblett 1998a), and materiality (Keane 2007) suggest that imbuing value in objects requires processes of detachment, objectification, commodification, and appropriation. Here folklorists might bring the perspectives produced in folk art studies to bear in exploring how the "natural" objects of alternative and complementary medicine (or mass-produced objects in clinical encounters, such as pharmaceuticals and medical technologies) are made, circulated, administered, and ingested. If many anthropologists, sociologists, and science studies scholars focus on observing bodies in such restricted contexts as examination rooms, counseling sessions, and surgical pavilions, folklorists can critically study a broader range of forms of embodiment and objectification and how they get reified into bounded sets of ratified and stratified bodies and objects. In addition to documenting the narratives that find little room for expression in spaces dominated by biomedical professionals, folklorists can look critically at narratives that recount what took place in clinical encounters as they are performed in other spaces for family members, coworkers, neighbors, classmates, and friends. In response to accusations of noncompliance or self-medication, folklorists can document how people make complex decisions about how to reposition pills, candles, herbs, and other objects recommended by healers—including those acquired in virtual marketplaces. Accusations of noncompliance and self-medication (Nichter and Kamat 1998; Das and Das 2006) can provide starting points for exploring discrepant ideologies and practices of embodiment, objectification, materiality, and animacy (Chen 2012).

4. Practices of knowledge production/circulation/reception. Here Menéndez's characterization of the multiplicity of forms of medical knowledge (*saberes médicos*) provides a crucial point of departure. Rather than focusing on forms of knowledge that are privileged in clinical medicine, folklorists can examine broader economies of knowledge production—including their own—that bear on their chosen topic and see how they interrelate; to be sure, this is one of the strengths of recent work on folk medicine. Here again, it is crucial to avoid reproducing such oppositions as lay versus expert, thereby casting scientific understandings uncritically, and then documenting "folk," "popular," or "vernacular" conceptions in terms of how they depart from "expert" practice. Medical social fields are organized in terms of communicable models, ideological constructions of how knowledge is produced, circulated, and received (see chapter 3). Communicable models that focus on knowledge about health and disease, which I refer to as biocommunicable models, inform siting and subjectifying practices by locating the production of legitimate knowledge in particular places and subjects, its circulation in others, and its reception in others still. Biocommunicable models often project complex—frequently inverse—relationships between the circulation of discourse and pathogens. As I explore in the next chapter, pandemics prompt public health officials to repeat endlessly that only widespread reception and assimilation of biomedical knowledge on the part of "the public" can disrupt the circulation of microbes. New biomedical knowledge is imagined as emerging in leading laboratories and clinics; circulating through medical journals, public health campaigns, the news media, the internet, and doctor-patient conversations; and being received by laypersons—if they are paying attention and not resistant. Nevertheless, biocommunicable models are multiple and dynamic, and folklorists can explore their complex intersections and track how forms of diagnosis and treatment, narratives, and technologies are used in constructing highly unequal—and sometimes lethal—politics of medical knowledge.

Here a relational and critical focus is particularly crucial. Everyone produces, circulates, and receives knowledge about the body, health, and disease. A major contribution of folkloristic work on healing can be to document other biocommunicable models that cast nonspecialists as knowledge *producers*. Mind you, those associated with alternative modalities can be just as hierarchical; Indigenous healers in Venezuela with whom I worked saw authoritative knowledge about the diseases they treated as being produced only in their own dreams and clinical interventions, circulating properly only through what they told patients and community members, and requiring passive forms of reception and compliance that resemble those demanded by their physician counterparts (Briggs 2008). A long history of interest in poetics and performance can position folklorists to challenge ways that the politics of knowledge produce and embody deep inequalities of race, gender, sexuality, disability, and nation.

Guiding Principles

A new folkloristics of health will provide a key locus for advancing research on several of the issues that I have addressed in preceding chapters. One reason is that dominant communicable models project medical and scientific knowledge as what Latour (1987) refers to as immutable mobiles, capable of traveling anywhere without losing their force or needing modification. Once again, Bowker and Star (1999) point to the complexity of producing this illusion, given that circulation requires both mutations that result from entanglements with the ideologies, practices, technologies, objects, and naturalcultural relations that proliferate in particular sites and efforts to shore up the seeming objectivity and stability of such things as categories and statistics by stripping them of overt traces of these indexical histories. The productivity of exploring gaps between models and practices of circulation is evident in a great deal of recent work in folkloristics, such as that by Deborah Kapchan (2007), Kirshenblatt-Gimblett (1998b), and Philip Scher (2002), as well as in adjacent fields (Feld 2000; Goodman 2005; Myers 2002). A number of scholars, including Regina Bendix (2018), Jane Goodman (2002), Stefan Groth (2012), Valdimar Hafstein (2004, 2018b), Kirshenblatt-Gimblett (2006), Peter Nas (2002), Scher (2002), and Martin Scherzinger (1999), have focused on the way that international organizations, such as UNESCO and WIPO, seek to regulate the circulation and commodification of intangible cultural heritage. It would be helpful to bring similar attention to issues of scale, mobility, and bureaucratization to folkloristic research on health.

Recent work has tracked the extent to which pills, germs, bodies, technologies, and epistemologies—including those framed as cutting edge as well as those defined as traditional or alternative—are on the move. The notion of global assemblages (Collier and Ong 2005; Sassen 2006) points to how subjectivities and objects defined as global or local come together in complex and variable ways in particular spaces, moving through specific sorts of grooves (Tsing 2005) and encountering obstacles (Lakoff 2005). A number of scholars have documented narratives and other cultural forms that purport to track how objects, body parts, technologies, diseases, and diagnostic categories circulate globally (e.g., Cohen 1998; Petryna 2002; Pigg 2001; Scheper-Hughes 1996). Folklorists could analyze how poetic and performance features help constitute and challenge both pragmatics and ideologies of mobility. This work might be guided by three principles:

1. (Im)Mobilities. Rather than simply competing with other scholars to be the master cartographers of medical globalization, folklorists should keep the objects, ideas, and people on their maps closely tied to analyses of how notions of (im)mobility get produced. Even as concepts of authenticity (Bendix 1997) seem to require that "alternative" medical practices and epistemologies be rooted in particular places and in seemingly bounded territorial communities, those framed as modern and biomedical seem naturally to circle the globe. Folklorists could thus excel in documenting how subjectivities, bodies, medicines, technologies, cultural forms (narratives, songs, gestures, forms of bodily decoration, etc.), and practices (of diagnosing, treating, counting, knowing, speaking, writing, and reading) intersect and how their melding confers what seem to be intrinsic forms of value, mobility, and immobility.

2. Inhabitations. The critiques by Nichter and Kamat (1998), Das and Das (2006), and Menéndez (2005) of notions of self-medication that I mentioned above suggest how cultural forms get attached to competing ways of inhabiting spaces and subject positions—taking the same pills can be read as the sign of a model patient or of a noncompliant self-medicator. Folklorists can take the lead in seeing how treatments, technologies, narratives, forms of interaction, and constructions of the body are differentially inhabited. As the literature I outlined at the beginning of this chapter suggests, folklorists have a great deal to offer in tracing how health-related modes, practices, and objects construct and get attached to particular subjectivities and subject positions.

3. Boundary-work. Forms of mobility and inhabitation are shaped by and shape the boundaries that seem to contain or at times obstruct these complex interrelations, hiding some from view and elevating others to hypervisibility. Folklorists and medical anthropologists were recruited for a central role in constituting biomedicine, shoring up its borders, and reifying its politics of knowledge by serving as boundary workers who could separate science from superstition, knowledge from belief. A key principle for reorienting work in folklore and medicine is thus to see how boundaries are made, who makes them, who crosses them, and which "boundary objects" (Star and Griesemer 1989) provide means of both recognizing boundaries and translating across the social worlds they define. Since the time of John Aubrey in the seventeenth century, folklorists have been quite skilled in both constructing and crossing social boundaries; honing reflexive skills can reposition them as ethnographers and analysts of boundary-work.

I will admit that I am asking a lot. "Traditional" epistemologies and practices are imbricated everywhere with forms that are framed as modern and biomedical. Tracking even something as simple as a visit to the doctor for a respiratory infection involves a complex, heterogeneous array of sites, subjectivities, bodies, objects, and forms of knowledge. As I have suggested, folklorists have long been experts in dealing with heterogeneity and complexity, in locating people, objects, places, and cultural forms that often get erased or oversimplified. The four practices and three principles I proposed are intended to suggest how folklorists can embrace rather than become paralyzed by this complexity and heterogeneity; they can also aid us in critically analyzing how reifications are produced and circulate without simply reproducing them. It seems crucial to see what the neighbors are saying, to better familiarize ourselves with contemporary work in medical anthropology, sociology, and STS to see what new landmarks have emerged and what gaps and blind spots remain, even as we draw on analytic skills that constitute folkloristics.

One thing that might help here is a name change. I suggest casting these efforts under the rubric of "the folkloristics of health." *Health* points beyond a focus on disease to embrace notions of prevention and well-being in general. It embraces clinical and public health dimensions, expanding folklorists' attention beyond medicine to epidemiology and public health policy. Crucially, it builds on calls by Hufford, O'Connor, and others to explore the shifting, sometimes tense relational boundaries that constitute multiple lay and official epistemologies and practices. Lastly, the term does not start from a seemingly separate empirical domain, but rather suggests that health-related research is and must be a vital part of the discipline.

If what I am proposing seems challenging, I suggest that we keep the potential fruits in mind. Work conducted during the last two decades provides stunning evidence of how research on folklore and health can shatter the glass ceiling that confined it to realms of cultural difference and barred it from offering more trenchant critiques of biomedical and scientific power. A broader agenda for this area of research, one that positions it in dialogue with work being conducted in other disciplines, holds the potential for re-placing the field of health research as a major source of insight into issues and analytical frameworks that can inform folkloristics in general. By demanding our rightful place among contemporary approaches to bodies, healing, and disease, we can make even deeper contributions to the intellectual and institutional standing of the discipline in the academy—and to the public folklore of health.

This chapter has consisted of a proposal, and its rhetoric has been largely programmatic. Chapters 9 and 10 provide concrete illustrations of the sort of research I have in mind. Chapter 9 focuses on how journalists, public health officials, researchers, and audiences create narratives of epidemic diseases. Chapter 10 takes us back to Delta Amacuro in order to explore how deeply plants were woven into the fabric of opposing ways of approaching healing and disease and how they clashed during the mysterious epidemic. That chapter will accordingly extend the approach that I have outlined here by suggesting that a new folkloristics of health must include nonhuman actors and perspectives.

NOTES

1. For examples, see Clifford 2013; Feld 2000; Goodman 2005; Hafstein 2004, 2018b; Kapchan 2007; Kirshenblatt-Gimblett 1998a, 2006; Nas 2002; Scher 2002; and Silverman 2012. Nestor García Canclini ([1990] 1995) has pointed to the importance of techniques for co-producing traditionalities and modernities in constructing forms of nationalism and political formations in Latin America.

2. I take the notion of practices here largely from Pierre Bourdieu ([1972] 1977), as additionally informed by Michel de Certeau (1984) and work in critical geography (Lefebvre [1974] 1991) and linguistic anthropology (Hanks 1996).

3. See Tangherlini 1999 on the incorporation of critical geography in folkloristic analysis.

8

Moving beyond "the Media"
From Traditionalization to Mediatization

THIS CHAPTER PARALLELS THE PREVIOUS ONE BY PROPOSING an alternative framework for reorienting a line of research, even as it shifts to a new domain. My goal here is first to disrupt common perspectives on "folklore and the media"—or, alternatively, between folkloristics and media studies—and then reorient work in this area. In my bid to banish the phrase "folklore and the media," I argue that its use requires first creating a boundary between folklore and "the media" and then pretending to bridge it. If this binary fundamentally misunderstands both of these seemingly discrete entities, as I hope to establish, then adopting it as a fundamental premise relegates "folklore and media" discussions to a small niche on the outskirts of both disciplines. Rather, my hope is that what follows will foster new ways of reconfiguring folkloristics and media studies in general.

In order to steer clear of the entrenched folklore/media binary, I suggest that it is crucial to reconceptualize the underlying terms and frameworks that guide folkloristics and media studies in such a way as to highlight remarkably parallel theoretical turns that each has undertaken in recent years. This move, I argue, positions them not as autonomous, unrelated disciplines but as complementary perspectives on processes that are deeply imbricated. I draw on the notion of traditionalization to shape my discussion of folkloristics and on mediatization in reconfiguring media studies. I explore how these terms developed and the advantages they offer to rethinking the folkloristics–media studies nexus, but it might be useful to indicate briefly what I mean by them right up front. Reconfiguring work by Hermann Bausinger, Dell Hymes, Richard Bauman, and others, I define *traditionalization* as a process through which a broad range of cultural forms—not simply those explicitly commodified, popularized, or invented—are constructed so as to link them to the emergence of similar forms in the past. Such links may be explicit ("My mother used to tell this story when I was young") or implicit, as when a personal narrative regarding a recent event is marked by familiar generic elements. Traditionalization can thus saturate cultural forms with affects and patterns of expectation that structure—without determining—how audiences engage with them. *Mediatization*, on the other hand, springs from the work of Spanish-Colombian media studies scholar Jesús Martín Barbero and such European figures as Nick Couldry, Andreas Hepp, Stig Hjarvard, and Knut Lundby. Rather than starting with a priori separations of "the media" from what are projected as distinct social spheres (such as politics, religion, or folklore), mediatization traces processes that unfold across a wide range of sites, actors, technologies, ideologies, and practices—many of which seem to have little to do with "the media."

I argue that traditionalization and mediatization, even as they are frequently cast as opposites, are co-constitutive, producing much of the social worlds we inhabit through their complex imbrication. I use two major examples in advancing this argument. The first is the Grimm brothers' *Kinder- und Hausmärchen*, which seems to lie squarely in the realm of traditionalization. Attempting to disrupt commonsense definitions and boundaries, I use the Grimms to illustrate mediatization. Chapter 9 will bring the perspective on folklore and media that I develop here together with the proposal for a new folkloristics of health that I advanced in chapter 7 by looking at the mediatization of the 2009 "swine flu pandemic." News coverage of an influenza epidemic would seem to constitute a quintessential example of modernity and mediatization, but I use it to explore traditionalization. Suggesting that sophisticated analytics and ethnographic techniques are required to analyze complex connections between traditionalization and mediatization, I use these concepts in proposing a framework intended to stimulate research in this area, interest folklorists in digging more deeply into media studies, and suggest to scholars of mediatization that they can draw important analytics from folkloristics.

PERSPECTIVES ON FOLKLORE AND "THE MEDIA"

Interest in the relationship between folklore and media stretches from the discipline's seventeenth-century prehistory through the present. In order to rethink this issue, I begin by critically exploring orientations to folklore-media relations that continue to structure ways that folklorists undertake research in this area. I accordingly outline five perspectives as a preamble to devising a new point of departure.

A first perspective is older than folkloristics as a discipline; it established a frame of *opposition and mutual exclusion* between folklore and media. A good starting point is provided by the quote from John Aubrey that I provided in chapter 2, where he identified printing, books, and gunpowder—along with the dissemination of literacy among "the ordinary sort of People"—as the death knell for folklore, including "Old-wives Tales," "Fables, and stories of Robin-good-fellow and the Fayries" (1972:290). Here the folklore/media binary involves a construction of orality as a primordial sphere of face-to-face interaction that literally embodies traditional, preconscious modes of thinking, talking, singing, making, and being. This approach, which still has resonances today, casts mediatization as a constitutive outside, a residual category projected as not-oral and not-traditional through its objectification in modern technologies and ontologies. This binary formed a key way that the opposition was constructed between a preexisting traditional, premodern social world and a newly emerging realm of modernity (Bauman and Briggs 2003). Centuries later, Richard Dorson (1976:5), unlike Aubrey, did not see the mere presence of "the mass media" as inevitably leading to folklore's demise, but he (in)famously suggested that when folklore becomes "fakelore"—involving popularization, commercialization, and "the mass media"—it ceases being the "real folklore" that constitutes folkloristics' proper object.

A second perspective casts the folklore/media binary as one of *domination*, projecting media organizations and technologies as appropriating, exploiting, and demeaning folklore. Criticism of Walt Disney fairytale films looms so large here that we might almost call it Disneyfication. Domination involves not just absorbing folklore content into popular media but producing a dominant text that is homogenizing, distorted, inaccurate, and oversimplified, thereby displacing primordial features of oral transmission and performance by reducing variation and contextualization (see, for example, Koven 2003; Russo 1992; Tucker 1992). In an extensive discussion of "folklore and the media" that complicates this binary, Linda Dégh (1994:23) nevertheless accused "the media" of creating a "homogenizing effect of uniform information and the mass-marketing of stories" that "systematically enculturates the citizens of the world, turning them into the consumers of identical cultural goods by creating a symbolic egalitarian social order that supersedes segmentation by national boundaries." Note how Dégh spatializes the folklore/media boundary, depicting the former as intrinsically national in character while "the media" constitute global conglomerations that do not recognize national boundaries. This perspective involves technological determinism, the attribution of agency to media technologies, forms, and logics and associated processes of commodification and circulation, without taking into account active processes of reception (see Hall 1980; Martín Barbero [1987] 2003). Feminist folklorists classically critiqued how Disney films take "uninspiring" Grimm heroines and make them seem so lacking in will, awareness, and agency as to "seem barely alive" (Stone 1975:44). Foregrounding class relations, Jack Zipes (1979) views the Grimm brothers as having appropriated proletariat and peasant oral culture; mediatizing and commodifying fairytales provided a key mechanism for transferring subaltern symbolic capital to the bourgeoisie.

A third perspective could be called, following Sylvia Grider (1981), *symbiosis*. She suggested that television programs and movies provide children with narrative content that they transform into creative and complex narratives, which she calls "media narraforms." The suggestion is that folklore and media spheres continue to be defined by distinct aesthetic patterns and contextual features even as content passes between them. This process now frequently unfolds through social media. I have, for example, frequently seen my family members receive jokes via group text messages or WhatsApp, perform them face-to-face and/or through cell or video calls, and recirculate them through different media platforms, all in the space of quotidian exchanges taking place in a single morning.

A fourth, *imbrication*, was encouraged by Alan Dundes's (1980:17) classic suggestion that new communication technologies augment the creation and circulation of folklore, "becoming a vital factor in the transmission of folklore and . . . providing an exciting source of inspiration for the generation of new folklore." Here, a folklore/media binary with sharp boundaries gives way to consideration of much more complex and consequential forms of interaction and projections of convergences between what are cast as previously separate domains. Imbrication has become a dominant theme in studies of digital folklore. Trevor Blank (2012:12) argued, for example, that "it behooves folklorists to acknowledge that there is significant overlap in the distinguishing characteristics, contextual functions, and methods of dissemination between both face-to-face and virtualized venues of vernacular expression." He argued that digital media compromise the autonomy of folklore and of media along multiple dimensions. Robert Glenn Howard suggests that the internet, like folklore, embodies features of an anti-institutional vernacularity, thereby blurring the folklore/mass media distinction; individuals "participate in creating a telectronic world where mass culture may dominate, but an increasing prevalence of participatory media extends into growing webs of network-based folk culture" (2008:192; 2012). Studying the virtual world of Second Life, Tom Boellstorff (2011) suggests that online and offline domains interact in such a way that virtual forms of embodiment shape people's senses of their own bodies and vice versa. In formulations that adopt this perspective, the folklore/media opposition sometimes resurfaces in implicitly evolutionary terms, associating folklore historically with a preexisting oral, embodied realm that increasingly is transformed by mediatization, the latter frequently equated with "new" technologies.

Finally, some scholars have argued for a *strong mediatization* view of folklore, suggesting that both popular and scholarly conceptions of oral folklore have been (re)configured by mediatized representations. In his prescient 1961 book *Folk Culture in a World of Technology*, Hermann Bausinger suggested that technologies have shaped folk culture for centuries; indeed, folk culture is not an artifact of a separate, autonomous, rural social world but is "a well-calculated part of modern mass culture" ([1961] 1990:xii). He argued that published collections of German folk songs from the fifteenth and sixteenth centuries provided an ahistorical standard of valuation that shaped both scholarly and popular engagements with folk culture. Tying the emergence of what are considered classic oral folklore genres to elite print cultures, Susan Stewart noted that, like proverbs, ballads, and fairytales, the epic "is a distressed and antiquated genre from its very inception as a literary form" (1991:76). In work on early gramophone and phonograph recordings, Richard Bauman suggested that media technologies helped produce our very sense of oral, live performance, how it is perceived and experienced, by consuming recordings of political speeches, minstrelsy, and other forms (Bauman 2004, 2010, 2016; Bauman and Feaster 2005). This mode of linking folklore and media dispenses with any sense of separate—let alone autonomous—spheres. I later turn this perspective around in looking at how traditionalization, in turn, can fundamentally shape mediatization.

Important differences separate these five perspectives; the last two would seem to be more in line with most contemporary folkloristics. Nevertheless, I would assess them as all falling short of providing a sufficient analytic foundation. To varying degrees, all begin with a priori, largely commonsense notions of folklore and "the media," going on to map how distinct objects, sites, and processes are brought—through technological, social, and political-economic dimensions—into interaction. What I think is necessary is to turn the question on its head, asking not how folklore and media intersect but how their interrelations produce what comes to be understood as folklore and "the media."

A basic limitation of these perspectives is how they reflect rather old-fashioned, problematic ways of thinking about disciplines. In the nineteenth and early twentieth centuries, a sort of formula emerged for constructing disciplines and their claims to authority and autonomy. A first step was to locate an object that existed out there in the world, one that had not yet been claimed by other disciplines. A second step framed a set of practices as providing the only authoritative means to locate, collect, and analyze this object and to defend the discipline's objects and methods against any competing claims, including by other scholars and laypersons. Thus, anthropology claimed culture, geography space, sociology society, and media studies "the media," just as folkloristics claimed folklore. Insofar as understandings of folkloristics and media studies reproduce boundary-work, studying "folklore and the media" will always be plagued by humpty-dumpty remedial efforts that promise to magically heal foundational separations.

Nevertheless, folkloristics and media studies have moved in parallel ways by questioning practitioners' former claims to dominate a single, a priori, bounded object. Accordingly, why base discussions of "folklore and the media" on obsolete and problematic disciplinary formulations that cast folkloristics and media studies as autonomous disciplines that focus on radically different, unrelated objects? In the following sections, I sketch how work on mediatization has challenged media studies' foundational disciplinary reifications, and I use traditionalization to examine folkloristics' recent transformations.

MEDIATIZATION

In an unusual case in which European theorists used Latin American research as a point of departure, mediatization scholarship sprang from a fundamental challenge that Spanish-Colombian researcher Jesús Martín Barbero issued decades ago. In order to dispense with media-centrism, he rejected a priori concepts of "communication" and "the media," suggesting that "we had to lose sight of the 'object' in order to find the way to the movement of the social in communication, to communication in process" ([1987] 2003:280; my translation). In shifting attention to an active process that he referred to as "mediation," he examined how radio, television, and other media helped produce and were shaped by such constructs as society, the state, the people, and race.

The Dangers of Technological Determinism and Symptomatic Technology

Another way—also potentially valuable for folkloristics—that mediatization perspectives challenged commonsense assumptions is in rejecting what Raymond Williams (2003) called "technological determinism" and "symptomatic technology." The first, exemplified by Castells's (1996) *The Information Age*, reifies media technologies as possessing historical agency, as *producing* social, cultural, and ideological change. The second projects a particular technology as if "it were a byproduct of a social process that is otherwise determined" (Williams 2003:6), such as casting a particular digital technology as a symptom of neoliberalism. Following Williams here can spark important critiques of the technological determinism that structures a good deal of thinking about folklore and media, particularly digital media, in which a new technology is projected in causal terms as transforming folklore. Dundes's valuable suggestion that "technology . . . is providing an exciting source of inspiration for the generation of new folklore" (1980:17) nevertheless echoes this sort of technological determinism.

Shifting Definitions of Mediatization

Particularly relevant for rethinking folklore/media issues is the stress in mediatization research on how "the media" relate to other social fields, such as politics (Strömbäck 2008), religion (Hepp [2011] 2013; Couldry and Hepp 2013), and health (Briggs and Hallin 2016). Similar to the five folklore/media perspectives outlined above, mediatization researchers have conceptualized these relationships in various ways. Some early formulations embraced a domination logic, starting from binary definitions and then projecting how media organizations or "media logics" (Altheide and Snow 1979) dominated other spheres. Jesper Strömbäck, for example, projected four phases of media/politics mediatization, suggesting that in the fourth phase "the media and their logic can be said to *colonize* politics" (2008, 240; emphasis in original). Hjarvard (2013:2) characterized mediatization as referring to "how social institutions and culture processes have changed character, function, and structure in response to the omnipresence of the media." Recent work by Couldry, Hepp, and Lundby rather suggests that mediatization should not be defined formally and ahistorically as a singular, homogeneous thing but rather as a locus of critical perspectives. Rejecting a singular "media logic" that determines reception or dominates other domains (Couldry 2012; Couldry and Hepp 2013, 2017; Hepp [2011] 2013; Lundby 2009) and the way that initial conceptions of mediatization reproduced "a model of a functionally differentiated society in which 'the media' are a specifically institutionalized society system" (Hepp [2011] 2013:45), they stress the heterogeneity of mediatization and reject universalistic and evolutionary perspectives.

An example might suggest the value of rethinking folklore in terms of mediatization. Faced with diminishing US markets for tobacco products after the fatal effects of smoking were finally publicly confirmed, multinational corporations pushed more vigorously into Latin America (Stebbins 2001). In Venezuela, a massive marketing campaign faced a major obstacle: enactment in 1981 of prohibitions on television and radio advertisements for cigarettes. British American Tobacco (BAT) therefore invested massive sums in mediatizing folklore. The Bigott Foundation, the philanthropic wing of BAT's Venezuela subsidiary Bigott Cigarette Manufacturing, sponsored television segments and a glossy magazine, *Revista Bigott*, that celebrated Venezuelan folklore, and it funded "Popular Culture Workshops" that brought children into contact with purportedly disappearing national traditions. As David Guss (2000) and Yolanda Salas (2003) have richly documented, this effort conjoined the mediatization practices of folklorists, folk artists and performers, advertising firms, officials from tobacco and broadcast corporations, children, and audiences in producing a folkloric nationalism. The foundation funded research by folklorists, sponsored conferences, and published scholarly research. Given that cigarettes and smoking could not be directly traditionalized or mediatized, use of the Bigott name and logo in association with mediatized folklore forms generated a positive affective connection to the company and its products. This massive mediatization process thus juxtaposed a host of widely dispersed practices in producing stunning visual, auditory, and tactile forms through what was constructed ideologically as a nonpolitical and noncommercial process—traditionalization. The result was not simply the insertion of a preexisting folklore into "the media" but, in a country that had embraced a modernity afforded by massive income from petroleum extraction, the coproduction of a mediatized national folkloric tradition.

The Importance of Practice, Ideology, and Form in Analyzing Mediatization

As this example suggests, defining mediatization requires distinguishing how *processes of mediatization* involve dimensions of practice, ideology, and form. With regard to *practice*, mediatization involves assemblages of sites, organizations, logics, technologies, and forms of practice that stretch across domains (framed as media, religious, political, folkloric, medical, etc.), not simply elements that inhabit domains explicitly defined as part of "the media." These heterogeneous practices produce complex aesthetic *forms* that invite affective responses of pleasure, fear, familiarity, distance, pity, and so forth. An emphasis on form builds on the work of Georg Simmel, further elaborated by media scholars David Altheide and Robert Snow (1979). Apart from—and even sometimes in contradiction to—content, Altheide and Snow stressed "format," meaning "how material is organized, the style in which it is presented, the focus or emphasis on particular characteristics of behavior, and the grammar of media communication. Format becomes a framework or a perspective that is used to present as well as interpret phenomena" (10). Like Deleuze and Guattari ([1980] 1987), mediatization scholars foreground questions of *ideology*, of the variable ways that media forms, technologies, and practices are constructed and invested with or divested of value. Nevertheless, agents engaging in mediatization processes often project these heterogeneous assemblages ideologically as occupying distinct cultural fields, reproducing the category of "the media" along with such domains as folklore, health, and politics; I provide an example in chapter 9.

TRADITIONALIZATION

In previous chapters, I traced how in the closing decades of the twentieth century folkloristics itself became an object of critical scrutiny. I noted that starting in the 1950s with the work of Américo Paredes, assertions of scholarly distance, the ability to objectively document processes that others could only enter as interested subjects, were challenged by people who did not occupy the position of the "modern subject"—a purportedly disembodied figure that elite, white, European or North American, heterosexual, adult, able-bodied men seemed to naturally embody. The discussion similarly tracked how folklorists' former focus on a single, bounded, disciplinary object gave way to emphasis on heterogeneous, complex practices enacted collectively and often competitively by multiple actors, including bureaucrats, activists, corporations, laypersons, media professionals—and folklorists.

From Tradition to Traditionalization

"Tradition" has too long and complex a history in folkloristics to permit even a cursory outline, but I note two opposing tendencies.[1] One retains tradition's position as the central object of folkloristics and an element of social life that is out there in the world as a form of "communal property" (Noyes 2016; see also Bronner 2011). The other, often inspired by Hobsbawm's (1983) work on the "invention of tradition," casts tradition as a problematic construct created by elites (including folklorists) to naturalize such dominant constructions as those of people, history, and nation (see, for example, Handler and Linnekin 1984). Bausinger suggested an alternative perspective nearly six decades ago by drawing attention to an active social process of "traditionalizing" cultural forms. Even as laypersons reached selectively into the past in choosing elements to traditionalize, folklorists played a key role in traditionalizing forms through what they collected and modes of representation and analysis ([1961] 1990:64, 71). For Bausinger, traditionalization was both invented—that is, it was the product of continual interventions into folk culture—and actually existing, providing a key element through which people perceive and embody cultural forms.

In his 1974 American Folklore Society presidential address, Dell Hymes described traditionalization "not simply as naming objects, traditions, but also, and more fundamentally, as naming a process" (1975:353); he placed it at the center of folkloristics and social life. Describing traditionalization as "a universal need," he argued that scholars, too, traditionalize elements and periods of their own disciplinary histories. In this essay Hymes did not, however, build traditionalization into a framework for rethinking folkloristics, nor did he indicate how and where to look for examples of traditionalization. In a number of works, Richard Bauman pushed traditionalization in the direction of an orienting framework for the field, arguing, "Tradition, long considered a criterial attribute of folklore, is coming to be seen less as an inherent quality of old and persistent items or genres passed on from generation to generation, and more as a symbolic construction by which people in the present establish connections with a meaningful past and endow particular cultural forms with value and authority. Thus the focus of attention is the strategic process of traditionalization" (1992a:128). Traditionalization, for Bauman, involved individuals' efforts to reflexively fashion cultural forms—and thereby themselves—through invocations of meaningful pasts as well as through collective constraints on who and what could be traditionalized and how that could be done (see also Bauman 2004).

Traditionalization vis-à-vis Folklorismus, Folklorization, Folkloresque

Traditionalization overlaps with several concepts that highlight the sorts of forms that Dorson tried to expunge as "fakelore." "Folklorismus" (Bendix 1988a) pointed to the generation of cultural forms in popular, commercial, and touristic contexts by appropriating traditional models. John McDowell, noting Paredes's (1974) use of the term *folklorization* (2010:183), suggested that "a consensus has formed implicating folklorization as a processing of local traditions for external consumption." He argued that the folklore/folklorization boundary is neither sharp nor linear; the emergence of "spaces where processed tradition loops back upon local artistic practices" suggested to him that scholars err in thinking that folklorization necessarily entails "the alienation, stagnation, fossilization, and ultimately, corruption of folk practices" (2010:185, 184). Michael Dylan Foster and Jeffrey Tolbert (2015) proposed "folkloresque" to identify the appropriation of images, characters, and themes from folklore in literature, film, and other media. Like the rich literature on heritage, these formulations provide a highly useful means of bringing out dimensions of power, materiality, embodiment, and commodification that were less explicit in Hymes's and Bauman's work on traditionalization.

Traditionalization provides tools for analyzing the reifications and objectifications that folklorismus, folklorization, and folkloresque identify, but also includes phenomena not explicitly commodified, popularized, or invented. As such, traditionalization does not reproduce binaries separating "popular" and "traditional" forms nor suggest that traditionalized forms necessarily bear a "metacultural" relationship of distancing and detachment—to invoke the process that Barbara Kirshenblatt-Gimblett (2006) identified for heritage. Traditionalization can bring into a single framework the sorts of cultural forms formerly privileged by folklorists as well as invented traditions, revivals, "the use of tradition as a mechanism of social control," and "the idea of folklore itself" (Bauman 1992b:32). This move opens up possibilities for seeing all folklore as mediatized, not just forms whose mediatization is strikingly evident. The example of the Grimms below will develop this point.

Traditionalization, Temporalization, and (De)Politicization

Bauman and Briggs (1990:77, 78) suggested that "the process of traditionalization" is "part of the symbolic construction of discursive continuity with a meaningful past. Attention to such processes locates performances, texts, and contexts in systems of historical relationship." In retrospect, this temporal projection requires revision to transform traditionalization into a broader analytic framework. Extensive research on temporalization practices (see, for example, Koselleck 2004) emphasizes that fashioning pasts simultaneously produces presents and futures. Moreover, such relations create gaps—senses of disconnectedness—as much as feelings of connection and intimacy (Briggs and Bauman 1992). As Bausinger ([1961] 1990:71) noted, forging historical links can distance actors from proximal histories even as it fosters connections with distal pasts.

I first grasped the complexity of temporalization practices as associated with traditionalization in research on New Mexican Spanish-language folklore (1988). The frame *Decían los viejitos de antes* . . . (The old folks of bygone days used to say . . .) projected what Bausinger ([1961] 1990:64) called "a continuous process of transmission and handing down," which he characterized as the center of "earlier stages of folk culture." Nevertheless, these performances also produced historical *dis*continuities associated with conflicts with Indigenous peoples, expropriation of land and labor by White elites, and legacies of accommodation and resistance. Traditionalization constructed discrepant "traditional futures" (Clifford 2004), inviting audiences to engage in *retraditionalization* processes that would reclaim grant lands and cultural forms rather than acquiescing to further erosion of communal symbolic and material capital. Legends of a lost gold mine countered racist images of poor, unsophisticated peasants by recovering the disappeared history of a nineteenth-century resident whose wealth and influence reached deep into Mexico, thereby traditionalizing a potential source of venture capital, so to speak, in the form of a vast cache of gold and silver (Briggs and Vigil 1990). These past-future projections sought to structure the present, including demands that I position myself either as an agent of gringo colonialism or an ally in anti-racist struggles.

Traditionalization can be profoundly depoliticizing, as revealed by collaborations between folklorists, anthropologists, museum professionals, touristic entrepreneurs, politicians, artists, writers, and administrators of heritage regimes to cast Native American, Latinx, and Indo-Hispano communities in New Mexico into segmented, exotic cultural pasts unaffected by colonialism or racism. This example highlights the need to attend to how materialities, gender, sexuality, race, disability, and other dimensions of power shape traditionalization; it also brings to mind Hymes's (1975:354) call "to analyze critically the consequences of traditionalization." As traced in chapter 4, a locus classicus of the depolicizing power of traditionalization lies in folklore collecting by British colonial administrators and missionaries in South Asia, where traditionalization cast "natives" as irrational, premodern, superstitious, and in need of British colonial paternalism (see Cohn 1996; Raheja 1996). Traditionalizing the projected violence of colonial subjects and transforming the violence of colonial rule into the embodiment of rationality and progress depoliticized South Asian resistance to colonial rule, particularly in the wake of the 1857 insurrection. Traditionalization thus became a marker for Indigenous, colonial, and postcolonial subjects who were incarcerated by culture (Appadurai 1988), trapped in a folkloric "imaginary waiting room of history" (Chakrabarty 2000:8). Traditionalization can, however, also repoliticize cultural forms: rumor and legend sometimes cast colonial overlords as magically and murderously extracting blood or other bodily fluids of the colonized (Naithani 2001; White 2000). Traditionalizing past conflicts can also repoliticize grievances, paving the way for genocide.

FROM MEDIATIZATION TO TRADITIONALIZATION

Now it is time to connect traditionalization and mediatization. As I noted, striking parallels are evident in how these notions enabled folklorists and media studies scholars to rethink their disciplines. In both cases, these concepts confronted contradictions and epistemological limitations engendered by constructions of folklore and "the media" as singular, totalizing, actually existing objects, defined in a priori terms as central disciplinary foci. Further, in addition to shifting from objects to processes and emphasizing their heterogeneity, scholars in each discipline emphasized the diversity of roles, registers, logics, material resources, and interests that shape cultural forms. Mediatization unfolds in campaign headquarters, government offices, churches, corporations, research centers, NGOs, and spaces—many now mobile—in which people receive and retransmit media forms, as much as in television and radio studios, newsrooms, Google, and publishing houses. Traditionalization is similarly enacted in classrooms, scholars' offices, tourism bureaus, advertising agencies, UNESCO headquarters, recording studios, and street corners, in how people now play to their cell phones as much as to television and press cameras or folklorists' recording devices. Finally, both of these notions responded to analytic challenges that emerged when discipline-based perspectives and practices confronted the need to grasp how folkloric and media forms are deeply entangled with other social fields. Traditionalization and mediatization by definition never exist in isolation but only in relation to processes defined as being beyond folklore and "the media." Thus, both mediatization and traditionalization provide ways of retaining a measure of disciplinary boundary-work and simultaneously facilitating the boundary crossing needed to grapple with the complexity of social life. I will return to this point below. A central advantage of seeing folkloristics through the lens of traditionalization and framing media studies through mediatization is that both emphasize reflexivity and objectification in parallel if distinct ways.

Thus far, I have tried to make a case for reorienting studies of folklore and "the media." I argued that recent reformulations of folkloristics and media studies created a new basis for bringing them more fruitfully into dialogue and pointed to how notions of traditionalization and mediatization can provide productive points of alignment and comparison. Given that neither *traditionalization* nor *mediatization* are catchall terms referring to all of social life, I return now to my previous distinction between form, ideology, and practices in order to specify how they can be of analytic and methodological value.

FORM

With regard to *form*, the most important formal dimension of traditionalization involves genre. Briggs and Bauman (1992) suggested that genre is less a matter of stuffing content into prefabricated packages than the inflecting of discourse in such a way as to produce particular patterns of expectation and response, what we might call *genrefication*. Repetition, parallelism, sound symbols, and other forms of verisimilitude, reported speech, gestures, and movements of the head and body are crucial elements.[2] Bauman and Briggs (1990) stressed intertextuality, in which formal features evoke prior patterns or performances. A video documenting a Venezuelan festival, for example, traditionalizes the event as the replication of past festivals; the Bigott Foundation's "Popular Culture Workshops" presented children with cultural forms through practices of temporal reflexivity that mapped their features onto what were characterized as continuous processes of transmission, as enacted by authentic folk performers. Use of the term *text* should not, however, erase the importance of bodily, sensory, material, environmental, and affective engagements, including with nonhumans. Poetic, visual, embodied, and other formal dimensions are powerful because they seem to inscribe traditionalization on the sensory surfaces of forms, thus forging connections in the realm of what Raymond Williams (1977) referred to as structures of feeling, more felt than consciously formulated. (Recall from chapter 5 my discussion of the power of entextualization in subject formation.) Formal elaboration becomes, in Bauman's (1992a:128) words, "a quality of traditionality that is considered to inhere in a cultural form conceived of as akin to a persistent natural object."

Joining mediatization theorists in rejecting technological determinism, folklorists can similarly emphasize both the hegemony invested in dominant forms, practices, and ideologies and the agency emerging from active processes of reception. Rather than constituting a machine that produces particular responses, formal dimensions provide affordances (Gibson 1997) that facilitate particular forms of listening, movement, affect, and interaction with objects and nonhumans without precluding others. Form is an affordance akin to the way the handrail on a staircase in a public space encourages people to grasp it in order to prevent a fall, without excluding possible contact with children's posteriors, skateboards, and bicycle locks. Emphasizing form provides a crucial point of contact with media studies, which has extensive literatures on visual dimensions, sound and voice, temporality (including seriality and the layering and disruption of linearity), music, and more. I further explore this connection below.

Ideology

Ideological dimensions also loom large as we link mediatization and traditionalization. Deleuze and Guattari ([1980] 1987) stressed that the impact of technologies does not accrue simply to technological features but is mediated by ideologies, ways people construct them, and by political economies. The term *ideology* has many meanings; I use it not to signal some free-floating intangible or distorting lens but to indicate active varieties of *ideological labor* that operate on a continuum from not fully articulated structures of feeling (Williams 1977) to central features of political platforms used by fascist, democractic, and communist governments alike. "Metacultural" estrangement (Kirshenblatt-Gimblett 2006) and "heritage consciousness" (Scher 2016) are thus particular forms of the ideological labor of traditionalization. As noted above, for three centuries traditionalization has been the central form of ideological labor for producing subjects who seem outside the reach of modern rationality and hygiene, just as mediatization—reified in particular technologies from printing to the newest mobile phone, self-driving car, or "smart" appliance—has been cast as the sine qua non of modernity. Nevertheless, both types of ideological labor contain contradictions that simultaneously create their opposites: consuming commodified traditionalities (such as reading fairytales to children) became a marker of modern subjects, just as producing traditional subjects, forms, and spaces became a key requirement for fashioning modern, multicultural states. Key to such ideological labor is the creation of chronotopes (Bakhtin 1981), projecting some temporalities and spaces as origin points for traditionality (such as the US's Appalachia or Karelia in Finland); others—such as Silicon Valley—become ground zero for making modernities.

Practice

A third analytic is *practice*. Bourdieu's ([1972] 1977) use of the term is particularly instructive, drawing attention to deeply rooted patterns of thinking, making, interacting, and embodying ("habitus") as well as how each encounter with the world requires adaptation and innovation. The media studies notion of remediation (Bolter and Grusin 1999), the way "old" media practices get recycled for use with "new" ones, suggests how we frequently adapt aspects of familiar communicative practices while engaging with "new" technologies. Literatures on video games (Boellstorff 2008; Miller 2008), on how intimate relations are severed among college students (Gershon 2010), the way cell phone use often coexists with face-to-face interaction (Campbell and Kwak 2011), and on digital folklore (Blank 2012) suggest that practices are seldom divided into separate folkloric and media repertoires.

Documenting mediatization and traditionalization requires attention to how complex, multifaceted, and widely distributed ideologies, forms, and practices are (re)produced, circulated, and received. Ethnographic documentation of instances in which traditionalization and mediatization practices converge or are held far apart, as illustrated below, offers a potentially fruitful venue for transforming work on "folklore and the media."

MASTER MEDIATIZERS OF TRADITION: THE BROTHERS GRIMM

To illustrate this framework, I present two cases. One focuses on a classic example of mediatized folklore, the Grimms' famous *Kinder- und Hausmärchen* (*KHM*), while the other scrutinizes a sphere that embodies mediatization and seems to defy traditionalization. The latter example, which I develop in chapter 9, details the overnight creation of a mediatized pandemic. Despite its ideological concentration on newness, I point to how traditionalization made this possible. The first case invites folklorists to rethink a familiar story by contemplating how mediatization produced a template for traditionalization. The "swine flu" example rethinks two modern domains (journalism and medicine) through the lens of traditionalization. The reason I spend more time developing the second case is that the first, that of the Grimms, builds on a considerable body of scholarship that is familiar to most folklorists, including work that I presented previously with Richard Bauman (Bauman and Briggs 2003, chapter 6). I do not, on the other hand, presume that most readers will be conversant with how journalists, public health officials, researchers, and clinicians mobilize quite different disciplinary backgrounds and forms of practice in collaboratively constructing narratives that project epidemics.

Jacob and Wilhelm Grimm projected a particular set of practices as integral to studying folklore: leaving the space of the city, traveling to the countryside, locating genuine bearers of folk narratives and other forms, inscribing oral performances, selecting authentic forms, and carefully editing them. The Grimms deemed these practices an effort "to collect these tales in as pure a form as possible," claiming that "no details have been added or embellished or changed" ([1812/1819] 1987:210). Three features are crucial. First, these practices were organized from start to finish as parts of a specific mediatization process, designed to produce a mediatized product. Second, the prescribed practices were dispersed in time and space, requiring the assistance of a diverse range of actors that included narrators, intermediaries, editors, printers, publishers, booksellers and, we would presume, other nonhuman actors, such as horses. Third, their practices were organized around a semiotic construction that I have referred to as the ideology of metapragmatic transparency (Briggs 1993b), involving both the construction of separate and opposing oral versus literate spheres and practices of transcription and editing that purportedly reproduce "essential features" of oral performances with "fidelity" and "genuineness" through particular features of written and printed texts. Withering criticism by Jack Zipes (1979), Maria Tatar (1992), and others branded the Grimms as traitors, arguing that their discursive practices fell short of the very model they celebrated. Ironically, such diatribes point to the power of the traditionalization-cum-mediatization model the Grimms enshrined; these critics did not seem to realize that metacommunicative transparency is an ideological construction that will *always* be contradicted by traditionalization and mediatization practices. Not only did the *KHM* reflect capitalist, literary, and technological (printing) dimensions that did not spring directly from the "dearest fragrance" and "native adornment" of folk transmission and performance, but the Grimms' model of mediatization was centrally involved in producing a globally dispersed sense of the oral and traditional, its feel and appeal.

The role of mediatization in shaping formal features of the *KHM* suggests how intimately traditionalization and mediatization are connected. Editorial practices undertaken between the manuscript version and subsequent editions included inserting direct discourse (putting words into characters' mouths), personal names, and proverbs; weaving fragments into seemingly unified narratives; augmenting linear plot structures; and adding symmetrical repetitions. The result was recurrent formal patterns that came to be the sine qua non of the fairytale genre, producing a type of form-feeling (Sapir 1949) that influenced other scholars' collection and editorial practices and how consumers buy, read, and listen to the tales. The selection and editing of texts was oriented toward the commodified endpoint, that is, producing books for use in bourgeois nurseries and other contexts.[3] Wilhelm Grimm states in the second edition's preface, even as he universalizes the whiteness of his projected youthful audience as embodying "the same purity that makes children appear so wondrous and blessed to us; they have the same bluish-white, flawless shining eyes": "in this new edition, we have carefully eliminated every phrase not appropriate for children" ([1812/1819] 1987:217).

These features have been extensively scrutinized in terms of traditionalization. The thought experiment I propose is reading the *KHM* as an *icon of mediatization*, as producing forms that naturalized mediatized subjects (narrators, heroines, readers, and listening children), objects (the *KHM* and, later, fairytale theme parks, Disney movies, costumes, and so forth), practices (of transcribing, translating, publishing, reading, theatrical and filmic enactment, etc.), and the very mediatization process the Grimms were creating. They globalized this process by encouraging translations of the *KHM*, now in over seventy languages, and urging folklorists in other countries to use the Grimms' model to produce formally similar tale collections.

Ideological dimensions of the Grimms' mediatization process were particularly developed in *KHM* prefaces. These pre-texts presented origin stories that spatialized and temporalized sources and mediatized products as linear, one-way movements from rural to urban spaces. Bausinger ([1961] 1990) anticipated Raymond Williams's (1973) *The Country and the City* by examining how a separation of urban and rural realms was ideologically produced through a reciprocal, interactive process of ruralification and urbanization. The *KHM* joined popular magazines, fiction, and later film as mediatized forms that helped create this seeming spatial-social gap. Prefaces further provided ideological affordances that invited certain interpretive and affective responses to formal features. The Grimms simultaneously denigrated other traditionalization-mediatization practices, such as those undertaken by Johann Gottfried Herder, Achim von Arnim, and Clemens Brentano, and rendered still others invisible.

A great deal of the ideological force of the Grimms' traditionalization-mediatization strategy lay in the interface between form and content in the tales themselves. Feminist folklorists have revealed how the *KHM* construct gender and sexual inequalities, casting folk culture as having a patriarchal base and inserting and extracting direct discourse so as to fashion good, quiet, and passive heterosexual girls and bad female figures—like witches and stepmothers—whose extensive quoted speech revealed their evil subjectivities. Tatar (1992:24) suggested that the Grimms' editorial practices paved the way for later gender stereotyping in Disney films. Ann

Schmiesing (2014) argued that the tales constructed abled and disabled bodies in complex and consequential ways. In short, the Grimms' layering of traditionalization and mediatization has had lasting effects on the power of traditionalized media forms to shape perceptions of bodies, spaces, temporalities, and subjectivities.

One of the most remarkable aspects of the *KHM* is how the Grimms used dimensions of form, ideology, and practice to project a magical amalgamation of traditionalization and mediatization that largely dominated folkloristics through the middle of the twentieth century and still lurks around the discipline's edges. The model they crafted also continues to provide the infrastructure for practices of traditionalization in many popular folklore texts, touristic enactments, heritage regimes, folkloric theme parks, folk art markets, and much more, even as feminist and LGBTQ+ movements produce forms—such as feminist fairytales and homoerotic YouTube remakes of Disney fairytale movies—that open up chasms between traditionalization and mediatization and explore alternative strategies for linking them.

Even as traditionalization and mediatization can be projected as perfectly coterminous, as in the Grimms' case, they can also be cast as diametrically opposed. Héctor Beltrán (2012) presented a wonderful example of a San Francisco Bay Area healing ceremony that featured a practitioner characterized as a traditional Mayan shaman. When one of the working-class (im)migrant participants asked to record the ceremony on his cell phone, the middle-class sponsor replied, "Everybody turn off your cell phones. No audio or video recording, please." Kalim Smith (2007) compared two contrastive types of performances held in the Kumeyaay Nation near San Diego. *Nightfire* was performed on a stage between the Viejas Casino and Outlet Mall; loudspeakers narrativized common Native American stereotypes through a script concocted by a Hollywood firm, with computer-synchronized smoke, lights, and water. The use of actual Kumeyaay words or cultural elements was prohibited. Contrastively, a genre called bird singing, a sacred form that connects the living and the dead, cannot be recorded or written down, nor can bird songs be taught to outsiders. Note how these examples project a double, contradictory relationship between traditionalization and mediatization. In bird singing and the healing ceremony, traditionalization requires ideologically projecting a space that exists prior to and independently of mediatization, from which it must be carefully protected. This injunction nevertheless affords a central role to media ideologies in traditionalizing these forms, defining genres and performances vis-à-vis a negative inversion of ways that mediatization is ideologically constructed.

CONCLUSION

Since I have argued that mediatization fundamentally shapes both folklore and folkloristics, the issues I addressed here have implications beyond research that explicitly focuses on "folklore and the media." In the course of disrupting familiar approaches to folklore/media relationships, I have reconceptualized folkloristics and media studies by fashioning the concepts of traditionalization and mediatization into tools for drawing attention to how disciplinary underpinnings have been transformed in important and compatible ways. This move opened up avenues for going beyond juxtaposing autonomous and potentially incompatible premises—or worse, grafting frameworks from one discipline onto commonsense notions about the other—to create bases for new types of engagements. Given that there are important limits on what can be accomplished in one programmatic essay, I would like to conclude by pointing to additional possibilities.

Let me begin by mentioning two areas in which folklorists have created especially promising bases for research on traditionalization and mediatization. One involves the mediatization of religious forms and experiences, a subject explored by both folklorists and media studies scholars. In highlighting the centrality of photography for witnessing miraculous apparitions, Daniel Wojcik (2009) analyzed how ideological constructions of photography and spirituality are entwined in producing forms that shape practices for ritually interacting with otherworldly beings. Robert Glenn Howard's ethnography of online Christian fundamentalist groups documented enclaves whose creation is shaped as deeply by mediatization practices as by biblical literalism, spheres in which "sharing knowledge creates a community" (2011:11). "Mega-churches" and other facets of the global expansion of evangelical Christian churches rest on extensive practices of mediatization. Charles Hirschkind (2006) analyzed the centrality of listening—rather than speaking—in shaping Muslim selves and subjectivities, particularly through the audition of cassette tapes of Islamic sermons.

A second opening emerges from the extensive literature on heritage. Kirshenblatt-Gimblett (2006) has suggested that heritage regimes are "metacultural," inflecting traditionalization as folklorization (Hafstein 2018a). Bendix (2018:8) suggests that heritage regimes revolve around "construing culture as property." Accordingly, how do the varieties of reflexivity and objectification that mediatize heritage—including news coverage, commercial recordings of "authentic" and "folklorized" songs, *National Geographic*–type publications, YouTubes, social media, promotional videos accompanying UNESCO Representative List of Intangible Cultural Heritage nominations, and webpages—traditionalize forms in ways that facilitate their incorporation into heritage regimes? As Hafstein's (2018a:134; 2018b) work suggests, mediatization enters these scenes in multiple ways, including, ironically, lamenting the threat of "increased media coverage" to the authenticity of forms whose traditionalization has been thoroughly mediatized. Philip Scher documented an example in which Trinidadian carnival participants were criticized on television and in newspapers for displaying interest in mediatization. In a reporter's words, "Mostly women, many members took a long time to move on as they played to the television and press cameras" (2002:475). Diverse actors in heritage regimes, including scholars, tend to focus on mediatization only when it gets ideologically positioned within "the media," thereby missing how the dispersal of mediatization practices across multiple sites, logics, materialities, bodies, and forms of power engenders the fundamentally mediatized and metacultural character of "heritage labor" and "heritage consciousness" (Scher 2016). Heritage research could benefit from ethnographic explorations of UNESCO press and media production practices, journalists assigned to "culture" or "lifestyle" beats who cover festivals and performances, advertising companies that make promotional videos, and the production of selfies and cell phone videos that now constitute the everyday life of consuming heritage, thereby illuminating the role of mediatization in shaping heritage regimes. Ways that different actors forge competing ideologies and practices of traditionalization and mediatization would be particularly interesting.

My goal here is not to attempt to determine the arenas of mediatization and traditionalization that will figure in future research. Indeed, the idea is rather to invite documentation and analysis of a broad range of different sites and modes of mediatization that appear in folklorists' research areas. Similarly, all of us are engaged in practices of traditionalization and mediatization; reflecting on our own lives would thus provide excellent arenas for critical reflection and analysis. Additionally, it is now commonplace to invite students in folklore classes to scrutinize their own media practices. This chapter might provide a prompt for pushing classroom discussions and student papers in productive directions by expanding the focus from describing new mediatized objects to analyzing emerging forms, practices, and ideologies of traditionalization and mediatization. Such exercises will reveal fascinating examples that the analysis I have provided cannot adequately encompass, thereby opening up new analytical possibilities; as usual, good pedagogy can spark creative research. These lines of investigation would expand the preliminary analysis I have presented here by looking comparatively at the different ways that traditionalization and mediatization unfold.

More broadly, forging deeper engagements between folkloristics and media studies can show how folklorists can craft more robust disciplinary futures. In suggesting what this sort of analysis can offer to ongoing discussions of folkloristics' futures, I would like to make clear what I have *not* done here: I have not argued that folkloristics and media studies are or should become one. Defining folkloristics not through possession of a bounded, unique, actually existing object but rather through processes of traditionalization in which multiple actors, including folklorists, engage and explore complex relations with other social processes and disciplinary frameworks pushes the discipline beyond ostrich-in-the-sand claims to autonomy. Investigating similarities and differences in how folkloristics relates to other fields can transform premises and open up new modes of inquiry. Cross-training, in which graduate students become proficient in at least one other field, seems particularly valuable; indeed, intersections with linguistics, anthropology, literature, ethnomusicology, performance studies, literature, and ethnic studies have long provided sources of critical insight and creativity.

I have thus tried to show how folkloristics can—and I think must—have its disciplinary cake and eat it too, that it can best make unique contributions to broader scholarly and public debates precisely by using serious study of other processes and disciplinary traditions to gain deeper insight into its own premises and modes of inquiry. Demonstrating such contributions is crucial for constantly reinvigorating the discipline and for proving to deans and funding agencies that vibrant, well-funded academic and public folklore programs are valuable. The price of success, as Martín Barbero's challenge suggests, is the hard work required to "lose sight" of entrenched disciplinary objects in order to discover how the bodies, technologies, materialities, and ideologies that they purport to represent are continually brought into being. Given both widespread anxieties about the omnipresence of mediatization and the scholarly and political power of ongoing efforts to construct—and often blame—a seemingly autonomous and bounded domain of "the media," by exploring traditionalization and mediatization folklorists can offer invaluable perspectives on the contemporary world and renew their disciplinary foundation.

NOTES

1. For recent overviews, see Bronner 2011 and Noyes 2016. On traditionalization, see Mould 2011.

2. Here again, vast bodies of literature are relevant, including the Russian Formalists and Prague School theorists, importantly Jakobson (1960), along with Hymes (1975), Tedlock (1983), Bauman (2004), Hill (1995), Nuckolls (1999), and more.

3. See Bottigheimer 1987; Tatar 1987; and Zipes 1979.

9

Germ Wordfare
The Poetic Production of Medical Panics

I BEGIN WITH AN APOLOGY AND A PROMISE. IN chapter 7 I laid out a call for a new way of approaching folkloristics. There I wondered out loud why recent advances in research on folk medicine do not seem to have broken folk medicine out of its enclave: it seldom figures centrally in broad disciplinary debates or gets recognized as making the sorts of theoretical or methodological contributions that are credited to scholars of, say, narrative, folk song, riddles and proverbs. I laid out a framework that, I hope, can help focus theoretical issues and further innovative research. In chapter 8, I similarly examined a broad range of ways that folklorists have addressed relationships between folklore and media. I proposed abandoning the commonsense category of "the media," using the concepts of traditionalization and mediatization to suggest a new approach. Here's the apology: both chapters were largely programmatic, laying out ideas about what sorts of perspectives and problems *might* be most productive. I offered, however, few specifics and only one extended example (that of the Grimms) that might clarify what I have in mind or demonstrate its potential value.

This chapter picks up where the previous two leave off. It provides an example of what I have termed the new folkloristics of health by looking at how familiar elements, including practice, performance, and poetics, emerge in a domain that lies at some distance from the sorts of sites, topics, and persons generally studied by folklorists. It also advances the argument presented in chapter 8 by looking at what seems to be a quintessentially mediatized and modern arena—news coverage of health—as an example of traditionalization. The example I develop here pertains to one of the most pressing problems of our day. A pandemic is a quintessentially modern object: its alarming temporality of sudden eruption and frightening trajectory seemingly erupts naturally from its biological nature as a "new," "novel" type of virus or other pathogen. News stories about pandemics similarly attract audience interest and market value precisely because they are new, satisfying the central journalistic criterion of "newsworthiness." "Breaking stories" in particular juxtapose and reify journalistic and "real world" temporalities—reported by journalists even as the events unfold. Continuing the reversal that led me to analyze the Grimms' Brothers tales as examples of mediatization, however, here I analyze the making of a news story that ideologically frames its content—an account of a new virus and an unfolding pandemic—by looking at how its formal features and complex practices juxtapose different logics, sites, and professional roles through processes of rehearsal and performance that exhibit striking features of traditionalization. Beyond illustrating the type of research that, I think, is afforded by the frameworks I presented, I want to suggest how productive it can be to join distinct analytic perspectives in folkloristics and to bring them into dialogue with ideas emanating from other disciplines, here journalism and media studies, performance studies, medical anthropology, and science-technology-society studies.

PERFORMING BIOSECURITY

An additional goal of this chapter is to show how useful the study of poetics and performance can be in critically analyzing the contemporary world by focusing on what has emerged in recent years as a major concern: the proposition that evolving viruses and other microbes constitute one of the greatest threats to humankind. Indeed, "preparedness" planning for epidemics has become a central policy preoccupation, reshaped public health policies, and rationalized massive public expenditures. In addition to bioterrorism—the use of microbes, perhaps genetically engineered to make them more lethal—as weapons of mass destruction, one of the most prominent targets of biosecurity panics has been influenzas and other infectious diseases. I concentrate here on the 2009 pandemic of H1N1, first known as "swine flu," especially on how it became a global health nightmare in just twenty-four hours in April 2009.

The reason I have selected this epidemic rather than more recent events—such as outbreaks of Ebola in West Africa starting in 2013 or the COVID-19 (coronavirus) epidemic that is continuing even as I write in 2020—is that I was able to conduct the sort of extensive textual and ethnographic research that is required to fulfill the research strategies I proposed in chapters 7 and 8. Media studies and journalism scholar Daniel C. Hallin and I collected all stories published about H1N1 in five US newspapers

(*USA Today*, *The New York Times*, the *San Diego Union-Tribune*, the *Atlanta Journal-Constitution*, and the *New York Post*) and analyzed them qualitatively and quantitatively. We used the comments sections of newspaper, radio, and television websites and other sources to track internet and social media discussions. We also interviewed journalists reporting for media ranging from local newspapers and radio and television stations to national network television and *The New York Times* (*NYT*). We interviewed city, county, state, and national public health officials, epidemiologists, other researchers, and clinicians. We also conducted ethnography whenever possible, including in biosecurity "exercises" that came in the wake of H1N1.[1] This chapter suggests why going beyond textual analysis to look ethnographically as well at how disease stories and other media narratives are produced and circulate is crucial. At the same time, both pandemics and discourse about them enter into complex histories and epidemiological cartographies, so I begin by sketching what surrounds H1N1 and COVID-19.

Scholars working in anthropology and science and technology studies (STS) have argued that concerns with biosecurity represent a major global epistemic transformation. Andrew Lakoff (2017) traced a recent shift in "normative rationality" from a focus that emerged in the nineteenth century on "population security," centered on the calculation of risk for regularly recurring problems, to "vital systems security," which uses a logic of "preparedness" in anticipating pandemics and other threats that are impossible to predict or calculate. He stressed the role of tabletop or scenario-based exercises in which participants simulate catastrophic events. Lakoff suggested that their primary purpose was pedagogical: to convince officials of the need to merge public health and security concerns in placing catastrophic disease outbreaks at the top of policy agendas. (Later in the chapter, I analyze a different way that these "exercises" have shaped biosecurity discourse.) Studying H5N1 or avian influenza in Indonesia, on the other hand, Celia Lowe (2010) argues that a pervasive logic based on "vital systems security" was less apparent there than a concern with "multispecies clouds," including viruses and birds but also bodies, narratives, and politics, that were transformed through unpredictable, coincidental, and often nonrational interactions. Here I focus on what was widely hailed in the United States as demonstrating the success of biosecurity infrastructures: the rapid response to the emergence of a "new" virus, a novel strain of H1N1, or "swine flu."

How can studying poetics and performance shed new light on these issues? Anthropologists and STS scholars seem to position themselves as what Paul Rabinow (2008), borrowing from Niklas Luhmann, characterized as second-order observers looking over the shoulders of scientists and other professionals as they make first-order observations. Social scientists thus imbue their work with a sense of authority and urgency by positioning themselves in the spaces and times in which new knowledge is projected as being produced. As Donna Haraway (1996) has pointed out, a danger here is that retelling a scientific story will further reify the same characters and settings, thereby directing attention away from other actors and narratives. Interest in how stories are made, circulated, and received might, on the other hand, position scholars at what might seem to be the opposite and less prestigious end, looking less at how new viruses evolve and vaccines are developed than at how narratives about them are fashioned. What I want to argue here, however, is that these are not contrastive, opposing sites but different dimensions of a widely dispersed mechanism for creating what seem to be new viral/narrative objects. Although few readers of this book were probably sickened by SARS in 2003, we were all infected by how it circulated in multiple media forms (see Lee 2014). Suggesting that students of poetics and performance are particularly qualified to solve the mystery of how these "new" medical crises are made, I want to look in detail at how a powerful "swine flu epidemic" narrative was produced so quickly.

Research by leading performance studies scholar Diana Taylor on the archive and the repertoire is of value here. Complicating the opposition between archival memory as stable, decontextualized, and authoritative versus the emergence of ephemeral, nonreproducible knowledge in performance, she examines how the grandmothers, mothers, and children of the disappeared in Argentina performed their relationship to their murdered relatives by wearing their photographs on their bodies. In what she refers to as "the DNA of performance," Taylor (2003:168) argues that these activists used photos "to bring together the science (DNA testing) and the performative claims in transmitting traumatic memory." Here I go on to ask how scientific objects are performatively constructed in the first place. What would happen if we denied the prior and separate existence of scientific sites from places where representations are made and circulate? What ways might emerge of looking at how objects get made, who gets credit for making them, what counts as scientific knowledge, who produces it, and how credit is given or denied for playing one's proper role in circulating it? A number of medical anthropologists and other scholars have analyzed the deeply performative character of practices for bringing claims about DNA into being and how scientists, patients, consumers of DNA testing kits, and others inhabit them. Thus, rather than either going "upstream" to explore places where scientific objects are seemingly made or "downstream" to sites that are projected as loci for acts of representation, I go on to challenge this problematic spatialization and the boundary-work that underlies these ways of configuring scholarly projects.

MAKING THE "SWINE FLU PANDEMIC" STORY

On April 23, 2009, national television news broadcasts and *The New York Times* presented short, routine stories reporting a Centers for Disease Control and Prevention (CDC) conference call discussing seven US cases of "swine flu." Twenty-four hours later, however, "swine flu" was the lead story on television news broadcasts and the focus of a major story in *The New York Times* (which appeared in the print version the following day). In coverage whose intensity was sustained over months, "the swine flu pandemic" became one of the leading news stories of 2009. Here is the text of the April 24, 2009, story on *CBS Evening News*:

> KATIE COURIC (HEREAFTER KC): And good evening, everyone. There's growing concern tonight about an outbreak of swine flu right next door in Mexico, concern that it will spread here and around the world. Mexican officials took extraordinary steps today to try to contain the virus, closing public buildings in Mexico City. This new strain has killed at least twenty people in Mexico and made more than a thousand sick. At least eight cases of the virus are reported here in the United States. Sandra Hughes begins our coverage tonight.
>
> SANDRA HUGHES (HEREAFTER SH): Fear is running high as the death toll rises in Mexico's capital city. The worried line up for testing, their faces covered with masks. The government in this city of 20 million closed all public places, including schools, in a desperate attempt to stop the spread of this strain of flu, never seen before.
>
> RICHARD BESSER (HEREAFTER RB): Our concern has grown since yesterday.
>
> SH: With more than 1,000 people sick in Mexico and eight recent cases in the US concentrated in two border states, two near San Antonio, Texas and six near San Diego, California, US health officials are watching this outbreak closely. More than 600,000 people cross the US-Mexico border each day, and the CDC fears it's too late for containment.
>
> RB: As a precautionary step, the CDC is working to develop a vaccine seed strain specific to these recent swine influenza viruses in humans.
>
> SH: Normal swine flu transmission is through contact with pigs. US researchers want to know how the American patients, who seem to have all recovered from the disease, got it when none is believed to have had any contact with pigs.
>
> WILLIAM SCHAFFNER: Well, this begins to look like a new influenza virus strain that could do a lot of mischief around the world.
>
> SH: Now officials are also concerned tonight because they have discovered that this strain that has killed so many in Mexico is in fact the same strain to sicken people here in the US, Katie.

KC: Sandra Hughes; Sandra, thanks very much. Meanwhile, Dr. Jon LaPook is our medical correspondent, and Jon, first of all, what are the symptoms of swine flu?

Jon LaPook (hereafter JLP): Well, it's similar to the regular flu, so fever, aches, and pains, cough, headache, and sometimes you get nausea, vomiting, and diarrhea. What's very important, people tend to confuse those symptoms with the symptoms of the common cold, which are much milder and generally from the neck up.

KC: Alright, and how is it treated?

JLP: Fortunately, this strain seems to be very sensitive to the commonly used flu meds, so Tamiflu and Relenza. The key thing, you need to take those medications, they best work if taken within forty-eight hours of symptoms, which is all the more reason to know what your symptoms are, talk to your doctor if you get them.

KC: And that's not in short supply, we should mention.

JLP: There's lots of it, lots of it on the shelf, no reason to stockpile.

KC: Alright, and how serious do you believe is this outbreak?

JLP: Well, the CDC and the WHO is taking it seriously, they're sending teams of people all over the place, and I find that very reassuring, they are all over this. And a little bit of a reality check, Katie, in Mexico the health minister told us today that the death rate seems to be leveling off. And in the United States there have been eight cases, but all of them recovered, only one required hospitalization. So, there's reason for concern but absolutely, positively no reason to panic.

KC: Alright, Dr. Jon LaPook; Jon, thank you so much.

For television, which generally presents simpler stories than "quality" broadsheet newspapers, this is a remarkably expansive and complex narrative. As on CNN and the other two national news networks, this was the lead story, indicating the producers' sense of its newsworthiness. It is a package, meaning that it includes segments featuring the anchor, a reporter sending footage from another location, and a segment with Dr. Jonathan LaPook, a board-certified physician in internal medicine and gastroenterology at New York-Presbyterian Hospital and CBS's medical correspondent. Its production in a twenty-four-hour period is a remarkable feat. We get a geography of the disease in two countries, an outline of government policies, public reactions, the virus's genetic profile, symptoms, and treatment, including antivirals and vaccine development. Each subsequent news broadcast, newspaper article, and social media post extended this swine flu cartography.

CBS not only located the virus in Mexico but used footage of US Immigration and Customs Enforcement (ICE) agents walking beside long lines of cars crossing from Mexico into the United States, as reporter Sandra

Hughes narrated: "More than 600,000 people cross the US-Mexico border each day, and the CDC fears it's too late for containment." Although CNN and the three major television networks soon dropped this theme—in the face of US health officials' insistence that immigration would not be a major factor in spreading the virus—anti-immigrant social media and contributions to comments sections continued to sound this theme, which also got more sustained play on the conservative Fox News Network. (Fox initially called H1N1 a bacteria; by April 25, Fox correctly termed it a virus, but mistakenly claimed, "The good news is this: the US is stockpiled with an antibiotic that kills the virus.") Nevertheless, the narrative developed on April 24 was remarkably stable until heated debates about H1N1 vaccine emerged in August. The epidemic, soon to be a pandemic, became the major focus of public health authorities worldwide. Substantial public expenditures, including for antivirals and vaccines, were seemingly unavoidable once this medical/mediated object emerged. How health journalists and public health officials "handled" the pandemic came to be seen by these professionals as a model for preparedness discourse. It would thus seem valuable to figure out how this powerful performance is structured and how it got constructed so quickly. As we will see, a long-standing process of traditionalization provided the infrastructure for producing the narrative and triggering its massive uptake.

The broadcast created what we could call, following M. M. Bakhtin (1981), *an epidemic chronotope*, involving carefully crafted dramatic movements between different types of spaces, actors, objects, and types of narrative authority. It begins with a powerful framing or keying device, one that opens every national network news evening broadcast: the program's musical intro, a zooming of the camera from above the studio, with the anchor poring over a text and the title and logo of the broadcast and day's date visible, followed by the standard greeting: "And good evening, everyone." This visual, textual, and auditory poetics have highlighted her performative role as anchor; Couric shifts tone immediately in the story's lead: "There's growing concern tonight about an outbreak of swine flu right next door in Mexico, concern that it will spread here and around the world." Like narratives in general, these broadcasts do not simply report but make events. The position of each story in the broadcast signals the significance of the events under construction: lead story position signals that an event is projected as the most significant to have occurred that day in the world. The studio is a master space of narration, dominated by a narrative voice that is so valued and recognizable that it commands impressive salaries: Couric reportedly earned $15 million annually. Nevertheless,

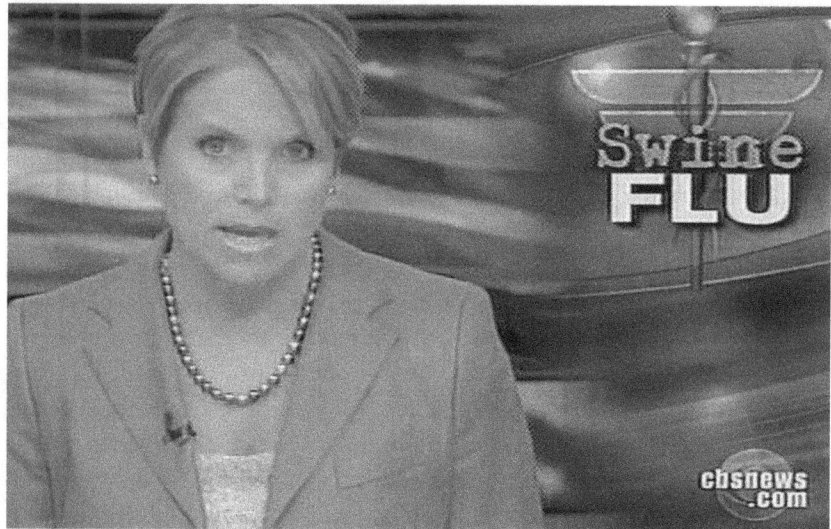

Figure 9.1. CBS anchor Katie Couric, April 24, 2009, *CBS Evening News*

professional ideologies suggest that journalists "report" events that are made by other actors: "swine flu" is projected as already an actually existing object whose objective status is signaled by its appearance as a text alongside Couric (see figure 9.1).

Television news broadcasts revolve around movements between what is projected as the central space of narration and chronotopically distant locations in which events unfold. Their narrative structures thus require the doubling of journalistic performers to include correspondents who take us to what is constructed as the indexical origin of stories. The story is a complex account of people, viruses, animals, and actions in two countries, and Hughes is magically able to take us to what are projected as the three primordial times and places of the epidemic chronotope, moving from Mexico City to the border crossing to San Diego. Hughes was certainly not in Mexico City, and she probably never crossed the border that day, but, as the network's Los Angeles–based correspondent, she could journey to San Diego to produce footage in time to meet the East Coast deadline for the day's *Evening News* broadcast. Television news relies on the power of the visual, auditory, and the verbal to create montages that produce the illusion that audiences are actually watching the events unfold, with correspondents as witnesses. Hughes seems to be observing fear and chaos in "*this* city of 20 million"; her voice-over makes her appear to stand alongside ICE agents as they scrutinize passengers (see figure 9.2); then she appears in San Diego,

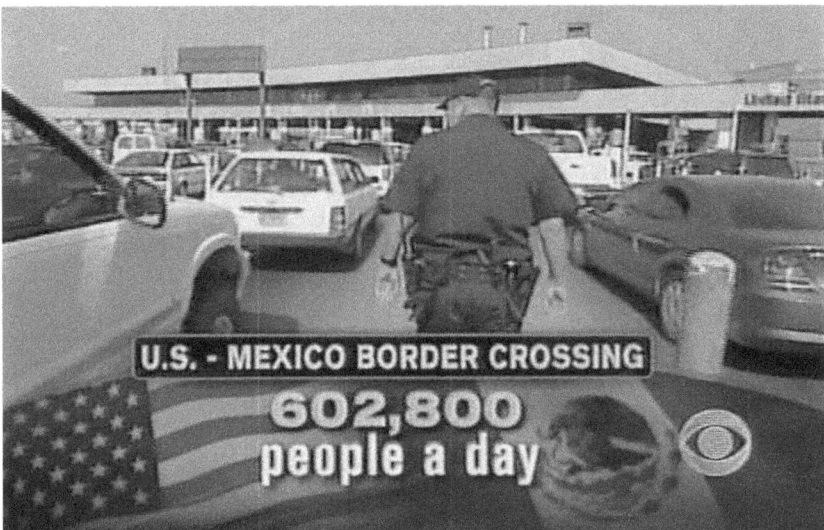

Figure 9.2. ICE agents scrutinize crossers at US-Mexico border

the point at which "this strain that has killed so many in Mexico" has just arrived "to sicken people here in the US."

By this point in the broadcast, we have already met two additional performers. As the acting director of the Centers for Disease Control and Prevention (CDC), Richard Besser had professional stature and official status; he would seem to naturally appear in an on-camera press conference (see figure 9.3).[2] Our ethnography suggests, however, that his presence reflected less epidemiological facts on the ground than performance strategies. On the previous day, unusual flu cases were present in Texas, California, and Mexico. Nevertheless, Besser decided to inform journalists via a telephone conference call with Dr. Anne Schuchat, director of the National Center for Immunization and Respiratory Diseases. Using a subordinate official and not providing visuals practically ensured that journalists would not turn "swine flu" into a major story. Indeed, *The New York Times* and national television news broadcasts presented low-key stories in spaces that signaled their lesser importance. In a March 3, 2012, interview with Daniel Hallin, Besser told us about his decision: putting a subordinate on a conference call on April 23 signified that "it was still looking kind of small"; with the press conference the following day, however, "it got bigger, it quickly made it to the level of me, as the acting director." Besser framed this shift as based on "one of the principles we use in communication, is you kind of escalate depending on the response you want to get."

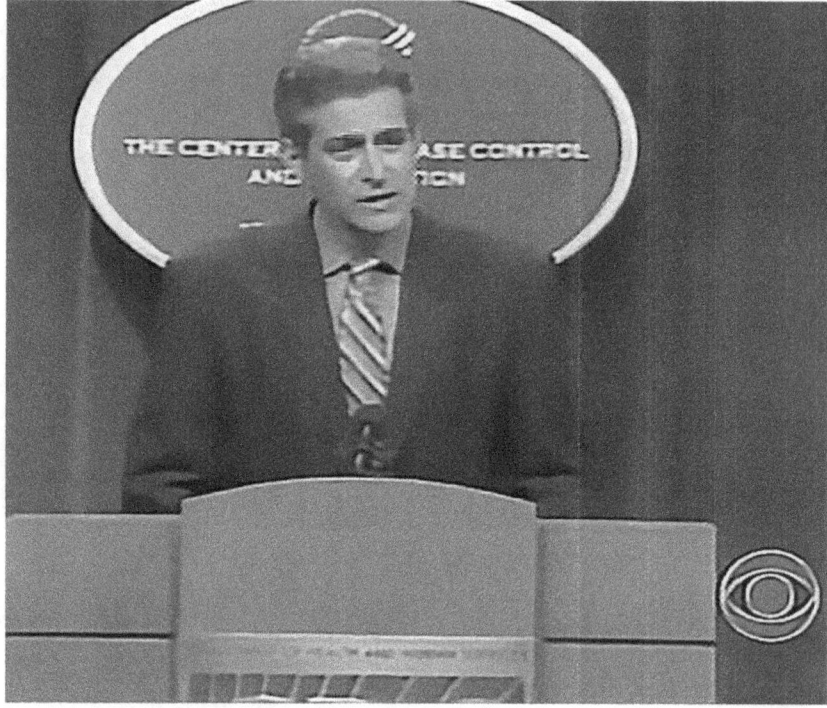

Figure 9.3. Acting director Richard Besser at CDC news conference

In other words, Besser consciously constructed what was taking place as an event, marked its seriousness, and positioned the CDC as a central player in its future by staging a particular type of performance. Moreover, who is Besser? After graduating from the University of Pennsylvania Medical School, Besser completed a residency in pediatrics at Johns Hopkins before becoming a CDC epidemiological intelligence service officer. He later returned to the CDC, heading its emergency preparedness branch for four years before becoming its acting director in January 2009. Interestingly, in addition to being a pediatrician and epidemiologist, Besser was a television commentator while teaching at UC San Diego's medical school in the 1990s; after leaving the CDC, he became ABC's chief health and medical editor.

What about the ominous-looking Dr. William Schaffner (see figure 9.4)? A key figure in health news stories is the medical expert, a clinician or bench scientist presented as a specialist on the topic. I have interviewed US, Latin American, European, and Asian health journalists, and one of the first things they all display as a sign of their stature is their archive of contacts with health experts, selected due to their prominence in their

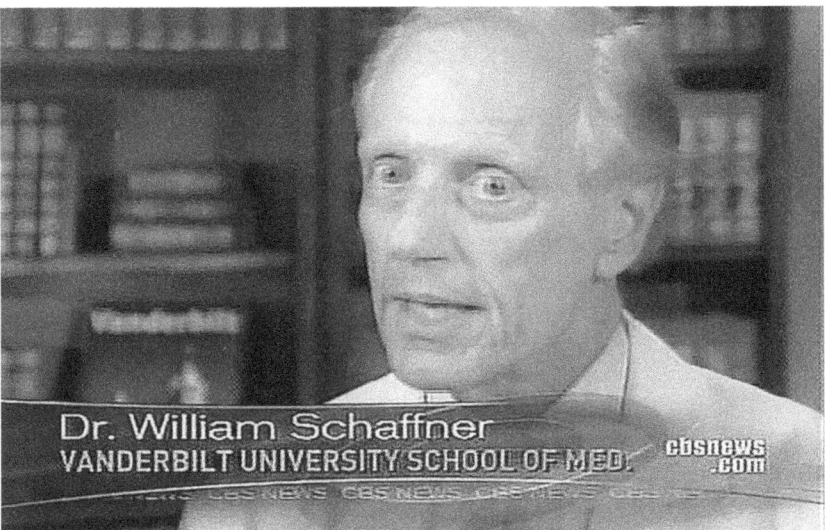

Figure 9.4. Dr. William Schaffner performs a sound bite

fields of specialization and the prestige of their organizations. But let me turn this equation around: what percentage of such "experts" become regulars on national network news? Answer: relatively few. Becoming a regular "source" requires competence with respect to several performance criteria, the development of which is generally boosted by media training that enables "experts" to perform in ways that please journalists.

First, you need to provide reporters with material on nearly any question they ask. If you say, "That's really outside my range of expertise," you are very unlikely to receive another inquiry from journalists, who count on getting material rapidly and reliably from "sources." Becoming "an expert" requires awareness of and compliance with journalistic temporalities, which differ from television to print to social media. If you do not anticipate journalists' deadlines, responding in time for them to submit their story, you get dropped.

Second, media training warns about taking a "cold call" from a reporter. If the phone rings and a journalist says, "Hi, I'm Denise Grady of *The New York Times* and I'm calling to ask what you think about Moderna's plans to start testing coronavirus vaccines on children ages 12 to 17," we are urged to say: "Sorry, Denise, I'm with a student. What's your deadline? Could I call you back in an hour?" Hang up, look up the facts, craft a sound bite, then return the call, repeating your sound bite multiple times in the interview, saying nothing that the reporter could use instead of your sound bite, lest your

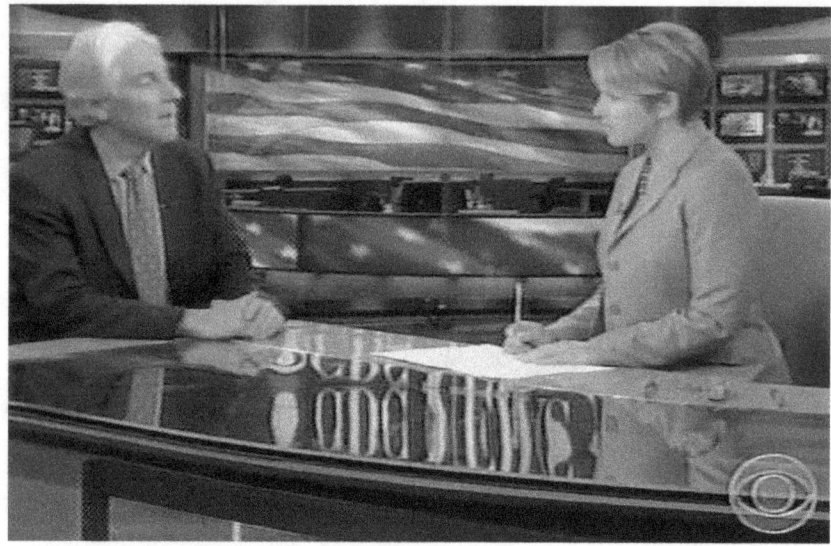

Figure 9.5. Dr. Jon LaPook with anchor Katie Couric

off-the-cuff comment become your inadvertent sound bite! An entire lecture would not exhaust the complex poetics of the sound bite, which, media trainers tell us, must be novel, short, gripping, and clear, meaning that you need to embody professional authority and emotional engagement and use a "lay" register. (White coats and medical school office settings help the visuals for television.) What does Schaffner say? "This begins to look like a new influenza virus strain that could do a lot of mischief around the world."[3]

Even as Besser and Schaffner help reinforce Couric's anxious tone and her projection of the actual existence and future threat of H1N1, neither Atlanta (the CDC's location) nor Nashville (where Schaffner teaches) become part of the chronotopic cartography of H1N1 epidemic spaces. The television news "package" rather requires a return to the narrative center of the studio and a conversation between correspondent and anchor taking the form of a split-screen dialogue, a rather fascinating format in which the appearance of a co-performance by two interlocutors is visually, verbally, and acoustically orchestrated by a vast off-camera team. Some participants, like LaPook, perform two performative roles, correspondent and expert. For medicine and public health, this dual role is increasingly played by physician-journalists who serve as medical correspondents or editors for CNN and the three major networks. Jon LaPook is thus not an outside "specialist" but, on camera and in studio, forms part of the *CBS Evening News* team (see figure 9.5). Initially cast as a clinician who lists

H1N1 symptoms and treatment procedures, he shifts to a public health role in urging viewers to monitor their symptoms and see their doctors if they seem flu-like—leaving aside the millions of US residents without health insurance who lack access to "their doctors." The warning about stockpiling antivirals, thereby highlighting what has become a key way of defining "the state" in the biosecurity world, occasions LaPook's shift to an epidemiological role in projecting the course of "this outbreak." His performance points toward rethinking of Bauman's (1977) classic characterization of the relationship between competence and performance. LaPook shifts skillfully between performing his competence as a leading television journalist, even as it requires him to embody his role as a clinician and his ability to project epidemiological futures; foregrounding his status as *Dr.* Jon LaPook helped Couric orchestrate the contribution of his complex performance in mediatizing "the H1N1 pandemic."

LaPook validates the biosecurity regime by echoing Besser's claim that the CDC and WHO have assumed their proper role in producing epidemiological knowledge, which he projects as "very reassuring." A seemingly contradictory message thus juxtaposes the need for "concern" with the emphatic statement that there is "absolutely, positively no reason to panic." Couric's role is crucial. The physician-journalist projects authority and confidence (doctor knows best), but she or he can also lead lay viewers to feel distanced. The anchor thus stands in for us audience members. Note that the information presented that same evening by NBC's chief science correspondent Robert Bazell was much more complex, tracing the genetics of the virus, comparing it to the 1918–1920 pandemic that killed "some 50 million people worldwide" and to other flu viruses, and mentioning vaccine issues and biosecurity plans. Anchor Brian Williams thus takes the role of lay viewers, providing a simplified summary and asking for a commonsense projection of what might come next: "And Bob, for the rest of us, you say this is a new virus, the old shot doesn't protect against this, is this a case of and now we wait?" This "us" projects anchors and audiences as laypersons who may have trouble understanding scientific knowledge. Williams's projection of his role in co-producing the narrative would accordingly seem to cue lay audience member as to how they are being interpellated, a role that Besser projected in his news conference (which, more later).

The swine flu story also introduced other classes of actors. Crowds in Mexico City are captured in images that echo Sandra Hughes's statement "The worried line up for testing, their faces covered with masks." SARS and avian flu had already established this quintessential costume component for influenza epidemics (see figure 9.6), which later became a controversial bodily

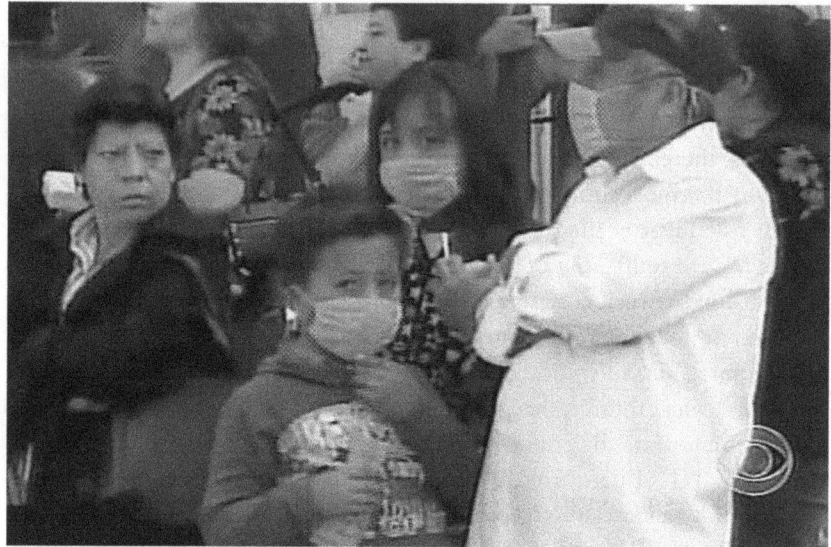

Figure 9.6. Mexican crowd and face masks

focus of the politicization of the COVID-19 pandemic in the United States. These images opened up a role for laypersons as taking precautions and waiting for diagnoses, tests, vaccines, and words of reassurance from governmental health professionals. The assignment of roles in the narrative also crossed species, recruiting pigs to play their part in the swine flu drama (see figure 9.7). NBC recruited a broader nonhuman cast of characters, including chickens, pigs, and viruses (seen through electronic microscope images).

Even as the roles were differentiated between anchor, corresponding journalist, medical editor, clinician, virus researcher, virus, pig, and chicken, a number of features linked their performances. First, a shared leitmotif of the epidemic chronotope was a temporal construction of the virus as "new." Besser suggested in his press conference that the CDC's actions were prompted by "a new influenza virus that has the potential to cause significant human illness." In the CBS story, Couric's "this new strain" was immediately echoed by reporter Hughes: "this strain of flu, never seen before." Medical researcher Schaffner's sound bite ties newness directly to projected global health consequences: it "could do a lot of mischief around the world." The newness trope connects laboratory results, epidemiological information, clinical medicine, vaccines, and immunology, tying people's immune systems to their communicative receptivity. Newness, of course, is also a major factor in determining newsworthiness. Newness brings the distinct temporalization practices of journalism, virology, epidemiology,

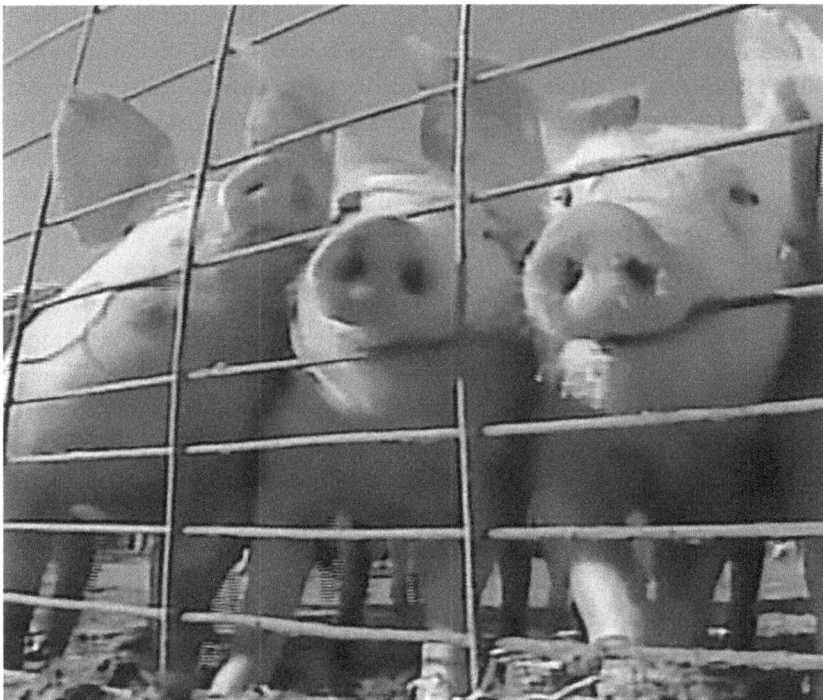

Figure 9.7. Pigs appearing in the CBS broadcast

public health, and clinical medicine into alignment, turning "swine flu" into a boundary-object that fosters translatability and sparks shared "concern."

Second, let us return to communicability, cultural models that project how knowledge about health is produced, circulates, and is received, first discussed in chapter 3. For infectious diseases, the term biocommunicability captures the complex relationships between the circulation of pathogens and discourse. Hughes's segment thus links H1N1 viruses crossing the US-Mexican border with CDC monitoring and her own reporting, validating the latter. A long-standing, widely distributed model projects creation of authoritative knowledge by biomedical professionals in leading hospitals, labs, and public health offices, its circulation by clinicians, health educators, and journalists, and its passive assimilation by lay audiences. The broadcast reinscribed this linear, hierarchically ordered model by projecting a new H1N1 informational circuit. Besser positioned the CDC as having inaugurated a process of producing information, not only in the United States but internationally, augmented by Mexican health officials, the WHO, and other public health agencies; LaPook makes this new communicable cartography explicit and affectively positive.

The CDC promised a continual stream of information through a new website and daily press conferences; Besser noted in the interview with Hallin that he made himself available for each morning and evening national news broadcast and provided a CDC spokesperson in response to each media request. Nevertheless, in the course of remarks delivered at an April 26, 2009, briefing in the White House, Besser warned that the virus was moving faster than biomediatization practices, producing a disjuncture: "Because of this speed in which things are progressing, you will find. . . . some inconsistency and we will work to minimize that."[4] In his April 24 press conference at the CDC, Besser projected this cartography into the future and assigned roles, it seems, to everyone: "I think that's important that people are paying attention to what's going on." President Barak Obama validated this communicable trajectory in a press conference of April 29: "And I think that we have to make sure that we recognize that how we respond—intelligently, systematically, based on science and what public health officials have to say—will determine in large part what happens." I return to the massive gap between the biocommunicable trajectories evident in the Obama administration's H1N1 discourse and that performed by Trump for COVID-19 below.

Third, in a study of the H1N1 pandemic, Theresa MacPhail (2010) stresses a rhetoric of uncertainty by which virologists and epidemiologists placed the unpredictability of the virus at the center of public health planning. Indeed, in their initial H1N1 statements, these performers emphasized the trope of uncertainty. Besser stressed in his CDC press conference, "I want to acknowledge the importance of uncertainty. At the early stages of an outbreak, there's much uncertainty, and probably more than everyone would like. Our guidelines and advice [are] likely to be interim and fluid, subject to change as we learn more." This theme dominated the entirety of the sound bite performed by NBC's expert, Dr. Michael Osterholm of the University of Minnesota, during its April 24, 2009, broadcast: "We really are in a very difficult position right now where we have much more uncertainty than certainty, and unfortunately that uncertainty all bodes poorly if we demonstrate ongoing transmission." This was the bottom line that scientific reporter Bazell gave in answer to the anchor's request for information accessible to "the rest of us": "It's the worst situation for public health, because all you can do is wait." Note that this uncertainty seems to be a natural, inevitable result of the virus's unpredictability.

Finally, affect was thus crucial. The anxious movements of pigs, chickens, and crowds was echoed in the words of professionals. NBC presented another sound bite from Besser's press conference: "This is something we are worried about, and we are treating very seriously." His countenance and body posture echoed the "worried" and "serious" character. Couric's frame for the segment linked the global spread of viruses to the theme of anxiety: "There's growing concern tonight about an outbreak of swine flu right next door in Mexico, concern that it will spread here and around the world." Hughes immediately starts with this theme: "Fear is running high as the death toll rises in Mexico's capital city." Besser later projected this global affective cartography in his remarks at the April 26 White House press briefing: "People around the country and around the globe are concerned with this situation we're seeing, and we're concerned as well." Journalists seemed to justify imbuing their reports with strong affect by projecting it as a reflection of their sources' affective stances, as in NBC anchor Williams's opening statement, "You can tell by the tone of federal officials, what they are saying, on and off the record, that they are concerned about a new strain of flu."

Although this rhetoric framed H1N1 as a quintessentially modern object, we should not be entirely persuaded by claims of newness. Wald (2008) and Lee (2014) examine how the content of "outbreak narratives" is traditionalized as it circulates from epidemic to epidemic, disease to disease, and genre to genre. My interest is particularly in how dimensions of form, ideology, and practice traditionalize these narratives, specifically in the role of traditionalization in the production and the the specific contours of a quintessential modern artifact: the health news story. The formal features of the CBS broadcast were traditionalized using the narrative conventions of television news broadcasts and specifically the genre of medical news stories. Moreover, I would be remiss if I stopped here and did not consider how narrative material moved across time and genre. The NBC broadcast featured shots of laboratory workers in space suits, samples in petri dishes, fancy diagnostic equipment, and heavy doors that seal off spaces containing highly lethal pathogens. Does this sound familiar? News stories replayed what had become a rather stable feature of popular culture, amplified by such bestsellers as Robert Preston's (1994) *The Hot Zone: The Terrifying True Story of the Origins of the Ebola Virus*. The April 24, 2009, newscasts relied on the tropes of fictional filmic narratives: germ thrillers from *The Andromeda Strain* to *Outbreak* to *Contagion* contributed these formal features to the epidemic narrative repertoire. The opening scene of the Hollywood blockbuster *Outbreak* turned these scenes—along with electron microscopic images of viruses and maps projecting the spread of viruses—into central features of popular cultural imaginaries (see figure 9.8). Here scientific performance practices migrate into fiction and then into medical news, thereby shaping responses to epidemics. We have been trained as audience members

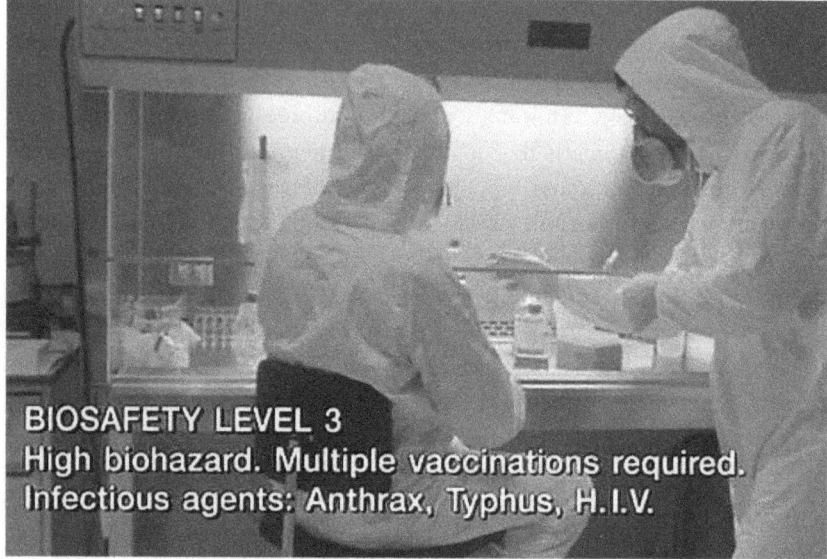

Figure 9.8. Shot of high-security laboratory in opening scenes of *Outbreak*

to respond affectively to the visual, musical, and auditory clues that accompany narratives regarding new epidemics. In these stories, public health officials, researchers, reporters, people in public spaces, and seemingly even pigs and chickens all perform this anxiety.

REHEARSING INFLUENZA

Making the swine flu pandemic story in just twenty-four hours involved a complex set of practices distributed among a range of different professionals and placed into juxtaposition, involving the modes of siting, subjectification, embodiment, objectification, and of the production, circulation, and reception of knowledge that I laid out in chapter 7. Nevertheless, the analysis so far represents only part of the story of the construction of the H1N1 narrative, in that it freezes it in time—as beginning on April 24, 2009—precisely in accord with the temporalization practices that health officials and reporters projected. If we remember Richard Schechner's (1985:36) definition of performance—"never for the first time"—and emphasis by Bauman (2004) on the centrality of rehearsal, then a more powerful account of performing epidemics can emerge.

Dan Hallin and I were able to interview many of the individuals who played a key role in constructing the US "swine flu pandemic" story. One thing that they stressed in reflecting on this coverage, which they considered highly successful, was that it was not their first time participating in influenza outbreaks. They often mentioned work on SARS and avian flu as affording knowledge not only of influenza outbreaks but of interactions between public health agencies, journalists, researchers, and laypersons. And prior to the H1N1 performances lay a powerful set of rehearsals. Besser noted succinctly that "a lot of us had been trained in risk communication," a relatively new realm of public health practice and academic research referred to as "crisis and emergency risk communication," which has become a regular part of training for public health officials in local, state, national, international, and nongovernmental agencies. These performances reflected to a remarkable degree the principles codified in the CDC's *Crisis and Emergency Risk Communication: Pandemic Influenza* manual and the associated course. An extraordinarily elaborate ideological or cultural construction of language, the manual constructs pandemic temporalities and "risks" at least as much in communicative as in clinical and epidemiological terms. A central focus of the manual pertains to projecting affective responses on the part of laypersons and, for public health professionals, "expressing empathy and caring." The unpredictability of viruses requires "uncertainty being experienced" (CDC [2006] 2007:11). Given that "the public hates uncertainty" (17), empathically sharing this affective/biomedical position links health professionals, journalists, researchers, and publics, thereby, according to the manual, engendering calm and trust in officials. Voilá! It comes as small surprise that journalists and health officials made extensive use of the "uncertainty" trope in H1N1 discourse. MacPhail (2010) suggests that virologists and public health officials produced "strategic uncertainty" as a key part of the scientific rationale for their interventions into research and public policies. My analysis suggests not only that uncertainty is a key artifact of the mediatization process but that its rehearsal predated the 2009 pandemic.

Several pieces are still missing. How could a range of professionals have collaborated in producing a story so quickly, one that remained relatively stable? Besser directed the CDC's Emergency Preparedness and Response Division for four years before becoming its acting director. He noted that CDC personnel "had been thinking about pandemics and disasters, you know, all the time." His division had prepared materials to be used in the case of a pandemic; they had to be "modified, because we'd been planning for bird flu, and this was pig flu, but, that's very different from starting with an unknown infection where you may not have materials." Millions of dollars were spent on sponsoring "exercises" or "scenarios" for schools, local governments, state and national agencies, and other entities. Besser continued: "We had also been exercising around pandemic flu for years," and the CDC had given "states and locals . . . money to exercise on flu." These simulations involved military, health, and Homeland Security officials, virologists, clinicians, politicians, a range of other government workers, and journalists, all of whom collaborated in rehearsing performance practices. These efforts involved particular forms of entextualization, of creating discursive and material artifacts meant to be lifted out of these particular contexts and become available for recontextualization. They are embodied in mock news coverage that is produced in advance of the exercises, pieces that bear a remarkable resemblance to what becomes "the real thing." Beyond the participation of journalists in making these mock news bulletins and in the exercises themselves, officials recruit reporters to create stories that turn these simulations into news.

Lakoff suggested that scenario-based exercises promote a preparedness logic that has pervasively shifted thinking about health and security. I would suggest that we might see them as elaborate, sometimes massive rehearsals that permit synchronization of preparedness performance practices. As Besser put it, these exercises enabled the CDC to develop ongoing relationships with "a cadre of really good public health reporters," ones "that were covering the story really well, and we knew would get it right." Besser continued: "We had included reporters from some of the major media outlets in our exercises, so we could get a better sense of what things they'd want to know, what questions we might be hearing. That was very illuminating, and I think it helped us as well." Talk about performer-audience co-production! I would submit that these exercises constituted possibly the most extensive and massively funded rehearsal process in the history of the planet, with the possible exception of civil defense measures for nuclear war, and that what emerged on April 24 was their major debut and was massively consequential. During his news conference, Besser stated that "we still do not have enough information to give us any sense of the extent of spread of this virus, and the illness spectrum is not currently known." Nevertheless, just five days later, on April 29, President Obama declared in a news conference that "I've requested an immediate $1.5 billion in emergency funding from Congress to support our ability to monitor and track this virus and to build our supply of antiviral drugs and other equipment," and more funding was subsequently allocated. This traditionalization-mediatization regime realigned public health priorities and expenditures virtually without scrutiny or debate for a virus that turned out to be less lethal than most seasonal flus.

AUDIENCE RECEPTION, PARODIC AND OTHERWISE

It is worth asking what audiences made of all this. These stories invited performances of public affects and forms of embodiment. Viewers were asked to accept the discursive and biomedical authority of the CDC and other responsible authorities, as relayed through journalists' accounts of press briefings. Laypersons were asked to perform continually their sanitary citizenship (Briggs and Mantini-Briggs 2003), their inclusion in the body politic, through particular actions, which Besser and officials repeated endlessly: "Cover your cough or your sneeze, wash your hands frequently [generally failing to mention the most critical element—soap], and see your doctor if you have fever, cough," and so on. Besser told us that these early days of the epidemic formed "a teachable moment and people can take some action around preparedness," learning about preparedness plans and thinking about what they would do if, for example, their children's school closed. In short, "people" were asked to participate in creating possible futures that health officials and reporters projected; nevertheless, lay efforts were cast as reactive and thus not generally newsworthy. Laypersons did sometimes get to speak in news stories, but their role was usually confined to echoing the affects that journalists and officials modeled for them. To move beyond these spaces through displaying the wrong affects, from panicking to disbelief to contempt, or the wrong behaviors, such as "stockpiling" antivirals or going out in public with a respiratory infection, would seemingly position people as unsanitary subjects (Briggs and Mantini-Briggs 2003) who allow their individual bodies to become threats to the health of the social body and the body politic alike. Efforts at lay knowledge production would constitute threats to scientific logics, part of the irrational responses that, officials often told us, could pose a greater "risk" than the pathogens themselves. As I write these lines, the world is launching another massive global performance, now centered on coronavirus (COVID-19).

It does seem clear that infection rates from the *mediatized* virus were massive. The CDC was interested in the question of reception, so it funded the Harvard School of Public Health to conduct telephone surveys. On April 29, 77 percent of respondents reported that they were "following the news very closely" or "somewhat closely," while 22 percent were paying attention "either not too closely, or not at all." These figures were virtually unchanged on May 6. The comment section of news media, listervs, blogs, internet sites, and social media suggested that widespread circulation often resignified the discourses that officials had tried to prevent, from immigrant and Mexico bashing to conspiracy theories that asserted sinister

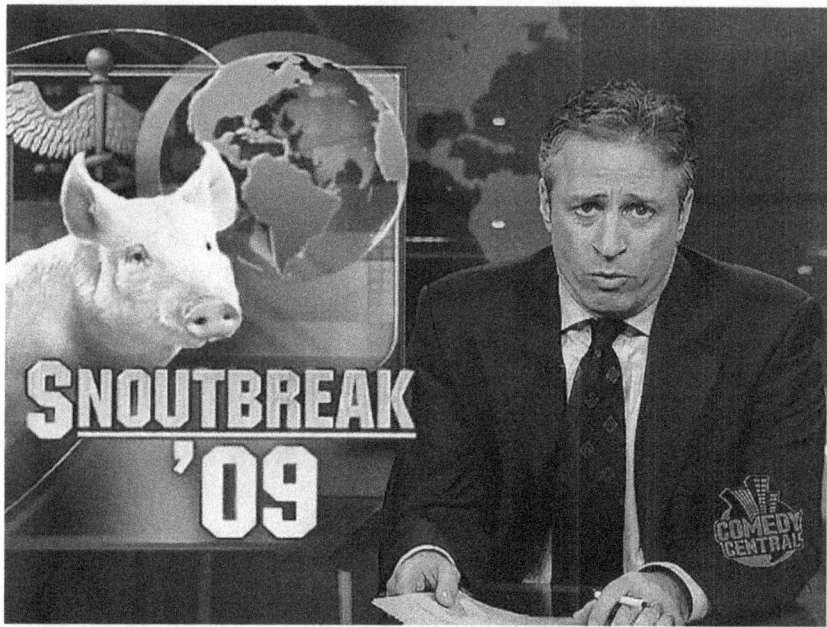

Figure 9.9. Jon Stewart's *The Daily Show* "The Last 100 Days" segment on April 27, 2009

origin stories for the virus, animating counter-performance spheres over social media. As Jon Lee (2014) points out, this interaction between medical discourse, health journalism, legends, and conspiracy theories involves complex relationships between mainstream news and a range of other media forms.

One of the most entertaining and analytically interesting responses emerging within "the mainstream media" came in an April 27, 2009, segment of Jon Stewart's *The Daily Show* (see figure 9.9). Joining two journalistic foci of the day, President Obama first 100 days in office and H1N1, Stewart broadcast a "The Last 100 Days" segment. He used faux reporting, segments from network and cable news broadcasts, and commentary to critically reproduce features I identified above as central to the performative construction of the epidemic. Stewart replayed images of vaccination, viruses, masks, and laboratory scenes with accompanying dramatic music in resignifying their semantic and affective content. He parodied journalists' projection of flu epidemiology in Mexico and the traffic in viruses to the United States, beginning with a news broadcaster voice and morphing into a parodic tone: "Now as you probably know, the outbreak began south of the border in Mexico, where it has claimed 149 lives so far, ranking it last on the list of things that can kill you in Mexico. Number one, of course, still bullet flu, mmm, bullet flu of course an airborne virus in Mexico. Now from what I understand, the virus has been mostly contained in Mexico, so I don't think that anything's coming across that border . . . unless it wants to." This statement crossed the border, as it were, between critiquing and reanimating Mexico bashing.

Continuing that "I haven't looked at the news for about two hours, so let's just see where we're at," Stewart replays maps that track the emergence of cases in US states and other countries, concluding with a map that turns all of Canada red. He interjects: "Uh, I like a good scare as much as the next guy, but for six mild cases of the flu you're going to turn 4 million square miles bright red?" After a few more clips of news coverage, interspersed with growing sarcasm, Stewart mocked affective dimensions of H1N1 coverage. In response to a clip that stated, with the backdrop of a world map, "Swine flu could wipe out tens of millions if it isn't stopped," Stewart responds: "Now that's the [bleep] scariest thing I've heard all week. Well, you've done it, I'm freaking out. Is there anything else you guys wanna add?" Stewart replays *CNN* and *Fox News* segments where journalists, including Anderson Cooper, suggest, "We don't want to freak anyone out." Stewart's sarcasm reaches its apex as he responds, "Do you even watch your own networks? You're the only reason we are freaking out!"

At the same time that Stewart and I focus on the same performative tropes, our analyses diverge. The second-person plural he uses pins the blame on mainstream journalists: "Do *you* even watch *your own* networks? *You're* the only reason *we* are freaking out!" (my emphasis). Journalists are branded as both creating fear and pretending to curtail it. What I have demonstrated, however, is that this contradiction is not the product of bad journalism but a foundational feature of preparedness performances, which are co-created by media and health professionals through training and exercises. The airborne bullet virus segment similarly faulted journalists for failing to accurately portray epidemiological patterns. Medical anthropologist Eduardo Menéndez criticized the Mexican press on the same point (Menéndez and Di Pardo 2009). The premise here is that the distribution and content of health news stories *should* perfectly match the distribution of causes of disease and death, morbidity and mortality. Stewart's critiques constituted responses to mainstream media that preserved their discursive borders; in suggesting that journalists had crossed the boundary between science and storytelling, his critique actually further reified this border and the subordinate status of journalists in public discourse about health.

But did the journalists get it wrong? Besser's press conference of April 24 deliberately sparked massive press coverage at a time when there were only eight US cases, none fatal. He suggested during our interview: "You only have one chance to get ahead of a new outbreak. You're going to start out very aggressive, and then only back off when you know it's safe to back off." Producing a mismatch between epidemiology and mediatization was thus intentional, a core feature of crisis and emergency communication strategies and therefore of preparedness. In comment sections of media websites, listervs, internet sites, and social media, critiques often portrayed boundaries between public health officials and journalists as illusory, as staged for political reasons. Once the focus of attention for both public health officials and journalists shifted in August to vaccines, both initial shortages of projected vaccine supplies (and thus "rationing") and the anti-vax networks opened up greater room for critical engagement with public health/journalistic performances. NBC's embedded physician, Dr. Nancy Snyderman, became a major focus of anti-vax tweets, listervs, and internet memes when she exhorted viewers on MSNBC's Morning Meeting on August 25, 2009, "This is one time, forget the conspiracy, listen to our government agencies, these guys are telling the truth. You know, there's no conspiracy here folks: just get your damn vaccine!" Social media replayed her statement over and over, turning her into a cartoon villain laughing at an unsuspecting populace.

CONCLUSION

My goal has been to portray the overnight production of the "swine flu pandemic" narrative as an example of traditionalization. Indeed, otherwise it would have been difficult to achieve the same degree of coordination and effectiveness so expeditiously. The visual, textual, and auditory poetics of the television news broadcast provided a means of empowering a master space of narration that nevertheless—given journalistic ideologies—purportedly did not create events but only "reported" them. These features allowed the story to seem to gush forth from the very spaces in which it was unfolding, the broadcast's narrative sequence mirroring the movement of dangerous pathogens. The specific subgenre, that of medical stories, made room for poetic performances of "sound bites" by mediatization-savvy "experts" and press briefings by health officials, designed precisely to reliably fill particular slots in the narrative, echoing the plot elements and affective projections of journalists in seemingly objective and authoritative voices.

Bauman and Briggs (1990) suggested that intertextuality looms large in strategies of traditionalization, projecting implicit or explicit relationships between formal, ideological, and/or practice features of unfolding events in relation to what are cast as prior acts. NBC linked the unfolding "swine flu" story to the nightmare narrative of "what happened in 1918," when the Spanish flu killed "some 50 million people worldwide," adding black-and-white photos of skeleton-like patients and rows of white crosses. Donald McNeil's April 24, 2009, *The New York Times* story (published in print the following morning) went further, invoking 1918, 1957, and 1968 H1N1 epidemics as well as 2003 Canadian SARS cases. Thus, even as the virus was constructed as new, about a present that was erupting into a frightening future, the "swine flu pandemic" narrative was positioned vis-à-vis a long trajectory of influenza horror stories. Projecting intertextuality forward, the April 24 stories set a pattern that followed in stories emerging nearly every day across media platforms, including some three to five stories daily in *The New York Times*, incrementally adding statistics on cases and deaths, maps showing the "spread" of the disease, statements of uncertainty and often alarm, official pronouncements on unfolding public health measures, and ubiquitous exhortations to wash your hands and stay home when sick. Thus, in formal terms, the H1N1 story, like other epidemic narratives, was highly traditionalized from the start. Its features provided affordances that, like a good fairytale, invited patterned sets of expectations and responses, ways of constructing subjects and objects, and patterns of affective engagement. The productivity of epidemic traditionalization has been extended to narratives of teen pregnancy, obesity, diabetes, and opioid addiction, among others. As work by Paula Treichler (1999), Priscilla Wald (2008), Briggs and Mantini-Briggs (2003), and others suggests, "contagion narratives" that emerge in multiple sites and genres have become so traditionalized that they powerfully shape what counts as a health-related event, how it is interpreted, what kinds of embodied responses it engenders, and the forms of knowledge, ignorance—and, often, stigma—it produces. My discussion of H1N1 suggests that unlearning powerful presuppositions regarding how these narratives are made and circulate requires going beyond textual analysis of narrative content (1) to examine their complex formal features and (2) to conduct ethnography as a means of seeing how widely dispersed and distinct actors, sites, and logics are pragmatically entwined, even as they get ideologically portrayed as separate and often opposing.

To be sure, other folklorists have examined traditionalization in relationship to journalism. Jan Brunvand (1981) created a cottage industry tracing how legends become news, their traditionalization beguiling journalists to construe them as events. Noting that "to date, the newspaper has proven problematic for the folklorist," Elliott Oring (2012:102) points to nine features that make newspapers "seem to be the very antithesis of folklore." Examining relationships between legends and newspaper stories, he suggests that the worldviews of folklorists more closely correspond to those of journalists than to people who circulate legends, thereby shaping the pejorative frame of disbelief that surrounds scholarship on legends. Russell Frank (2011) explores "newslore," folklore that emerges in dialogue with but outside journalism. Similarly, a robust body of literature focuses on medicine and health. Diane Goldstein (2004) has explored multiple ways that folk and biomedical understandings intersect, including in legends and health communication surrounding HIV/AIDS. Andrea Kitta (2012) brought a folklorist's perspective to pro- and anti-vaccine controversies. Briggs and Mantini-Briggs (2003, 2016), Farmer (1992), and others explore how epidemic narratives created by journalists and health officials can construct powerful stereotypes and turn them into foundations for official policies and practices.

I would like to suggest that scholars interested in traditionalization need to attend to processes of mediatization as well. Even as the H1N1 story relied on traditionalization, it also required ongoing processes of mediatization widely dispersed between sites (laboratories, public health offices, security and emergency preparedness agencies, clinicians, and living rooms, as well as newsrooms) that entangled what are supposed to be separate and sometimes opposed logics and forms of professional training (medical, public health, military, political, corporate, and lay, as well as journalistic). I have not argued here that these domains have merged. Indeed, the success of health news depends on producing the illusion that domains, perspectives, and practices are bounded and separate, as signaled by anchor Brian Williams's positioning of "the rest of us" outside the scientific realm and Stewart's "You're the only reason we are freaking out!," which place audiences outside of preparedness performance practices.

Drawing on the frameworks outlined in chapters 7 and 8, I have tried to extend calls to muster perspectives on poetics and performance in offering interventions into public debates, upsetting commonsense concepts and narratives. Going beyond the unpreparedness literature would suggest that reducing these complex phenomena to the emergence of a pervasive new logic is not enough: narrativity, poetics, and performance are as important as "preparedness" is created anew with the production of each poetically and affectively charged sound bite, in each performance—whether in a scenario-based exercise, a press conference, a television studio, a policy discussion, a media training, or on social media—and in each act of weaving them together. Thinking about performance requires reflecting on rehearsal, requiring the sort of extended and dispersed fieldwork that Hallin and I conducted on H1N1. Given that new epidemics are deeply imbricated with new communicative technologies and practices of "mining" them, we can learn a lot about performance/technologies connections by unraveling them.

We might return here to Taylor's distinction between the archive and the repertoire and her notion of "the DNA of performance." If we put the science in the archive and the performance in political, nonscientific practice, folklorists will be locked out of the relatively prestigious status of second-order observers of first-order scientific observers, which is not to say that this is the only space they should occupy. How "new" pandemics are framed, experienced, and woven into ongoing health inequities, the emergence of "new" diseases, cures, and pills, and how dollars for research, prevention, and treatment are allocated are all tied up with traditionalized/mediatized performances. The co-production of scientific/mediatized objects takes place not just "in the media" but in clinics, labs, governmental and non-governmental agencies, and clicks on computers and cell phones. If scholars of poetics and performance sell themselves as the owners of domains of vernacular misunderstandings or popular reworkings of scientific objects, they will remain not second but nth-order observers, so far downstream that they can only make weak claims on the flotsam and jetsam of the prestige, authority, and funding that seem to lie at the supposed source. If, on the other hand, folklorists, anthropologists, performance studies scholars, and other researchers demonstrate a unique ability to look critically and ethnographically at the performative practices through which new objects and subjects get made, they can demonstrate that rethinking the traditionalization of new objects can be just as revealing as new takes on what are traditionalized as old objects.

In this chapter, I have endeavored to provide a concrete illustration of the hard work of unlearning—analytic and ethnographic—that is required. I have joined Diane Goldstein and others in pushing folklorists to look beyond clinical medicine to include public health, going on to suggest that exploring dispersed practices of mediatization is also required to question the politics of knowledge that shape how projections of biomedical knowledge and popular misunderstanding get made, naturalized, and questioned. I might add that this border is being critically scrutinized both by racialized populations seeking to expose and uproot multiple forms of racist violence on nonwhite bodies and by politicians, mediatizers, and armed (re)producers of anti-science and anti-vaccination "conspiracy theories." Accordingly, developing new perspectives on precarious ways that bodies, diseases, cultural forms, knowledge claims, and demands for justice intersect constitutes a major and necessary contribution to efforts to prevent more pandemics, more lethal inequities, and more undemocratic futures.

CODA: COVID-19 AND THE REJECTION OF PANDEMIC PERFORMANCE

To what extent did these performance practices shape US government responses to the COVID-19 pandemic as it began during the Donald Trump presidency? Now the H1N1 visual poetics of the facemask have, as in the 2014 Ebola epidemic, been complemented by full-body protective gear. The same narrative chronotope drove daily narratives as readers and viewers watched maps, charts, and specialists track COVID-19's geographic "spread" and escalating numbers of cases and deaths. Some remarkable differences were, however, strikingly apparent. Rather than telegenic Besser, the CDC was led by Robert Redfield, who seems uncomfortable with journalists; on-camera press conferences with the director were replaced by telephone conference calls with subordinate officials. In contrast, Trump appeared on numerous occasions in press briefings on COVID-19, which would seem to suggest that he assimilated the CDC's Crisis and Emergency Risk Communication performance practices.

Nothing could be further from the truth. CDC "crisis and emergency risk communication" guidelines recommend that officials "don't over reassure," "acknowledge uncertainty," and "acknowledge people's fears." After putting aside warnings for over more than two months that extensive preventive measures would be required, Trump offered reassurance: "Take it easy. Just relax. . . . Relax, we're doing great. It all will pass."[5] Rather than performing the cautious script crafted by governmental health and media officials, Trump performed his intuitions that a vaccine would soon emerge and that the Food and Drug Administration had approved chloroquine for use with COVID-19 patients, prompting Anthony Fauci, director of the National Institute of Allergy and Infectious Diseases, to correct him in several news conferences. Journalists, who had long participated in the coproduction of pandemic discourse, persistently decried Trump's departure from biosecurity performance practices: "President Donald Trump just can't stop contradicting his own public health experts on the coronavirus outbreak" (see Lopez 2020). As the United States surpassed all other countries in COVID-19 cases and deaths, Trump's spirited rejection of public health measures and performance practices helped prompt the failure of his reelection campaign in 2020.

NOTES

1. Hallin and I published a book entitled *Making Health Public* that contains a chapter on the H1N1 pandemic (Briggs and Hallin 2016). This analysis focuses on different stories and raises a distinct set of issues concerning the relationship between traditionalization and mediatization.

2. For a transcript of the press conference, see https://www.cdc.gov/media/transcripts/2009/t090424.htm.

3. Schaffner's Vanderbilt University website states that "Dr. Schaffner is committed to communicating about medicine to the general public. He regards this as a teaching opportunity. As such, he often is invited to comment in local and national media on communicable disease issues, translating research advances and public health events into language that the public can understand" (https://www.vumc.org/health-policy/person/william-schaffner-md).

4. For a transcript, see https://obamawhitehouse.archives.gov/realitycheck/the_press_office/Press-Briefing-On-Swine-Influenza-4/26/09.

5. For a transcript of this conference see Rev 2020.

10

From Progressive Extractivism to Phyto-Socialism
Trees, Bodies, and Discrepant Phytocommunicabilities in a Mysterious Epidemic

IN THIS CHAPTER, I CONNECT MICHAEL MARDER'S (2013) thoughtful book *Plant-Thinking* and a mysterious epidemic in a rainforest of eastern Venezuela. I bring them into dialogue through the notion of phytocommunicabilities, ways that plants, humans, and other species produce and exchange knowledge and materialities (see Schulthies 2019). My goal is neither to use Marder to explain rather inexplicable deaths nor to provide an empirical supplement to his philosophical reflections. Rather, diverse means by which residents attempted to figure out what was killing scores of children and young adults critiqued dominant understandings of plant-human entanglements at the same time that they complicated projections of totalizing contrasts between opposing ontologies by revealing how multiple, heterogeneous modes of plant-thinking and plant practices emerged. I explore how residents turned a debate about plant-human–other nonhuman relations into a political project designed to transform the Bolivarian socialist revolution by placing human-plant relations at its center, proposing what I will refer to as phyto-socialism. This example rethinks how "progressive extractivist" (Gudynas 2012) policies of left governments in Latin America—their continued reliance on capitalist exploitation of nonrenewable resources—have sparked clashes with Indigenous populations. Exploring competing ways that phytocommunicabilities were mobilized in tracing mysterious and fatal connections between trees, bats, chickens, sawmills, houses, healers, and pathogens can spark new insights into these complex philosophical, political, environmental, and ethnographic issues.

Marder argues that "the figure of the plant (which, like a weed, incarnates everything the metaphysical tradition has discarded as improper, superficial, inessential, and purely exterior) furnishes the prototype for post-metaphysical being. Plants are the weeds of metaphysics: devalued, unwanted in its carefully cultivated garden, yet growing in-between the classical categories of the thing, the animal, and the human" (2013:90). Rather than simply critiquing the philosophical marginalization of plants, Marder reflects on the productive quality of plant lives in stimulating new ways of thinking that are noncognitive, nonideational, nonimagistic. Commenting on Aquinas, Marder notes that "to get in touch with the existence of plants one must acquire a taste for the concealed and the withdrawn, including the various meanings of this existence that are equally elusive and inexhaustible" (28). Bringing plants into the picture thus challenges metaphysical assumptions by expanding understandings of embodiment, consciousness, and agency. In concert with anthropologists, Marder suggests that plant-thinking helps us avoid linear and teleological pitfalls. Respecting each plant's unique existence, he argues, can overcome the foundational reduction of individual plants to species, a "cognitive plucking" of abstract qualities embodied in a name and a location in a global taxonomy (5). This last point can contribute to work that goes beyond deconstructing taxonomy to explore the complex ways that notions of species are produced, deployed, and challenged and better equip us to exploit multiple ways of attending closely to particular nonhumans, humans, and their interactions (see Goldstein 2019; Haraway 2008; Hartigan 2017). Marder opens up more wiggle room within what Eduardo Viveiros de Castro (2004) calls "Western naturalism" by finding philosophical places where plants have grown within Eurocentric perspectives, thereby helping us reconfigure established analytics.

Thorny philosophical problems remain, and ethnography has much to offer in addressing them. For Marder, "plant-thinking" turns plants into an external point of reference whose immanent characteristics provide the basis for destabilizing and reconfiguring human thinking. Marder characterized plants as "bereft of interiority" and argued that plants "are voiceless and consequently cannot address the other." Except for ways that wind and other elements act on them, "the silence of vegetation is unbreakable and absolute" (2013:73, 74). The "insurmountable resistance" offered by "the muteness of plants" (75) requires a philosophical approach designed to leave plants in "profound obscurity," to allow "plants to flourish on the edge or at the limit of phenomenality, of visibility, and, in some sense, of 'the world'" (9). There is a deep conundrum here. Using terms like *muteness*, *silence*, *voiceless*, and *address* to characterize what seem to be intrinsic properties of plants projects three centuries of dominant ideological or cultural constructions of human language and communication on plants. This *phytocommunicable anthropomorphism* seems so absolute that Marder circumvents his own call to attend to each plant's particular existence by evoking a single phytocommunicability that applies across species. Having used highly Eurocentric ideas about human communication to project the immanent properties of plants, Marder positions this phytocommunicable construction as a basis for rethinking human thought. Anthropologists have spent a lot of time critiquing Eurocentric constructions of human language and communication (Bauman and Briggs 2003; Keane 2007) and documenting other conceptions historically and ethnographically (Schieffelin, Woolard, and Kroskrity 1998; Kroskrity 2000). Ethnographic explorations of discrepant phytocommunicabilities hold great potential for deepening the plant turn in scholarly research and popular practice, for rethinking human-plant relations from multiple, including decolonial perspectives, and for challenging the anthropocentrism of work on language ideologies (but see Pennycook 2018).

Marder (2013:22) privileges sites where plants proliferate "in the density of the jungle," where vegetal life reaches such a saturation that its exuberance overwhelms conceptual categories and modes of explanation. The philosophical challenges presented by the Delta Amacuro rainforest are particularly interesting for two reasons. First, residents do not presume—as Marder suggests—that plants are wholly other to humans, that "we fail to detect the slightest resemblances to our life in them" (3); they rather project a history of interrelatedness and intimacy, one that continues to shape plant-human encounters. Second, rather than viewing plants through critical engagement with Eurocentric genealogies extending from the Greeks to Derrida, as does Marder (2013, 2014), or becoming incarcerated within ontologically isolated worlds of cultural difference, as anthropologists sometimes suggest, Delta residents' efforts to situate phytocommunicabilities as crucial battlefronts in an ongoing history of colonialism holds out possibilities for seeing how plants challenge oppositions between "Western naturalist" and "Amerindian perspectivalist" (Viveiros de Castro 2004) perspectives. Even as Venezuela's Bolivarian socialist revolution is once again threatened by internal and external forces exploiting its fundamental political-economic contradictions, Delta residents' imaginative program for transforming the revolution's naturalcultural base—fashioned even as they tried to figure out what was killing them—has much to teach us all about crafting ways of thinking and acting to save a dying planet.

CONTRACTORS, HOUSES, AND AN EPIDEMIC

In the Delta Amacuro rainforest of eastern Venezuela, most residents are classified as "indigenous members of the Warao ethnic group." The landscape does not fit a category of pristine nature: naturalcultural relations were shaped over centuries by harvesting palm trees, swidden farming, rubber tapping, missionization, logging, and palm heart extraction (Heinen and Gassón 2006). Muaina was carved out of the jungle on a small coastal island. As I suggested in my letter to Dr. Freud, before Hugo Chávez Frías became president, Muaina was founded by a leader of Venezuela's Indigenous social movement, Librado Moraleda. Endowed with charisma and remarkable intelligence, Librado joined the Movement toward Socialism Party as an adolescent and fashioned Muaina as an experimental design to create an Indigenous socialism that placed plants at its center. A century after rubber tappers brutally exploited trees and labor in the Delta (Heinen 1988), Librado spearheaded efforts to outlaw politically powerful palm heart factories and sawmills, arguing that they damaged the rainforest and brutally exploited workers. Remarkably, he succeeded. A book he wrote in the Warao language contained a chapter tracing the history of non-Indigenous exploitation of the Delta's environment and residents and the suppression of protest (Escalante and Moraleda 1992). A teacher, he entwined botany and local gardening techniques in the Muaina school's curriculum; in James Clifford's (2004b) words, he was building traditional futures.

As has been extensively documented, Chávez launched a "pink revolution" in Latin America, challenging decades of neoliberal policies that eroded public infrastructures and exacerbated social inequality (see Ellner 2014). Building on social movements and organizations formed long before Chávez took power (see Briggs and Mantini-Briggs 2009; Ciccariello-Maher 2013; Velasco 2015), a key focus was countering the marginalization of low-income and Indigenous populations through redistribution of political power and state income derived from exploiting oil, gas, and other "natural resources." After becoming president in 1999, Chávez counted on Librado's voice in shaping pro-Indigenous policies of the Bolivarian revolution and provided Muaina with material support. Librado obtained a grant to support experiments in blending traditional and modern horticultural practices; he chose Indalesio Pizarro, a healer who could talk to plants, to coordinate it (see figure 6.2, page 166). Knowing that he would soon die from cancer, Librado chose Mamerto, Indalesio's son (see figure 6.3), to become his successor, arranging for him to study at the Indigenous University of Venezuela, whose goal was similarly to forge traditional—and anti-racist—futures. When Librado died in 2006, his wife Olga became

Muaina's leader, a rarity in the lower Delta's male-dominated politics. Chávez's government allocated funds to build houses for Muaina residents designed to look like those of working-class Venezuelans on the mainland. Contractors brought stacks of particleboard to use for interior walls and a sawmill to produce boards for window and door frames, siding, vertical beams, flooring, horizontal supports for floors, and support beams for roofs. They hired Muaina youths to fell trees in the dense forest, haul them to Muaina, and mill boards. Mamerto was taking time off from his studies, and they employed him, along with younger brother Melvi.

Here we have a classic example of what Eduardo Gudynas (2012) refers to as "progressive extractivism." With reference to pre-Chávez eras, Fernando Coronil (1997) traced the centrality of oil in Venezuela, which provided not only the driving force of the economy but fundamental understandings of a petro-state and petro-citizens whose individual aspirations and collective identities were predicated on their relationship to what was imagined as the country's natural, oil-producing body. In the 1980s and 1990s, extractivism was inflected by privatization and austerity policies that undermined health and educational services and augmented social inequality. Chávez's election as Venezuela's president preserved extractivism, the massive exploitation of nonrenewable resources to generate revenues for state coffers, as the country's economic base but redistributed it in such a way as to favor low-income sectors. As later occurred in Bolivia and Ecuador, nationalizing oil and gas reserves resulted less in expelling foreign corporations than in renegotiating contracts on more favorable terms. Luís Angosto-Ferrández (2019:204) suggests that the central role of the commodification and instrumentalization of nature through extractivism continues to be "an organizing principle for social life" in Venezuela's Bolivarian revolution.

In all three countries, Indigenous populations formed bases of political support and constituted symbolic centers for socialist calls for justice. Continuing a trend initiated by "neoliberal" governments, such as in Colombia, new constitutions guaranteed political, territorial, and cultural rights to Indigenous populations. The Bolivian and Ecuadoran constitutions incorporated an Indigenous concept, *sumak kawsay*, which can be translated as "life in plentitude," as a basic principle, one that imbued the earth, the environment, animals, and plants with rights and envisioned harmonious, nonexploitative human-nonhuman relations. Nevertheless, progressive extractivist policies have largely sparked the rejection and sometimes suppression of Indigenous efforts to protect lands. Even Evo Morales's government often framed Indigenous environmental protests as naive efforts to undermine resource extraction and thus the collective good. Scholars have depicted Indigenous social movements and socialist governments as opposing forces, concluding that pro-Indigenous ideologies ironically legitimized oppressive practices with deep colonial roots (Anthias 2018; Hindery 2013; Postero 2017; Sawyer and Gomez 2012; Velásquez 2018). What unfolded in Muaina extends and complicates these debates.

Extraction per se was not centrally at issue in Muaina. Some of Venezuela's oil reserves, reportedly the largest in the world, lie in the Delta. Smaller fields in the northwest corner—the opposite side of the Delta from Muaina—have been exploited for decades, but exploration projects have not led to massive drilling in this ecologically sensitive region. Nor did the contractors clear-cut swaths of the rainforest for commercial exploitation; they, rather, selectively cut trees to produce boards for Muaina houses. Residents did not object to harvesting trees per se; they, too, fell trees to make houses. Their critical engagement with the contractors rather focused on issues of design and ways of interacting with trees to be cut.

Constructing houses in Muaina involves sinking beams into the mud and water and building log frames supporting palm roofs (figure 10.1). People sleep in hammocks slung from roof supports. What is crucial is that houses are open, allowing the breeze to blow through in a tropical environment; an exterior wall is often fitted with *temiche* palms on one or two sides to keep out rain. This design also facilitates staying in touch with neighbors and people in nearby settlements, seeing them go to their gardens, get firewood, and travel to the clinic or town. A simple gesture can bring a boat to shore if you want to ask for a ride. Open houses permit observation of government officials, doctors and nurses, contraband smugglers, mobile merchants, and the occasional anthropologist. Open houses afford interactions with the surrounding forest, including the plants, birds, and animals next to houses and in the dense forest behind. But the contractors built fully enclosed houses using boards produced by the sawmill for exterior walls and roofs and particleboard for internal walls (figure 10.2, page 270). Particleboard in a rainforest? Olga showed us where particleboards were decaying and mold grew inside still unfinished homes. "We told them that they wouldn't work, that they would fall apart, and that we couldn't live in houses like these, but they didn't listen."

Beyond arguing that the houses would be leaky and unbearably hot and would disintegrate rapidly, Muainans' objections more broadly questioned political and philosophical dimensions of the contractors' design. Keith Murphy (2015:32) uses theories of materiality, actor network theory, and semiotics to suggest that design is a "process, an active, almost teleological

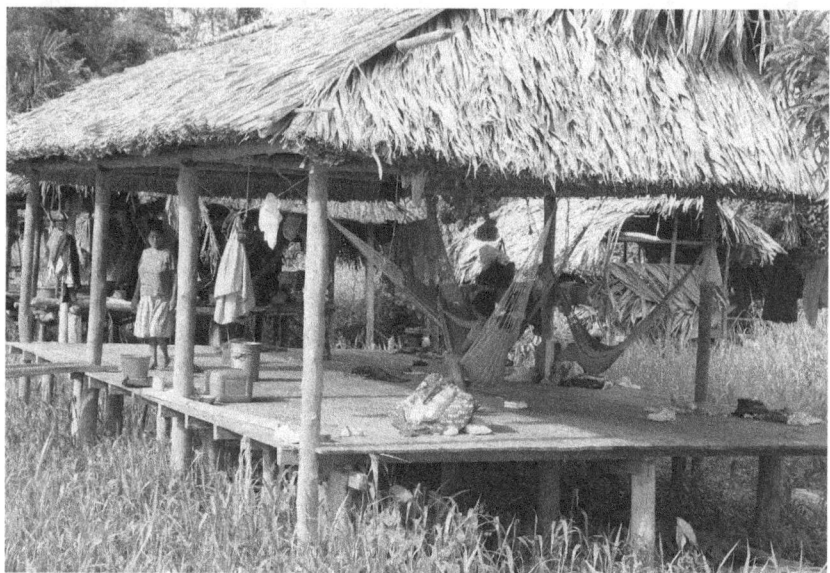

Figure 10.1. A Delta house

ordering of raw materials into some resultant thing" to produce "an intentional structuring of some portion of the lived world in such a way as to transform how it is used, perceived, or understood." Trees, both milled and pressed into boards on the mainland, would reshape people's identities. *Namubaka*, a person who lives in an enclosed house, is a derogatory term for a *criollo*, "a nonindigenous person." The felled trees would reshape the collective sensorium, the interlocking of senses across houses, transforming relations between people and other species.

SEX AND VIOLENCE IN PLANT-HUMAN RELATIONS: A MYTHIC HISTORIOGRAPHY

I do not want to suggest that this was only a dispute between humans centering on competing designs for exploiting plants. A clue that more complex human-plant relations were at stake emerged when Mamerto and Melvi asked the contractors to hire an older man "who knows the forest better." The person they had in mind was their father, Indalesio. The engineer refused, arguing that the young men knew the forest well. Indeed, they had spent years traveling up and down the rivers and walking through the forest, learning the names of species and their characteristics and getting to know the particular trees and other plants that guided travelers through

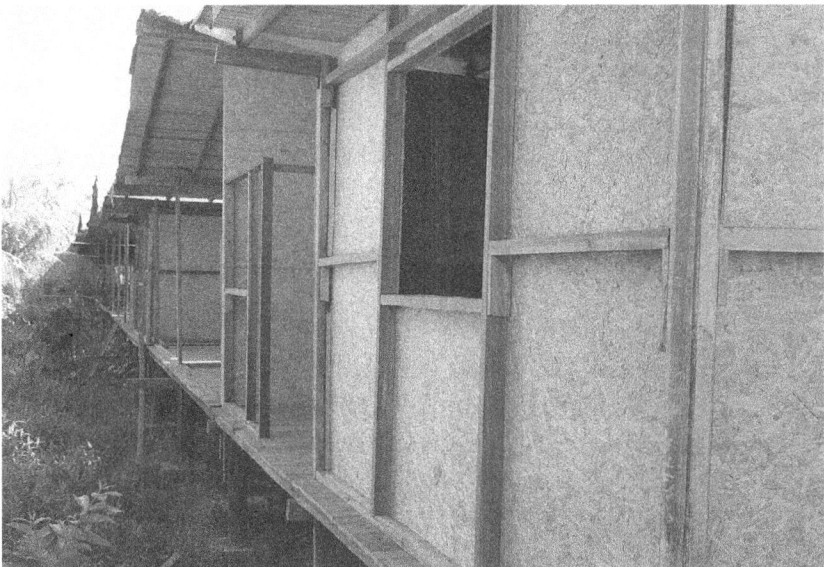

Figure 10.2. Houses built by the contractor in Muaina, unfinished but already decaying

mazes of small rivers and provided materials for hammocks, baskets, food, medicines, housing, and canoes. Mamerto and Melvi knew that their father, as a healer, had access to another type of phytocommunicability: he could access a deep history of human-plant intimacies that revealed how each were relationally constituted. Here the argument needs to move into a different register, a mythic one.

In June 1987, I was living with another remarkable individual, Santiago Rivera, in Mariusa, an area without stores, missions, or schools. Mariusans did not practice horticulture or Christianity, moved seasonally between forests and coastlines, spent months in moriche groves harvesting palm starch, and enacted an annual festival that uses plant power to prevent disease outbreaks. Santiago was largely monolingual in Warao. A master myth performer and builder of canoes, he was recognized as a powerful hoarotu healer and a fearless leader who challenged exploitation at the hands of politicians, bureaucrats, and business owners. He was one of the first of hundreds of Delta residents to die in the 1992–1993 cholera outbreak (Briggs and Mantini-Briggs 2003). Santiago often devoted nights to sitting around the fire with his sons and sons-in-law: gossiping, making plans, and teaching myths.[1] Santiago also instructed them on building canoes, so one night he told the myth of Daunarani, Mother of the Forest, which includes an account of the creation of the first canoe.

Long ago, before we existed, there were two women, sisters. They went off into the forest and found a moriche palm, cut it down, and began extracting its starch. As it was getting late, they returned home. When they came back the next morning, the starch had been extracted and was lying there, ready for consumption. When these events happened repeatedly, the women remained after dark to observe. A leaf from a neighboring palm reached down until it touched the cut that the women had made in the felled moriche trunk. The sisters ran over, grabbed the branch, and begged it to turn into a man; after much pleading, it did. The women married him, and the younger sister bore a son named Haburi.

One day a spirit found the man hunting in the forest, killed him, roasted his body, assumed his human form, and entered the women's home late that night. Throwing the roasted husband in front of them, he climbed into the man's hammock, telling the women to bring him his son. Looking at the meat, they recognized it as their husband's corpse: his penis lay on top. The women found a log that was about the child's size, placed it in the hammock, and fled with Haburi. Soon they could hear the spirit coming behind them. To slow his progress, one woman plucked a pubic hair, threw it in the path, and said, "You will become thorns." When the spirit grew near again, the other plucked a pubic hair, saying, "You will become knives."

The spirit was catching up, so they appealed to Frog, a medicine woman. Hearing Haburi cry, she let them enter her home. When the spirit demanded to see the women, Frog took a machete and killed him. Frog promised to watch Haburi while the women gathered tubers in the garden, but then stretched him, turning Haburi into a young man. Frog gave him a flute, bow, and arrow; he suddenly grew proficient. When the women returned, they found the handsome young man seductively playing the flute, but their child was missing. Frog tricked Haburi into thinking that she was his mother. Failing to recognize him, the two women had sexual relations with him. One day his uncles, the water-dogs, scolded Haburi, revealing Frog's trick. Returning home, Haburi told the women what had happened. Frog was furious. Trying to devise a means of escape, Haburi attempted to construct the first canoe; because he was using the wrong materials, each vessel sank. Eventually he used red and white *cachicamo* respectively for the canoe and the paddle. After the three escaped, the canoe was thrice transformed, first becoming a giant snake-woman, then the red cacichamo tree, then Daunarani, Mother of the Forest, who controls the spirits of all plants and possesses extensive powers (see Wilbert 2001).

Here trees, canoes, and humans come into being in mutually constitutive ways. Building a canoe enabled humans to escape a world dominated by dangerous, shape-shifting spirits and primordial scenes of incest. Humans become deeply identified with their canoes, virtually the only source of mobility in a region consisting of rivers and swamps. Daunarani, who imbues plants with agency and what we would call spirituality, emerges from Haburi's act of transforming trees into a canoe.[2] In other versions, Daunarani is heralded as the first wisidatu healer.

This diachronicity of plant-human relations is reenacted as a man becomes a builder of canoes, a *moyotu* (see figure 10.3). As Johannes Wilbert (1976) details, rigorous moyotu training takes the form of courting Daunarani and her daughters and involves sexual abstinence, tobacco smoke, fasting, and a dream journey to Daunarani's home via a giant snake, whose dangerous body provides the apprentice with a feel, literally, for the proper proportions of canoes. Building a large canoe requires particular forms of phytocommunicability. Craftsmen engage wisidatu healers to request Daunarani's permission to marry one of her daughters, a cacichamo tree. The two men approach the tree to see if the moyotu is pleasing to her; like a suitor, he adorns his body and serenades her with a conch trumpet. If she agrees, he promises to give her tobacco smoke and moriche starch to ease the violent transformation. Chanting becomes a communicable circuit that links the voices of builder and tree-woman in a sexualized exchange. Rain falling during this period is Daunarani's tears for the tree-woman (Wilbert 1996:73). A dream announces the arrival of the sky-snake, who inspects the work and demands moriche starch and tobacco. If the builder neglects any detail, children may die. Kathleen Barlow's and David Lipset's (1997) work in New Guinea suggests that Delta residents are not alone among peoples who rely centrally on dugout canoes in casting harvesting trees and converting them into canoes as primordial sites for crafting notions of gender and sexuality.

The myth and canoe-construction practices informed the workers' request for Indalesio's assistance. He could prepare a sort of environmental impact statement by asking Daunarani and her daughters for permission to harvest trees. Having managed Librado's horticultural project, he would have been the perfect translator between discrepant registers of plant-human relations. Denied his assistance, Mamerto and Malvi cut trees without asking permission. Then, in the middle of the project, Mamerto, his little brother Dalvi, and a cousin died from a mysterious disease, along with thirty-five people in other communities. The goal of my July 28, 2008, visit to Muaina was thus epidemiology, not ethnography: I was collaborating with Librado's brothers Conrado and Enrique, healer Tirso Gómez, nurse Norbelys Gómez, and Venezuelan physician Clara Mantini-Briggs in diagnosing a disease that

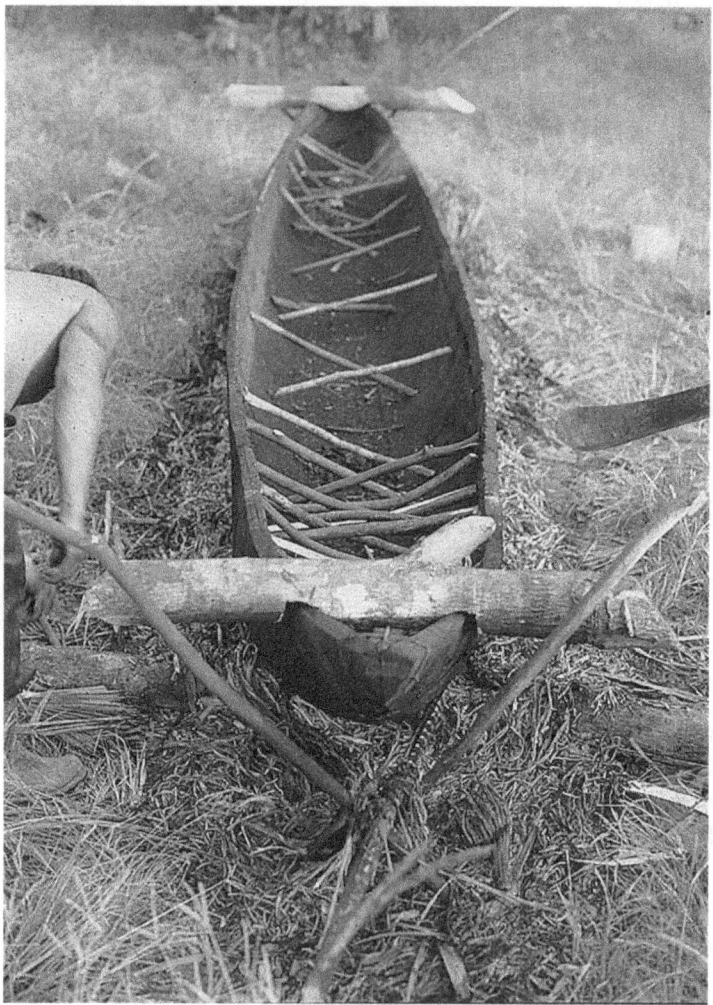

Figure 10.3. A dugout canoe under construction

had stumped clinicians and epidemiologists for a year.[3] Parents and other residents joined us in a meeting, held over the sounds of the sawmill and laments being performed for Mamerto, collectively searching for clues. Witnesses repeatedly spoke about the contractors, houses, and felled trees. No one voiced a simple, mechanical, cause-and-effect relation—that cutting the trees directly produced the deaths: participants knew that causation was more complex. Nevertheless, they saw the engineer's refusal to hire Indalesio and his design for the new houses as indexes of a problematic relationship between plants, humans, other species, power, and money.

A number of complexities faced the engineer. In selecting trees, he had to consider the anisotropic characteristics of species, meaning the properties that are evident as the wood is stressed in different ways. The vertical beams would bear substantial weight, so he needed wood with high compressive strength that would transmit energy downward, parallel to the grain. Floorboards, however, needed horizontal strength to prevent them from warping or breaking. He also considered how quickly different woods would dry and their hygroscopic properties, their propensity to absorb water and swell, important in a rainforest. By selecting the right kinds of trees and drying them properly, he could provide Muainans with the sorts of futures seemingly desired by Venezuelans who live in areas where forests have disappeared. His design would produce not just houses but modern socialist selves and a new naturalcultural-political world, transforming Delta residents' relationships to forests, rivers, gardens, education, sanitation, electricity, modernity, and one another.

A commission summoned the engineer to participate in the meeting. Muaina residents reiterated their demands to reconfigure the design process. The engineer projected himself as embodying the benevolent side of extractivism, as drawing on government funds in bettering the lives of Muainans by providing them with the same sorts of structures that were deemed to satisfy a socialist vision of Venezuelans' right to housing in the rest of the country. Reproducing anti-Indigenous stereotypes as reinflected through progressive extractivist logics, he saw Muainans as obstructing the project due to a superstitious understanding of nature. Residents' ideas about converting trees into houses were not entirely incompatible with the engineer's—for their own building projects, they select species that afford the strongest houses and resist fungi, pests, sun, wind, and water. Nevertheless, Muainans rejected the engineer's reduction of individual tree lives to chunks of wood with particular abstract properties, to their definition "only from the external standpoint of those who will impose their ends onto these essentially goalless living things" (Marder 2013:25). The failure to recognize a particular tree's singularity not only violated a sense of the ethical treatment of plants but endangered the humans who cut and used them. Muainans' protests were not articulated through NGO-speak, as "saving the rainforest"; they were less concerned with how many trees got cut and more with *how* they got cut and reinserted in human-plant relations. They wanted to include the agency of plants, including those living near the houses. They proposed what I would call a process of *phyto-design* in which the intimate relations that were ritually established with individual trees would be sustained throughout the process, granting them active roles in shaping the houses and the plant-human relations they afforded.

At the heart of the dispute lay discrepant projections of who produces knowledge about plants and plant-human relations, how this knowledge circulates, and how it is enacted materially—in short, contrasting phytocommunicabilities. For the engineer, knowledge about trees—embodied in abstract models and measurements—was produced beyond the Delta. His relationship to trees focused on calculating how many trees of which species and sizes were needed to produce the proper number and types of boards and how to train workers to mill them.[4] He demanded nearly exclusive rights to control phytocommunicable practices required for the project in Muaina, casting workers as merely capable of following instructions, not producing knowledge, and he left other residents and trees entirely out of the loop. Following a phytocommunicable model whose ontological base lay in the myth of Haburi, Indalesio saw trees, houses, canoes, and people as human-plant assemblages whose intimate sensorial, extra-sensorial (or "spiritual"), and agentive relations were the products of ongoing interactions with deep roots. For him, phyto-knowledge was produced by exchanges—both intimate and violent—between healers, moyotus, Daunarani, and her daughters. When people get sick shortly after cutting trees, wisidatu healers like Indalesio view such illnesses as signaling a phytocommunicable breakdown that must be quickly corrected.

BEYOND PHYTOCOMMUNICABLE BINARIES: WOMEN, BODIES, AND PLANTS

The debate would seem to be nicely captured by Viveiros de Castro's (2004) ontological opposition between Amerindian perspectivism and Western naturalism, as embodied in Indalesio's and the engineer's relations to trees. Stopping here, however, would reduce the story to a debate about plants enacted between men. Only men ratified as myth-tellers can relate the Haburi myth. Only men become canoe builders. With the exception of a few postmenopausal women, wisidatu healers are all men. Becoming a moyotu or wisidatu involves apprenticeship to a (male) master and a temporary separation from women, symbolized by sexual abstinence. It is a relationship between trees, tools, tobacco, "spirits," environments, *and men* that women witness without gaining direct access to what is said (and sung). The engineer and all of the other employees were men. Thus, ending our discussion with the confrontation between the engineer and the wisidatu would project phytocommunicabilities as revolving around a binary between competing male centers of power, reproducing ways that males use both plants and women to create male hierarchies and leaving us with narrow and problematic understandings of phytocommunicability. What is required, however, goes beyond assuming stable, preformed gender categories. Indeed, evidence from elsewhere in Greater Amazonia suggests that plant-human relations are key sites for producing notions of gender and organizing gendered relations. Anne-Christine Taylor (2001:51) suggests, for example, that Jivaroans envision vertical ties between parents and same-sex children through "the mode of propagation of the major cultivated plants, particularly manioc," complicating other Jivaroan modes of constructing gendered identities that liken boys to enemies and girls to half animals or prey. Indeed, connections between gender and human-plant relations raise complex philosophical and ethnographic questions.

In the Delta, girls move with their mothers through the forest as they walk or travel in small canoes to garden, gather firewood, and secure materials to weave baskets and hammocks. They watch and listen to their mothers as the latter see, smell, touch, pick, and listen to plants and voice their observations. Incrementally, girls become aware of names for plants, discern details of bark, leaves, fruit, and other parts, and identify smells associated with particular plants. They increasingly attend to sounds that plants make, indicating when curative possibilities are heightened or phytocommunicabilities have gone wrong, when plants have become angry and threaten phyto-aggression. Some trees can imitate a crying baby; if a woman hears this echoing effect, she will take the infant out of hearing range. If babies hear the tree's imitation, they may become suddenly ill, requiring a wisidatu to trace this pathological phytocommunicability, appease the tree with tobacco and song, and order it to leave the child's body. Rather than convergences between separate human and plant spheres, traveling through the forest reveals signs of the influence of people on plants and plants on people, constituting, in Laura Rival's (2016:38) terms, "the biophysical manifestation of a long history of human and environmental interactions."

Learning to heal with plants involves a constant, growing entanglement.[5] Myths and chants are woven into women's voices and bodies in the form of indexical traces that are entangled in words, actions, and materials as they travel through forests, gather reeds and moriche fiber, fashion them into baskets and hammocks (see Wilbert 1975), and mobilize plants' healing powers. These phyto-interactions do not simply access received bodies of knowledge but resignify elements of mythic texts and build archives that are lodged in women's minds and bodies and in the plants they sow, prune, and pluck as they become part of unique phytocommunicable circuits that connect patients, family members, other healers, nurses, and physicians. Here again, Marder's (2013:85) phyto-philosophy converges with that of *yarokotarotu*, phytotherapists, in viewing the plant as "a collective being," in seeing that "its body is a non-totalizing assemblage of multiplicities." Canoe builders and healers address the unified figure of a daughter of Daunarani, appealing to what they project as her sexual desire and appetite for tobacco smoke and palm starch, but the yarokotarotu's focus is on the distinct sensuous properties of leaves, stems or trunks, fruit, flowers, and other plant parts. A close friend of mine who served as a representative in the National Assembly laughed that distinguished visitors were astounded to see that her small house in town was surrounded by "weeds." She chuckled, "They don't know that I am a yarokotarotu and that I cultivate those 'weeds': they are my pharmacy!"

Girls hear healers sing to control invisible pathogens: nearly all have felt songs, tobacco trails, and the power of healers' hands move through their bodies. They grasp temporalities through plants, learning how their sensory and healing properties change through daily, monthly, and seasonal cycles. Girls connect their bodies to phyto-anatomy by using the same terms to refer to human and plant parts. They observe their mothers watch, smell, and touch human bodies and hear them comment on potentially problematic changes, pose diagnostic questions, offer allopathic and plant-based treatments, and make decisions about seeking additional care. As Theresa Miller (2019:90) details in sensitive ethnography conducted in northeast Brazil, these interactions go far beyond instrumentally exploiting plants for human ends; rather, "care and affection" become "the cornerstones of human-plant engagements." Cecilia Ayala Lafée and Werner Wilbert (2001:96) suggest that girls' fantasy play sometimes includes imaginative processes of diagnosis and phytotherapy. Men, of course, also interact with plants as they walk through the forest, prepare gardens, and travel in canoes; their attention is particularly drawn to trees that may be needed to build canoes or houses, thatch roofs, weave baskets and hammocks, provide fruit or other foods, and harbor game. Just as there is no singular Warao ethnobotany, women's and men's modes of interacting with plants are not stable, bounded, or homogeneous. As Rival (2016:78) suggests for Huaorani peoples, Delta residents use personal experiences with specific plants in building "highly sophisticated, highly empirical, and highly personal" plant-human relations.

Women feel and respect Daunarani's presence, even if they do not speak to her directly. They learn, in short, equally complex forms of phyto-communicability that are deeply woven into materialities and involve broad engagements with the sensorium. Most women gain substantial repertoires, estimated to include 100 plants, 45 illnesses, and 259 forms of phytotherapy (Werner Wilbert 1996:3; Ayala Lafée and Wilbert 2001:97). Individuals whose skill leads them to be sought out by persons beyond close family members gain wider recognition as yarokotarotu. Although their efforts involve complex diagnoses, trips into the forest, time-consuming interactions with plant materials, and extensive labors of care, there is little in the way of a recognized hierarchy of plant healers; they seldom receive compensation. Male healers generally consider women's knowledge to be inferior, ordinary, banal. Latin American medical anthropologist Eduardo Menéndez (1981) suggests that the positions of doctor and Indigenous healer are relational, defined through opposition and the subordination of the latter. Extending Menéndez's relational perspective, male healers elevate their knowledge by belittling that of yarokotarotu, drawing attention away from how phytotherapists produce notions of gender, humans, and health through entanglements with plants. Women's attunements to bodies and environments, in Natasha Myers's (2016) terms, "vegetalize our all-too-human sensorium."

Ten months before Mamerto died in Muaina, Odilia Torres faced her worst nightmare in Mukoboina, a smaller community thirty minutes upstream (see figures 10.4 and 10.5). Seven-year-old Yordi, her oldest, displayed "the same fever" that had killed two cousins. Touching his forehead, she noted that "he was really hot." Odilia immediately crossed the bridge to her parents' house. The grandmother, a skilled yarokotarotu, lay Yordi in her hammock, talked with Yordi and his mother, felt his forehead, smelled, listened, and looked.[6] Yordi had a fever, sore throat, cough; nevertheless, it wasn't a cold. Diagnosis and treatment were complicated by Yordi's sudden entrance into communicable cartographies that included the words of healers, nurses, doctors, and other Mukoboina parents about the "strange fever." Symptoms were not restricted to a single region of Yordi's body. The grandmother thus decided that bathing him in an infusion of mango leaves would be best, a sort of broad-spectrum treatment to address the cough, aching, and fever. She sent Odilia to the mango tree in front of her house to cut a large handful of young leaves, the ones most exposed to sun and rain and lacking blemishes or stains. The grandmother's house and the mango tree are visible in figure 10.6. As Odilia sat anxiously next to Yordi, her mother placed the leaves in a pot over the open fire in the kitchen structure behind the house. When the aroma reached its peak, she used a cloth to remove the leaves and poured the solution between two bowls until it cooled. The grandmother emptied the fragrant liquid over Yordi's body, making sure that it reached all surfaces of his skin, then wrapped him in a sheet to keep him warm.

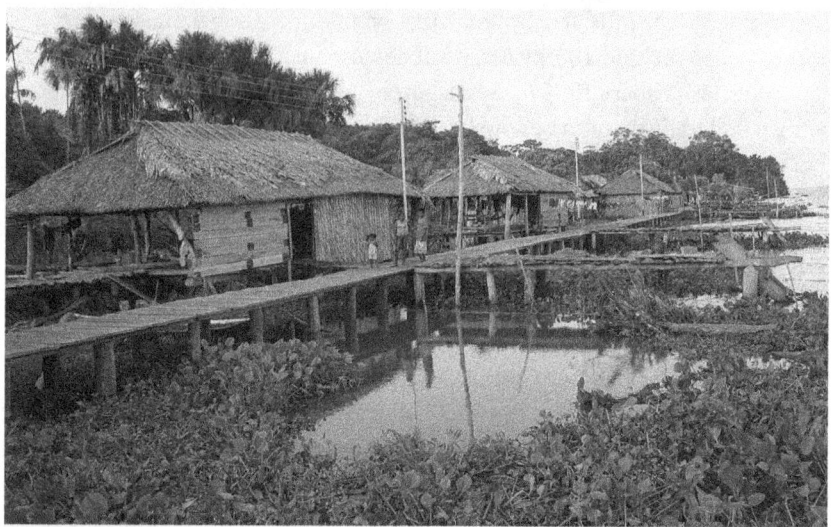

Figure 10.4. Mukoboina

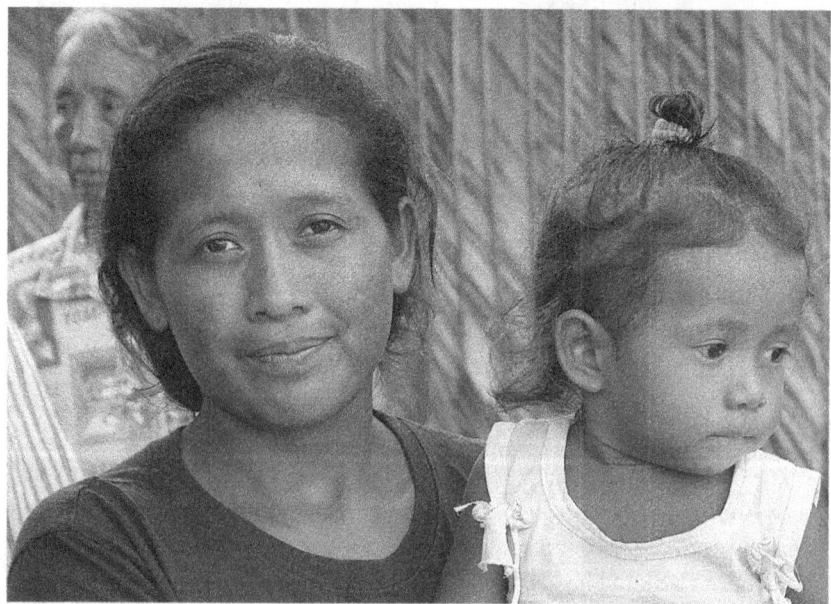

Figure 10.5. Odilia Torres and Yunelis

Odilia and her mother attempted to locate Yordi's illness within a broad sensorium. Experience as yarokotarotu had trained their olfactory abilities as they discerned how smells associated with each person changed as an

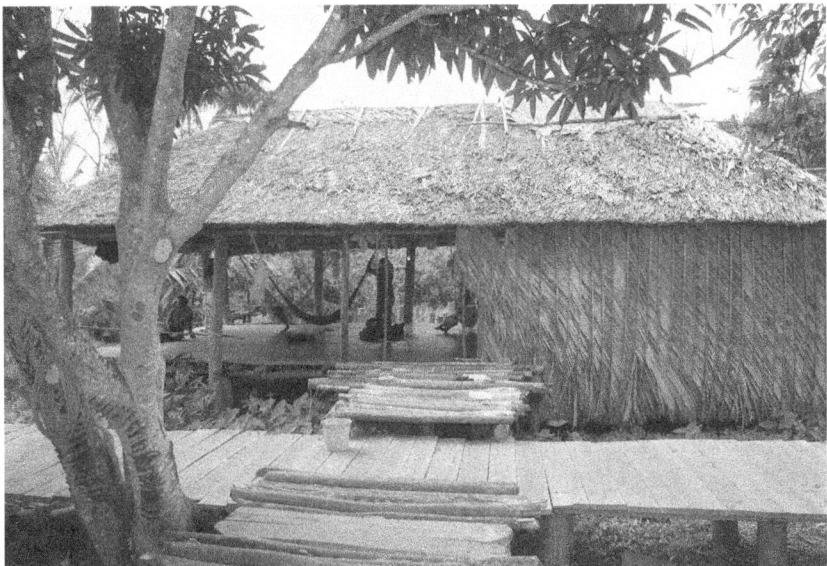

Figure 10.6. The grandmother's house, with the mango tree in the foreground

illness matches its specific fetid odor (see Werner Wilbert 1996). Likewise, each trip to the garden or forest provided them with another range of smells. The fragrance emitted by each plant afforded clues as to the diseases it could treat and revealed the curative agent itself; the smell was the outward manifestation of—to use our problematic categories—the curative and spiritual properties of a particular member of Daunarani's family. This phyto-sensorium was co-produced by people and plants as traveling through the forest connected women's bodies and senses with particular plants; focusing on smell had attuned them to how plants reach inside them, other plants, animals, and insects. Yordi's sweat and urine had a strange odor. The two women initiated an olfactory battle in which mango's fragrance would reach inside and hopefully drive the stench from Yordi's body.

The treatment did not diminish Yordi's fever. Knowing that the strange disease was killing children in just days, Odilia and her husband Romer Torres quickly moved on—appealing to the local wisidatu healer and then a series of doctors. The latter, unfortunately, were no more successful: Yordi died. Then Odilia and Romer lost Yordi's little brother a week later. Four-year-old sister Yomelis died in January from "the same fever," after being treated by healers, nurses, doctors, and specialists in urban hospitals. The parents' narratives and clinical examination of the last patient, Mamerto's wife, Elbia Rivas Torres, enabled Clara to offer a presumptive diagnosis of rabies. Most patients had been bitten nocturnally by vampire bats approximately a month and a half before developing symptoms, suggesting a route of transmission. Bats and viruses joined plants, houses, healers, and contractors in complex ways in making and sustaining an epidemic.

BEYOND BINARY PHYTOCOMMUNICABILITIES

Given that both Marder and Delta residents engage plants philosophically, the dialogue that I have tried to forge might interest them both. Insofar as Marder's goal "is not to erase plants' otherness but to bring them close" (2013:8), Delta residents could offer him a number of ways of thinking about how plants have always been close, ontologically, politically, materially, sensorily. Marder (53) suggests that "the plant that has no identity of its own secretly confers a plastic, malleable form upon life in its multiple instantiations and animates the grids of meaning, wherein other living beings operate." Male healers and the engineer would probably agree that plants hold secrets (and that only they can reveal them), but phytotherapists would push this formulation further to focus our attention on how individual plants and particular humans are constituted anew each day as people walk, paddle, garden, harvest, become ill, and heal. Marder's (2014:13) claim that "it is not silly to talk about plant experience so long as we specify that it is devoid of self-experience" might strike phytotherapists, moyotu, and wisidatu as nonsensical, given how carefully they attend to diverse ways of reading how plants signal their experiences in discerning an individual plant's disposition to cure or harm humans or its willingness to be transformed into a canoe or house.

My philosophical and ethnographic analysis has delineated how engagements with plants are—for Marder, phytotherapists, engineer, moyotu, and wisidatu alike—centered on issues of phytocommunicability. Even as my Delta interlocutors extend Marder's call to rethink the human through plant lives, they would argue that his account rests on a narrow phytocommunicable model, one that renders plants silent, mute, and voiceless. Delta residents are hardly the only ones to develop richer phytocommunicabilities. In her account of "the plant turn," Natasha Myers suggests that fascination with the lives of plants pushes scientists and laypersons to open up possibilities for rethinking both anthropomorphism and phytomorphism, adding that "it becomes increasingly unclear who is animating what, and what is animating whom" (2015:60). Hopis singing to corn in Arizona, performance artists staging phyto-encounters, matsutake mushrooms that forge commodity chains across a diversity of capitalist and noncapitalist logics (Tsing 2015), rebuilding communities around gathering ginseng on the margins of the violent landscapes of Appalachian coalfields (Hufford 2004), and people talking to their plants point to the many sites in which discrepant, unruly phytocommunicabilities emerge.

The clash between the engineer's reduction of the forest to raw materials and standardized houses versus myth performers', healers', and canoe builders' projections of intimate connections between plants and humans produced anger on both sides and never yielded compromise. At the same time that this situation suggests how opposing naturalist and multinaturalist perspectives (Viveiros de Castro 2004) can be complexly entangled (de la Cadena 2015), it points to the need to keep gender in focus in exploring how they are produced and distributed. Indeed, the discrepant phytocommunicabilities of male healers and the engineer share important features. Both claim distal sources of phyto-authority, of control over plant-human relations, as embodied in knowledge of mythic and ritual codes for communicating with plants or experimental data on the properties of woods and engineering standards. Each posits only one valid communicable circuit, which in both cases is linear, unidirectional, and positions male specialists as the necessary conduits for the production and circulation of knowledge about plants, at least those required for harvesting and building with trees. Both the engineer and healers projected any attempt to usurp their authority, any competing claims to generate or circulate knowledge about trees, as embodying ignorance and risking defective houses or fatal illnesses. Reducing their quarrel to phyto-dualism would obscure the similar ways that they construct and defend authority and power. Similarly, as important as gender is to this story, invoking an a priori gender binary as an analytic device would, I think, similarly fall short. Most men in the Delta are not wisidatu healers; they, too, are thus excluded from wisidatus' and moyotus' powerful phyto-pathways. Moreover, phyto-erudition is not distributed as a sort of homogeneous, bounded, codified body of knowledge that is rigidly linked to identity categories or the roles of yarokotarotu, wisidatu, or moyotu; practitioners rather fashion their own ways of thinking and relating anew each day as they interact with plants, dream, heal, and tell and hear myths.

Marder (2013:6) suggests that "countering environmental destruction must be a goal of any theorizing of plants." Events unfolding in Muaina in 2007–2008 point to the need for philosophical, political, and ethnographic depth and subtlety in taking up such challenges. Delta residents' demands to respect plant lives and sensibilities did not form a response to such altogether too familiar scenarios as massive projects to build dams, clear-cut forests, or position drilling rigs in backyards. A central concern was with human lives, and that is what brought me to Muaina. I did not return to the Delta in July 2008 with my own design, a research design, oriented toward producing theory for insertion into anthropological debates or environmental advocacy: I was recruited by Indigenous leaders who launched their own effort to stop an epidemic. Achieving a diagnosis where physicians, epidemiologists, and healers had failed nevertheless required a collective effort to unthink and rethink discrepant communicabilities, to discern how existing forms of knowledge production and circulation had failed. Like seeing a plant growing in a familiar space and realizing how its presence suddenly transforms one's relationship to a landscape, weeds came to disrupt the narrow clinical, epidemiological, and environmental perspectives that had thwarted diagnosis for a year.

I bring this essay to a close in February 2019, amid yet another crisis of Venezuela's Bolivarian socialist revolution. Extracting oil, gas, and other environmental "resources" remains the revolution's economic base (see Angosto-Ferrández 2019). Progressive extractivism requires drilling rigs and pumps, pipelines, tankers, markets, refineries, retail outlets, and complex circuits of foreign capital. These elements render revolutionary extractivism vulnerable to sabotage, economic fluctuations, and international sanctions, as well as draconian measures that the US government has recently adopted against Venezuela. Progressive extractivism's infrastructures include government programs for transforming oil and gas into houses, education, healthcare, and food for low-income Venezuelans on the one hand and the massive financial incentives—including high levels of corruption—that sometimes constrain elites from more active and effective attempts to seize political power from socialist governments. The Muaina housing project highlighted these two faces of extractivism. As many commentators have noted, extractivist infrastructures also include practices for producing nonhumans—even as they are ideologically cast as collective resources, rights-bearing subjects, or spiritual arbiters of ethical conduct—as resources whose violent commodification provides the only available means of securing collective human well-being.[7] These multiple contradictions have synergistically produced massive shortages of food and medicine and the exodus of millions of Venezuelans.

Before Chávez inspired a "pink wave" in Latin American governments, Librado Moraleda and other Delta residents were crafting a phyto-socialism that continues to challenge scholarly narratives, the capitalist Achilles' heel of progressive extractivism, and philosophical and ethnographic understandings of plant-human relations. Unlike invocations of sumak kawsay, their design for phyto-socialism never revolved around a single phrase or concept, one that can be easily decontextualized and recycled without stopping to consult with people who know its philosophical, mythic, and decolonial underpinnings. Not without their own contradictions, inequalities, and limitations, Delta phytocommunicabilities were produced anew each day, as much through bodily, material, and sensuous encounters as through esoteric songs and aesthetically and symbolically rich mythic performances. Phyto-socialism was not tied to a singular, bounded Indigenous ontology, one seemingly shared by all people classified as Warao, but continually fashioned in different ways through creative and critical engagements with plants, technologies, diseases, politicians, and histories. Phyto-socialism's infrastructures require phytocommunicable debates about how plants and humans affect and learn from and about one another as much as gardens, canoes, outboard motors, axes, trees, sago seedlings, and other plants. The conflict over deaths and house designs was not the first nor the last time that discrepant phytocommunicabilities clashed.

Delta residents help us see that phytocommunicabilities are more than arguments between people about how humans communicate with plants. Like Muaina residents' demands to include trees in designing houses, they actively position plants within explorations of the limits and the dangers that emerge as humans and plants constitute one another. I was working on this chapter in Northern California during the 2018 wildfire season that burned entire towns and caused some ninety deaths. Although I have no ready answers, what I learned from my Delta interlocutors does, however, at least prompt me, as toxic smoke enters my nostrils, lungs, and eyes and as I stare at charred forests, to listen/look/feel/smell/taste a bit more attentively to what plants might be telling us about the limits of our all-too-human designs.

NOTES

1. In previous essays (Briggs 1993a, 2000), I discussed two of these mythic performances, including the story of *my* origin, that is, of non-Indigenous peoples.

2. As Marisol de la Cadena (2015) suggests, such terms as *plants* and *spirits* are problematic placeholders that impose artificial simplifications on complex concepts.

3. For background on health systems in the Delta and on the mysterious epidemic, see Briggs and Mantini-Briggs 2016.

4. House construction itself was largely undertaken by carpenters brought from outside the Delta.

5. Werner Wilbert (1996; Wilbert and Ayala Lafée Wilbert 2011) provides detailed ethnographic documentation on phytotherapy.

6. Although the parents requested use of their real names, noting that they want people to know about them and their children, a few others, including Odilia's mother, were more reticent regarding disclosure of their names.

7. Among the many writers who have explored these issues, see Angosto-Ferrández (2019), Anthias (2018), Gudynas (2012), Hindery (2013), Postero (2017), Sawyer and Gomez (2012), Velásquez (2018), and Watts (2005).

Epilogue

I END WITH A LAMENT AND A PLEA. A major focus of this book has been on epidemics. As it nears publication in 2020, I am not tracking viruses or bacteria in the rainforest but "sheltering in place" in a California oak forest during the COVID-19 pandemic. I did not seek out an epidemic to research; indeed, I had sworn that I would never accept the psychic burden of investigating another. As with cholera and rabies, however, COVID-19 seemed to appear out of nowhere, and I similarly could not escape its demands to use my experience in exploring ways of sorting out a new tidal wave of complexities and uncertainties. And, for better or worse, COVID-19 seems to have taken all of the perspectives I developed in the preceding pages and thrown them, like a deck of cards, up into the air. Many of them still haven't landed. The ones that have become visible are not just sorted into novel arrangements but seem to have transformed into new suits. I close with a final reflection that pulls together my relation to epidemics, race, and the politics of knowledge.

When a devastating epidemic emerged in the Delta in 1992, regional health officials tried to cover up how cholera revealed the structural effects of the policies they had created. *Vibrio cholerae* is waterborne, and the oil-rich government had failed to provide potable water or sewage facilities. Epidemiologists only counted laboratory-confirmed cases, even as they failed to send test kits to makeshift rainforest clinics; some 500 deaths thus magically became 13, officially. In order to hide their culpability, public health officials crafted narratives that blamed "indigenous culture," suggesting that belief in spirits led people to reject doctors—even as thousands fled to the mainland, seeking medical assistance. When a mysterious disease killed thirty-eight children and young adults in 2007–2008, administrators used the cholera narratives to blame parents—suggesting that they might have fed their own children poisonous fish or fruit—even as officials tried to render the epidemic invisible. Rainforest residents told narratives that attempted to pinpoint the causes of these epidemics and traced how racism might have guided the pathogens' paths into Indigenous communities, thereby embracing vernacular forms of critical epidemiology. The circulation of lethal microbes thus went hand in hand with that of narratives that purported to explain why some people died and others lived. Mediatization mattered: who co-produced narratives and how competing stories circulated had real effects, helping shape policies and practices and, accordingly, who lived and who died in the epidemics and whether their aftermath would produce better health or more inequality and death.

COVID-19 could not provide a more striking example of what I have termed communicability. SARS-CoV-2 is a master of mobility, prompting "shelter in place" policies designed to limit its circulation even as COVID-19 discourse, including a plethora of conspiracy theories and shifting scientific findings, attempt to pin it down. Like the cholera epidemic, the daily emergence of new narratives is structured by the statistical drumbeat of numbers of cases and deaths; as with cholera in Venezuela, Trump administration officials decided to count only laboratory-confirmed cases and created systematic shortages of test kits. Like the lethal way that *Vibrio cholerae* and the rabies virus mapped racial inequality in Delta Amacuro, COVID-19 is, as I write, killing six times as many Blacks as whites in some US regions. The pandemic is thus making race virulently communicable—deepening the effects of systemic racism even as it provides highly visible venues for narratives that have long tracked its lethal effects. Then the killing of George Floyd by Minneapolis police officers on May 25, 2020, demedicalized COVID-19 deaths, placing them out of narrow biomedical case definitions and statistics and locating them within much larger and more long-term histories of US state violence against people of color.

In *The Ballad of Gregorio Cortez*, Américo Paredes (1958) showed how narratives of racialized state violence circulated in song, legend, news stories, and courtroom testimony and through what was at the time a new technology, the telegraph. Historian Monica Muñoz Martínez (2018) documented how Latinx families continue to perform narratives more than a century later about relatives lynched by Texas Rangers and white mobs between 1910 and 1920. Narratives told in US communities of color have long pointed to the coloniality of violence against Native American, Black, Latinx, Asian American, and immigrant communities, to their embeddedness in legacies of settler colonialism, genocide, slavery, and imperialism. Official histories nevertheless overlooked these events or at least lowered their profile and severed their historical connections. Now new economies of poetics and performance are emerging as cell phone videos and social media platforms turn "citizen journalism" into a force that cannot be so easily muted. Footage of the killing of George Floyd, Breonna Taylor, Ahmaud Arbery, Eric Garner, Oscar Grant, and many others reveals not only the brutal way they were murdered but the callous and sometimes explicitly racist attitudes exhibited by those who killed them. Links between these forms of racialized violence have suddenly become the most prominent debate in the contemporary United States.

How have narratives detailing the effects of everyday racism circulating in "ethnic media" and within Black, Latinx, and Native American communities been so effectively excluded from history books, policy debates, and much "mainstream" journalism? Such racist stereotypes as the threatening Black man, the overly fertile, welfare-mongering Black woman, brown bodies flooding across the US-Mexican border, and exotic but alcoholic Native Americans have been often—but not consistently—amplified by white politicians, journalists, and scholars, thereby providing whites with defense mechanisms for transforming stories of racial violence into confirmations of unequal social standing, or, at best, gruesome but easily forgotten exceptions.

Here I would like to return one last time to psychoanalyst Juan-David Nasio's suggestion that lives become entwined like the way "ivy covers a stone wall" (2004:20), "each attached to a specific aspect of that person that has touched us" (20). Our own being thus extends into others with whom we are connected just as their lives reach within us, leading to the intense pain identified by Freud when someone we love dies. Race, ethnicity, gender, sexuality, class, and disability deeply affect how this affective ivy grows, thus conditioning reactions to the death of others. Accounts of rape or harassment affect women who have experienced sexual violence, I am told, quite differently. Stories of the Holocaust similarly mean quite different things to Jews who have experienced anti-Semitism. Histories of genocide reach into Native Americans' everyday lives, just as accounts of lynchings, hate crimes, and police killings enter intimately into the feelings, thoughts, and actions of Black Americans. I write these lines cautiously, knowing that my words rest on stories I have heard, news articles, and academic studies, not personal experience. I acknowledge my privilege and the price of my safety.

The security footage and cell phone videos of a white Minneapolis police officer pressing his knee against George Floyd's neck for 8 minutes and 46 seconds as he pleaded, "I can't breathe," and even after he stopped breathing, have broken through the barriers that shape how stories of racial violence circulate between and within people. Arriving in the midst of the disconcerting feeling that a lethal virus might infect us at any moment and awareness of its harsh toll among Black Americans, videos of Floyd's murder seemed to have bypassed deeply rooted practices of racial Othering to enter the cracks and crevices of many white psyches in ways that demand changes in policies that devalue non-white lives. Ongoing protests are advancing a collective "work of mourning," in Freud's ([1917] 1957) terms, as pasts and futures, pain and rage fuse.

Poetics matters. Thousands of narratives entextualize both COVID-19 and police killings in competing ways, inscribing projections of causes and effects, perpetrators and victims in their recurring tropes, temporal and spatial features, ascriptions of agency, visual images, and acoustic effects. Ex-president Donald Trump sought to block these new possibilities for psychic and political connection by racializing SARS-CoV-2 as "the Chinese virus" and even "the kung flu," calling protestors "terrorists," and lauding police repression of protests as "beautiful." A Fox News / Trump tweets / conservative social media circuit not only cut interracial strands of ivy but pushed people within ideologically isolating walls of mediatization. But the potential of COVID-19 and Floyd's death for exposing intimate and often lethal relations between poetics and performance, psyches and the politics of mourning, traditionalization and mediatization, mobility and immobility, coloniality, and environmental destruction and multispecies sensibilities could not be so easily contained.

I conclude this lament with a plea. First, please use the analytics I propose in the preceding pages not as decontextualized academic models but as tools to assist you in your efforts to figure out how these processes intersect. This suggestion goes far beyond the specifics of this particular historical juncture. The preceding chapters have taken what are usually framed as separate research foci and analytical frameworks and explored how insights can emerge through unlearning their ideological and pragmatic infrastructures and tracing their connections. My hope is that you will unthink other premises and practices and find new links as you explore equally complex and intimate relations evident in other lines of investigation and real-world challenges. Second, don't just take my word for any of this. As pursuing business as usual becomes increasingly untenable, what are often deemed new voices and stories are reshaping debates taking place even in dominant public spheres. The illusion of newness is a product of practices of exclusion with long historical roots.

In short, it turns out that the mentors who can help us unlearn old paradigms and create more just policies and practices have been there all along. The efforts I have undertaken in the preceding pages to disrupt business-as-usual practices, scholarly and engaged, have suddenly been folded into the emerging landscape of a world on edge. In this book I have tried to perform a poetics that goes beyond liberal calls to listen to "marginal voices," which can constitute forms of appropriation that use humanistic camouflage to protect the status quo. My goal has rather been to outline a practice for finding a more diverse set of mentors, learning to listen to each, and joining dialogues capable of dismantling our most basic assumptions, crafting alternatives, and helping turn them into lived realities. The stakes are high, and the challenges are calling each and every one of us. Returning to the sort of more personal voice that addressed Dr. Freud, I thank you, my readers, for listening.

Acknowledgments

WRITING AN ACKNOWLEDGMENTS SECTION ALWAYS MAKES ME FEEL uncomfortable. Even with a project that unfolds during a distinct time frame, takes place largely in a specified geographical area, and pertains to a singular focus, I know that I will leave out someone who has made a crucial contribution—intellectual, financial, emotional, or textual—to the endeavor. Also, acknowledgments usually draw the familiar sorts of boundaries around research, leaving scholars and funding sources in, generally complemented by family members and friends, but excluding people who are denied the status of either researcher or "informant," especially the ones who perform the labor that makes a project possible. One of these boundaries separates humans from nonhumans, leaving nonhumans (except for an occasional favorite dog or cat) out of the origin story that gets told in acknowledgments. In this book, things are potentially much worse, because it not only spans forty years of research focused on a wide range of topics and diverse settings but takes me back to the people who shaped—starting in my childhood—the way I think, live, and work. Fortunately, a lot of the work of acknowledgment started right up front in the introduction. I thus want to reiterate here my thanks to:

- Señor Olguín, his horse, the dump rake, the alfalfa, and the rich brown irrigation water
- The beekeeper, his wife and, of course, the bees and their honeycomb
- Old Man Hawkins and his peach, apple, and pear trees (I'm leaving out his .22 short rifle)
- The Griegos
- Sigmund Freud
- Ludwig Wittgenstein
- John Donald and Harriet Robb and Nancy Robb Briggs
- Bill Briggs
- Rudolfo Anaya, my high school teacher
- Alfonso Ortiz

George and Silvianita López and their family

Aspen trees, penknives, and sandpaper

Córdova

Lands, landscapes, people, plants, rivers, art, and musics of New Mexico

E. Boyd and Marta Weigle

Gilberto Benito Córdova, my padrino

Enrique Lamadrid and Carlota Domínguez Lamadrid, my compadres

Julián Josué and Irene Vigil and Lilián Pacheco de Vigil

Dick Bauman

Beverly Stoeltje

Frantz Fanon

Américo Paredes

Lee Baker

Teodoro, Tomasa, Librado, Conrado, and Enrique Moraleda and Olga Pizarro

Tirso Gómez and Norbelys Gómez

Santiago Rivera and Sixta Pérez

Manuel Torres for teaching me how to heal

Maria Rivera, Odilia Torres, her mother, other Delta phytotherapists

Grieving parents in Mukoboina, Muaina, and other Delta communities

Florencia Macotera and Indalesio Pizarro

Johannes Wilbert, Werner Wilbert, and H. Dieter Heinen

W.E.B. Du Bois

Father Julio Lavandero

I thank *Vibrio cholerae* bacteria and rabies viruses for going away, and I ask them not to return

María Fernández, Anita Rivas, Florencia Macotera, and other Delta performers of lament

Herminia Gómez and her aunt and uncle

Héctor Romero, Belkis Ruiz Valderey and my beloved godson Pedro

My long defunct fifty-foot dugout canoe and its forty-horsepower Mariner outboard motor

The Delta's trees and rivers

Students from whom I have had the honor of learning over the past forty years

UC Berkeley students Elena Klonsky and Teniah Miller for help with preparing the manuscript and illustrations

Sadhana Naithani, for our collaborative project mapping intersections between folklore, folkloristics, and coloniality, and permission to reprint chapter 4

Michael Silverstein

All the mentors I don't have space to list here but who live within me nonetheless

Daniel Hallin

Ruth Goldstein

Becky Schulties

Jed Sekoff

Maureen Katz, for deepening my knowledge of psychoanalysis and reading part of the manuscript

Indiana University's Department of Folklore and Ethnomusicology, especially Diane Goldstein, for inviting me to give the Richard Dorson Lecture that prompted chapter 9

Elliott Oring and the Western States Folklore Society for inviting me to give the Archer Taylor Lecture, which started work on chapter 5

The National Science Foundation for a grant (BNS-8305386) that supported the research in New Mexico and grants from NSF's Law and Social Science Program and Cultural Anthropology Program for the work in Venezuela, including grant # 9979284, which funded my work on extractivism in the Delta

The Wenner-Gren Foundation for Anthropological Research for supporting fieldwork in New Mexico and Venezuela

The School for Advanced Research for the J. I. Staley Prize that provided the funds used for assisting in the rabies epidemic and for a Weatherhead Fellowship

The Lichtenberg-Kolleg at the Georg-August University of Göttingen for a fellowship

Regina Bendix

Margaret Mills

Galit Hasan-Rokem and Freddie Rokem

The *Journal of Folklore Research* (chapters 1, 2, 7, and 8), the *Journal of American Folklore* (chapter 3), *Studies in History* (chapter 4), *Western Folklore* (chapter 5), *Cultural Anthropology* (chapter 6), and *Ethnos* (chapter 10) for permission to reprint sections of or entire articles

Laura Gilpin, the Monterey County Agricultural and Rural Life Museum, the Colorado Springs Fine Arts Center, the Amon Carter Museum of American

Art, Barbara E. Fries, *CBS Evening News*, *The Daily Show*, Punch Productions and Warner Brothers for illustrations

Stefan Erasmi for figure 10

Rosa Norton for a beautiful and meticulous index

Rachael Levay, Darrin Pratt, Laura Furney, Robin DuBlanc, and Dan Pratt of Utah State University Press / University Press of Colorado and two wonderful reviewers

Gabriel, Amalia, Brielle, and Ian

Professor Gabriel Fries-Briggs for so much, including figure 4, and Hanna Mesraty and Malik Briggs-Mesraty

Feliciana and Clara for everything, always

References

Aarne, Antti, and Stith Thompson. 1961. *The Types of the Folktale: A Classification and Bibliography*. 2nd ed. FF Communications 184. Helsinki: Suomalainen Tiedeakatemia, Academia Scientarium Fennica.
Abadía, Edgar, Monica Sequera, Dagmarys Ortega, et al. 2009. "Mycobacterium Tuberculosis Ecology in Venezuela: Epidemiologic Correlates of Common Spoligotypes and a Large Clonal Cluster Defined by MIRU-VNTR-24." *BMC Infectious Disease* 9:122. https://bmcinfectdis.biomedcentral.com/articles/10.1186/1471-2334-9-122.
Abrahams, Roger D. 2005. *Everyday Life: A Poetics of Vernacular Practices*. Philadelphia: University of Pennsylvania Press.
Altheide, David L., and Robert P. Snow. 1979. *Media Logic*. Beverly Hills, CA: Sage.
Anderson, Benedict. (1983) 1991. *Imagined Communities: Reflections on the Origin and Spread of Nationalism*. Rev. ed. London: Verso.
Anderson, Warwick. 2006. *Colonial Pathologies: American Tropical Medicine, Race, and Hygiene in the Philippines*. Durham, NC: Duke University Press.
Angosto-Ferrández, Luís Fernando. 2019. "Neoextractivism and Class Formation: Lessons from the Orinoco Mining Arc Project in Venezuela." *Latin American Perspectives* 46 (1): 190–211.
Anthias, Penelope. 2018. *Limits to Decolonization: Indigeneity, Territory, and Hydrocarbon Politics in the Bolivian Chaco*. Ithaca, NY: Cornell University Press.
Anzaldúa, Gloria. 1987. *Borderlands/La Frontera: The New Mestiza*. San Francisco: Spinsters/Aunt Lute.
Appadurai, Arjun, ed. 1986. *The Social Life of Things: Commodities in Cultural Perspective*. Cambridge: Cambridge University Press.
Appadurai, Arjun. 1988. "Putting Hierarchy in Its Place." *Cultural Anthropology* 3 (1): 36–49.
Appadurai, Arjun. 1996. *Modernity at Large: Cultural Dimensions of Globalization*. Minneapolis: University of Minnesota Press.
Appadurai, Arjun, Frank J. Korom, and Margaret Mills, eds. 1991. *Gender, Genre, and Power in South Asian Expressive Traditions*. Philadelphia: University of Pennsylvania Press.
Arnold, David. 1993. *Colonizing the Body: State Medicine and Epidemic Disease in Nineteenth-Century India*. Berkeley: University of California Press.
Aubrey, John. 1862. *Wiltshire: The Topographical Collections of John Aubrey, F.R.S, A.D. 1659–70*. Edited by John Edward Jackson. Devizes, UK: Wiltshire Archaeological and Natural History Society.
Aubrey, John. 1972. *Three Prose Works*. Edited by John Buchanan-Brown. Carbondale: Southern Illinois University Press.
Austin, J. L. 1962. *How to Do Things with Words*. Edited by J. O. Urmson and Marina Sbisà. Cambridge, MA: Harvard University Press.
Ayala Lafée, Cecilia, and Werner Wilbert. 2001. *Hijas de la luna: Enculturación femenina entre los Waraos*. Caracas: Fundación La Salle de Ciencias Naturales.
Bacchilega, Cristina. 2007. *Legendary Hawai'i and the Politics of Place: Tradition, Translation, and Tourism*. Philadelphia: University of Pennsylvania Press.

Bakhtin, M. M. 1981. *The Dialogic Imagination: Four Essays*. Translated by Caryl Emerson and Michael Holquist. Edited by Michael Holquist. Austin: University of Texas Press.

Bakhtin, M. M. 1986. "The Problem of Speech Genres." In *Speech Genres and Other Late Essays*, translated by Vern W. McGee, edited by Caryl Emerson and Michael Holquist, 60–102. Austin: University of Texas Press.

Balibar, Etienne. 1995. "Culture and Identity (Working Notes)." In *The Identity in Question*, edited by John Rajchman, 173–96. New York: Routledge.

Barlow, Kathleen, and David Lipset. 1997. "Dialogics of Material Culture: Male and Female in Murik Outrigger Canoes." *American Ethnologist* 24 (1): 4–36.

Barral, Rev. P. Fr. Basilio. [1961]. *Guarao guarata: Lo que cuentan los indios Guaraos*. Caracas: Editorial Salesiana.

Barral, Rev. P. Fr. Basilio. 1979. *Diccionario Warao-Castellano, Castellano-Warao*. Caracas: Universidad Católica *"Andrés Bello."*

Basso, Keith H. 1996. *Wisdom Sits in Places: Landscape and Language among the Western Apache*. Albuquerque: University of New Mexico Press.

Bateson, Gregory. 1972. *Steps to an Ecology of Mind*. New York: Ballantine.

Bauman, Richard. 1971. "Differential Identity and the Social Base of Folklore." *Journal of American Folklore* 84 (331): 31–41.

Bauman, Richard. 1977. *Verbal Art as Performance*. Prospect Heights, IL: Waveland.

Bauman, Richard. 1992a. "Contextualization, Tradition, and the Dialogue of Genres: Icelandic Legends of the Kraftaskáld." In *Rethinking Context: Language as an Interactive Phenomenon*, edited by Alessandro Duranti and Charles Goodwin, 125–45. Cambridge: Cambridge University Press.

Bauman, Richard. 1992b. "Folklore." In *Folklore, Cultural Performances, and Popular Entertainments: A Communications-centered Handbook*, edited by Richard Bauman, 29–40. New York: Oxford University Press.

Bauman, Richard. 2004. *A World of Others' Words: Cross-Cultural Perspectives on Intertextuality*. Malden, MA: Blackwell.

Bauman, Richard. 2008. "The Philology of the Vernacular." *Journal of Folklore Research* 45 (1): 29–36.

Bauman, Richard. 2010. "The Remediation of Storytelling: Narrative Performance on Early Commercial Sound Recordings." In *Telling Stories: Language, Narrative, and Social Life*, edited by Deborah Schiffrin, Anna De Fina, and Anastasia Nylund, 23–43. Washington, DC: Georgetown University Press.

Bauman, Richard. 2012a. "'First Verses I Ever Knew': Américo Paredes and the Border Décima." *Journal of American Folklore* 125 (495): 5–22.

Bauman, Richard. 2012b. "Performance." In *A Companion to Folklore*, edited by Regina F. Bendix and Galit Hasan-Rokem, 94–118. Malden, MA: Wiley-Blackwell.

Bauman, Richard. 2016. "Projecting Presence: Aura and Oratory in William Jennings Bryan's Presidential Races." In *Scale: Discourse and Dimensions of Social Life*, edited by E. Summerson Carr and Michael Lempert, 25–51. Oakland: University of California Press.

Bauman, Richard, and Roger D. Abrahams, eds. 1981. *"And Other Neighborly Names": Social Process and Cultural Image in Texas Folklore*. Austin: University of Texas Press.

Bauman, Richard, and Charles L. Briggs. 1990. "Poetics and Performance as Critical Perspectives on Language and Social Life." *Annual Review of Anthropology* 19:59–88.

Bauman, Richard, and Charles L. Briggs. 2003. *Voices of Modernity: Language Ideologies and Social Inequality*. Cambridge: Cambridge University Press.

Bauman, Richard, and Patrick Feaster. 2005. "'Fellow Townsmen and My Noble Constituents!' Representations of Oratory on Early Commercial Recordings." *Oral Tradition* 20 (1): 35–57.

Bausinger, Hermann. (1961) 1990. *Folk Culture in a World of Technology*. Translated by Elke Dettmer. Bloomington: Indiana University Press.

Bausinger, Hermann. 1994. "Nazi Folk Ideology and Folk Research." In *The Nazification of an Academic Discipline: Folklore in the Third Reich*, edited by James R. Dow and Hannjost Lixfeld, 11–33. Bloomington: Indiana University Press.

Beltrán, Héctor, Jr. 2012. "*Echándole Ganas* across Borders: Narratives of La Frontera Sur from the Everyday into the Mainstream." MA thesis, Folklore Graduate Program, University of California, Berkeley.

Bendix, Regina. 1988a. "Folklorismus: The Challenge of a Concept." *International Folklore Review* 6:5–15.

Bendix, Regina. 1988b. "Of Names, Professional Identities, and Disciplinary Futures." *Journal of American Folklore* 111 (441): 235–46.

Bendix, Regina. 1997. *In Search of Authenticity: The Formation of Folklore Studies*. Madison: University of Wisconsin Press.

Bendix, Regina. 2018. *Culture and Value: Tourism, Heritage, and Property*. Bloomington: Indiana University Press.

Benjamin, Walter. 1968. *Illuminations*. Edited by Hannah Arendt. New York: Schocken.

Benjamin, Walter. 2003. "On the Concept of History." In *Walter Benjamin: Selected Writings*, translated by Harry Zohn, edited by Michael W. Jennings, 4:1938–40. Cambridge, MA: Harvard University Press.

Berman, Judith. 1996. "The Culture as It Appears to the Indian Himself: Boas, George Hunt, and the Methods of Ethnography." In *Volksgeist as Method and Ethic: Essays on Boasian Ethnography and the German Anthropological Tradition*, edited by George W. Stocking Jr., 215–56. Madison: University of Wisconsin Press.

Bettelheim, Bruno. 1976. *The Uses of Enchantment: The Meaning and Importance of Fairy Tales*. New York: Knopf.

Bhabha, Homi K. 1994. *The Location of Culture*. New York: Routledge.

Biehl, João. 2005. *Vita: Life in a Zone of Social Abandonment*. Berkeley: University of California Press.

Blache, Martha. 1988. "Folklore y cultura popular." *Revista de investigaciones folclóricas* 3:23–34.

Blank, Trevor, ed. 2012. *Folk Culture in the Digital Age: The Emergent Dynamics of Human Interaction*. Logan: Utah State University Press.

Blank, Trevor J., and Andrea Kitta, eds. 2015. *Diagnosing Folklore: Perspectives on Disability, Health, and Trauma*. Jackson: University Press of Mississippi.

Blommaert, Jan. 2010. *The Sociolinguistics of Globalization*. Cambridge: Cambridge University Press.

Blommaert, Jan, and Jef Verschueren. 1998. *Debating Diversity: Analysing the Discourse of Tolerance*. London: Routledge.

Boellstorff, Tom. 2008. *Coming of Age in Second Life: An Anthropologist Explores the Virtually Human*. Princeton, NJ: Princeton University Press.

Boellstorff, Tom. 2011. "Placing the Virtual Body: Avatar, Chora, Cypherg." In *A Companion to the Anthropology of the Body and Embodiment*, edited by Frances E. Mascia-Lees, 504–20. New York: Wiley-Blackwell.

Bolter, Jay David, and Richard Grusin. 1999. *Remediation: Understanding New Media*. Cambridge, MA: MIT Press.

Bottigheimer, Ruth B. 1987. *Grimms' Bad Girls and Bold Boys: The Moral and Social Vision of the Tales*. New Haven, CT: Yale University Press.

Bourdieu, Pierre. (1972) 1977. *Outline of a Theory of Practice*. Translated by Richard Nice. Cambridge: Cambridge University Press.

Bourdieu, Pierre. 1991. *Language and Symbolic Power.* Translated by Gino Raymond and Matthew Adamson. Cambridge, MA: Harvard University Press.

Bowker, Geoffrey C., and Susan Leigh Star. 1999. *Sorting Things Out: Classification and Its Consequences.* Cambridge, MA: MIT Press.

Brady, Erika, ed. 2001. *Healing Logics: Culture and Medicine in Modern Health Belief Systems.* Logan: Utah State University Press.

Breilh, Jaime. 2003. *Epidemiología crítica: Ciencia emancipadora e interculturalidad.* Buenos Aires: Lugar Editorial.

Brenneis, Don. 2006. "Reforming Promise." In *Documents: Artifacts of Modern Knowledge*, edited by Annelise Riles, 41–70. Ann Arbor: University of Michigan Press.

Briggs, Charles L. 1980. *The Wood Carvers of Córdova, New Mexico: Social Dimensions of an Artistic "Revival."* Knoxville: University of Tennessee Press.

Briggs, Charles L. 1986. *Learning How to Ask: A Sociolinguistic Appraisal of the Role of the Interview in Social Science Research.* Cambridge: Cambridge University Press.

Briggs, Charles L. 1987. "Getting Both Sides of the Story: Oral History in Land Grant Research and Litigation." In *Land, Water, and Culture: New Perspectives on Hispanic Land Grants*, edited by Charles L. Briggs and John R. Van Ness, 217–65. Albuquerque: University of New Mexico Press.

Briggs, Charles L. 1988. *Competence in Performance: The Creativity of Tradition in Mexicano Verbal Art.* Philadelphia: University of Pennsylvania Press.

Briggs, Charles L. 1992. "'Since I Am a Woman, I Will Chastise My Relatives': Gender, Reported Speech, and the (Re)production of Social Relations in Warao Ritual Wailing." *American Ethnologist* 19 (2): 337–61.

Briggs, Charles L. 1993a. "Generic versus Metapragmatic Dimensions of Warao Narratives: Who Regiments Performance?" In *Reflexive Language: Reported Speech and Metapragmatics*, edited by John A. Lucy, 179–212. Cambridge: Cambridge University Press.

Briggs, Charles L. 1993b. "Metadiscursive Practices and Scholarly Authority in Folkloristics." *Journal of American Folklore* 106 (422): 387–434.

Briggs, Charles L. 1993c. "Personal Sentiments and Polyphonic Voices in Warao Women's Ritual Wailing: Music and Poetics in a Critical and Collective Discourse." *American Anthropologist* 95 (4): 929–57.

Briggs, Charles L. 1996. "The Politics of Discursive Authority in Research on the 'Invention of Tradition.'" *Cultural Anthropology* 11 (4): 435–69.

Briggs, Charles L. 2000. "Emergence of the Non-indigenous Peoples: A Warao Narrative." In *Translating Native Latin American Verbal Art: Ethnopoetics and Ethnography of Speaking*, edited by Kay Sammons and Joel Sherzer, 174–96. Washington, DC: Smithsonian Institution Press.

Briggs, Charles L. 2005. "Communicability, Racial Discourse, and Disease." *Annual Review of Anthropology* 34:269–91.

Briggs, Charles L. 2007. "Mediating Infanticide: Theorizing Relations between Narratives and Violence." *Cultural Anthropology* 22 (3): 315–56.

Briggs, Charles L. 2008. *Poéticas de vida en espacios de muerte: Género, poder y estado en la cotidianeidad Warao.* Quito, Ecuador: Editorial Abya-Yala.

Briggs, Charles L., and Richard Bauman. 1992. "Genre, Intertextuality, and Social Power." *Journal of Linguistic Anthropology* 2:131–72.

Briggs, Charles L., Norbelys Gómez, Tirso Gómez, Clara Mantini-Briggs, Conrado Moraleda Izco, and Enrique Moraleda Izco. 2015. *"Una enfermedad monstruo": Indígenas derribando el cerco de la discriminación en salud.* Buenos Aires: Lugar Editorial.

Briggs, Charles L., and Daniel C. Hallin. 2016. *Making Health Public: How News Coverage Is Remaking Media, Medicine, and Contemporary Life.* London: Routledge.

Briggs, Charles L., and Clara Mantini-Briggs. 2003. *Stories in the Time of Cholera: Racial Profiling during a Medical Nightmare.* Berkeley: University of California Press.

Briggs, Charles L., and Clara Mantini-Briggs. 2009. "Confronting Health Disparities: Latin American Social Medicine in Venezuela." *American Journal of Public Health* 99 (3): 549–55.

Briggs, Charles L., and Clara Mantini-Briggs. 2016. *Tell Me Why My Children Died: Rabies, Indigenous Knowledge, and Communicative Justice.* Durham, NC: Duke University Press.

Briggs, Charles L., and Amy Shuman, eds. 1993. "Theorizing Folklore." Special issue, *Western Folklore* 52 (2–3).

Briggs, Charles L., and John R. Van Ness, eds. 1987. *Land, Water, and Culture: New Perspectives on Hispanic Land Grants.* Albuquerque: University of New Mexico Press.

Briggs, Charles L., and Julián Josué Vigil. 1990. *The Lost Gold Mine of Juan Mondragón: A Legend of New Mexico Performed by Melaquías Romero.* Tucson: University of Arizona Press.

Bronner, Simon J. 1986. *American Folklore Studies: An Intellectual History.* Lawrence: University Press of Kansas.

Bronner, Simon J. 1998. *Following Tradition: Folklore in the Discourse of American Culture.* Logan: Utah State University Press.

Bronner, Simon J. 2007. "Introduction: The Analytics of Alan Dundes." In *The Meaning of Folklore: The Analytical Essays of Alan Dundes*, edited by Simon J. Bronner, 1–50. Logan: Utah State University Press.

Bronner, Simon J. 2011. *Explaining Traditions: Folk Behavior in Modern Culture.* Lexington: University Press of Kentucky.

Brown, Michael F. 2003. *Who Owns Native Culture?* Cambridge, MA: Harvard University Press.

Brunvand, Jan Harold. 1968. *The Study of American Folklore: An Introduction.* New York: Norton.

Brunvand, Jan. 1981. *The Vanishing Hitchhiker: American Urban Legends and Their Meanings.* New York: Norton.

Burke, Kenneth. 1941. *The Philosophy of Literary Form: Studies in Symbolic Action.* Baton Rouge: Louisiana State University Press.

Butler, Judith. 1997. *Excitable Speech: A Politics of the Performative.* New York: Routledge.

Butler, Judith. 2004. *Precarious Life: The Powers of Mourning and Violence.* London: Verso.

Campbell, Scott W., and Nojin Kwak. 2011. "Mobile Communication and Civil Society: Linking Patterns and Places of Use to Engagement with Others in Public." *Human Communication Research* 37 (2): 207–22.

Canguilhem, Georges. (1966) 1989. *The Normal and the Pathological.* Translated by Carolyn R. Fawcett. New York: Zone.

Carr, E. Summerson. 2011. *Scripting Addiction: The Politics of Therapeutic Talk and American Sobriety.* Princeton, NJ: Princeton University Press.

Carr, E. Summerson, and Michael Lempert, eds. 2016. *Scale: Discourse and Dimensions of Social Life.* Oakland: University of California Press.

Carr, Gerald L., and Barbra Meek. 2013. "The Poetics of Language Revitalization: Text, Performance, and Change." *Journal of Folklore Research* 50 (1–3): 191–216.

Carvalho Neto, Paulo de. 1972. *Folklore and Psychoanalysis.* Translated by Jacques M. P. Wilson. Coral Gables, FL: University of Miami Press.

Castells, Manuel. 1996. *The Information Age: Economy, Society and Culture.* Vol. 1: *The Rise of the Network Society.* Cambridge, MA: Blackwell.

Castro, Aruchu, and Merrill Singer, eds. 2004. *Unhealthy Health Policy: A Critical Anthropological Examination.* Walnut Creek, CA: Altamira.

CDC (Centers for Disease Control and Prevention). (2006) 2007. *Crisis and Emergency Risk Communication: Pandemic Influenza*. Atlanta: CDC.
Chakrabarty, Dipesh. 1989. *Rethinking Working-Class History: Bengal, 1890–1940*. Princeton, NJ: Princeton University Press.
Chakrabarty, Dipesh. 2000. *Provincializing Europe: Postcolonial Thought and Historical Difference*. Princeton, NJ: Princeton University Press.
Chatterjee, Roma, and Deepak Mehta. 2007. *Living with Violence: An Anthropology of Events and Everyday Life*. New Delhi: Routledge.
Chávez, Alex E. 2017. *Sounds of Crossing: Music, Migration, and the Aural Poetics of Huapango Arribeño*. Durham, NC: Duke University Press.
Chen, Mel Y. 2012. *Animacies: Biopolitics, Racial Mattering, and Queer Affect*. Durham, NC: Duke University Press.
Cheng, Anne Anlin. 2000. *Melancholy of Race: Psychoanalysis, Assimilation, and Hidden Grief*. Cary, NC: Oxford University Press.
Ciccariello-Maher, George. 2013. *We Created Chávez: A People's History of the Venezuelan Revolution*. Durham, NC: Duke University Press.
Cicourel, Aaron V. 1992. "The Interpenetration of Communicative Contexts: Examples from Medical Encounters." In *Rethinking Context: Language as an Interactive Phenomenon*, edited by Alessandro Duranti and Charles Goodwin, 291–310. Cambridge: Cambridge University Press.
Clarke, Adele E., Jennifer Fishman, Jennifer Fosket, Laura Mamo, and Janet Shim. 2003. "Biomedicalization: Technoscientic Transformations of Health, Illness and U.S. Biomedicine." *American Sociological Review* 68:161–94.
Clifford, James. 1988. *The Predicament of Culture: Twentieth Century Ethnography, Literature, and Art*. Cambridge, MA: Harvard University Press.
Clifford, James. 1997. *Routes: Travel and Translation in the Late Twentieth Century*. Cambridge, MA: Harvard University Press.
Clifford, James. 2004. "Traditional Futures." In *Questions of Tradition*, edited by Mark Phillips and Gordon Schochet, 152–68. Toronto: University of Toronto Press.
Clifford, James. 2013. *Returns: Becoming Indigenous in the Twenty-First Century*. Cambridge, MA: Harvard University Press.
Clifford, James, and George Marcus, eds. 1986. *Writing Culture: The Poetics and Politics of Ethnography*. Berkeley: University of California Press.
Cocchiara, Guiseppe. 1981. *The History of Folklore in Europe*. Translated by John N. McDaniel. Philadelphia: Institute for the Study of Human Issues.
Cohen, Lawrence. 1998. *No Aging in India: Alzheimer's, the Bad Family, and Other Modern Things*. Berkeley: University of California Press.
Cohen, Lawrence. (2001) 2002. "The Other Kidney: Biopolitics beyond Recognition." In *Commodifying Bodies*, edited by Nancy Scheper-Hughes and Loïc Wacquant, 9–29. London: Sage.
Cohn, Bernard S. 1996. *Colonialism and Its Forms of Knowledge: The British in India*. Princeton, NJ: Princeton University Press.
Collier, Stephen J., and Aihwa Ong. 2005. "Global Assemblages, Anthropological Problems." In *Global Assemblages: Technology, Politics, and Ethics as Anthropological Problems*, edited by Aihwa Ong and Stephen J. Collier, 3–21. Malden, MA: Blackwell.
Conrad, Peter. 1992. "Medicalization and Social Control." *Annual Review of Sociology* 18:209–32.
Copeland, J. R. 1968. *Roads and Their Traffic, 1750–1850*. Newton Abbot, UK: David and Charles.
Coronil, Fernando. 1997. *The Magical State: Nature, Money, and Modernity in Venezuela*. Chicago: University of Chicago Press.

Couldry, Nick. 2012. *Media, Society, World: Social Theory and Digital Media Practice*. Cambridge: Polity.
Couldry, Nick, and Andreas Hepp. 2013. "Conceptualizing Mediatization: Contexts, Traditions, Arguments." *Communication Theory* 23 (3): 191–202.
Couldry, Nick, and Andreas Hepp. 2017. *The Mediated Construction of Reality*. Cambridge: Polity.
Crapanzano, Vincent. 1973. *The Hamadsha: A Study in Moroccan Ethnopsychiatry*. Berkeley: University of California Press.
Crapanzano, Vincent. 1981. "Text, Transference, and Indexicality." *Ethos* 9 (2): 122–48.
Csordas, Thomas J., ed. 1994. *Embodiment and Experience: The Existential Ground of Culture and Self*. Cambridge: Cambridge University Press.
Das, Veena. 2007. *Life and Words: Violence and the Descent into the Ordinary*. Berkeley: University of California Press.
Das, Veena, and Ranendra K. Das. 2006. "Pharmaceuticals in Urban Ecologies: The Register of the Local." In *Global Pharmaceuticals: Ethics, Markets, Practices*, edited by Adriana Petryna, Andrew Lakoff, and Arthur Kleinman, 171–205. Durham, NC: Duke University Press.
Daxelmüller, Christoph. 1994. "Nazi Conceptions of Culture and the Erasure of Jewish Folklore." In *The Nazification of an Academic Discipline: Folklore in the Third Reich*, edited by James Dow and Hannjost Lixfeld, 69–86. Bloomington: Indiana University Press.
De Certeau, Michel. 1984. *The Practice of Everyday Life*. Translated by Steven Rendall. Berkeley: University of California Press.
Dégh, Linda. 1994. *American Folklore and the Mass Media*. Bloomington: Indiana University Press.
Dégh, Linda, and Andrew Vázsonyi. (1969) 1976. "Legend and Belief." In *Folklore Genres*, edited by Dan Ben-Amos, 93–123. Austin: University of Texas Press.
De la Cadena, Marisol. 2015. *Earth Beings: Ecologies of Practice across Andean Worlds*. Durham, NC: Duke University Press.
Deleuze, Gilles, and Félix Guattari. (1980) 1987. *A Thousand Plateaus: Capitalism and Schizophrenia*. Translated by Brian Massumi. Minneapolis: University of Minnesota Press.
Derrida, Jacques. (1967) 1976. *Of Grammatology*. Translated by Gayatri Chakravorty Spivak. Baltimore, MD: Johns Hopkins University Press.
Derrida, Jacques. 1988. *Limited Inc.* Translated by Alan Bass, Jeffrey Mehlman, and Samuel Weber. Evanston, IL: Northwestern University Press.
Dick, Hilary Parsons, and Kristina Wirtz, eds. 2011. "Racializing Discourse." Special issue, *Journal of Linguistic Anthropology* 21 (S1).
Dirks, Nicholas B. 2001. *Castes of Mind: Colonialism and the Making of Modern India*. Princeton, NJ: Princeton University Press.
Dorson, Richard M. 1959. "A Theory for American Folklore." *Journal of American Folklore* 72 (285): 197–215.
Dorson, Richard M. 1968. *The British Folklorists: A History*. Chicago: University of Chicago Press.
Dorson, Richard M. 1969. "A Theory for American Folklore Reviewed." *Journal of American Folklore* 82 (325): 226–44.
Dorson, Richard M. 1971. *American Folklore and the Historian*. Chicago: University of Chicago Press.
Dorson, Richard M. 1972. "Introduction: Concepts of Folklore and Folklife Studies." In *Folklore and Folklife: An Introduction*, edited by Richard Dorson, 1–50. Chicago: University of Chicago Press.

Dorson, Richard M. 1976. *Folklore and Fakelore: Essays toward a Discipline of Folk Studies*. Cambridge, MA: Harvard University Press.

Dow, James R. 2008. "There Is No Grand Theory in Germany, and for Good Reason." *Journal of Folklore Research* 45 (1): 55–62.

Dow, James R., and Hannjost Lixfeld, trans. and eds. 1986. *German Volkskunde: A Decade of Theoretical Confrontation, Debate, and Reorientation (1967–1977)*. Bloomington: Indiana University Press.

Dow, James R., and Hannjost Lixfeld. 1994. *The Nazification of an Academic Discipline: Folklore in the Third Reich*. Bloomington: Indiana University Press.

Du Bois, W.E.B. (1903) 1990. *The Souls of Black Folk*. New York: Vintage.

Duchêne, Alexandre, and Monica Heller, eds. 2012. *Language in Late Capitalism: Pride and Profit*. New York: Routledge.

Dundes, Alan. 1965. *The Study of Folklore*. Englewood Cliffs, NJ: Prentice-Hall.

Dundes, Alan. 1980. *Interpreting Folklore*. Bloomington: Indiana University Press.

Dundes, Alan. 1987a. *Parsing through Customs: Essays by a Freudian Folklorist*. Madison: University of Wisconsin Press.

Dundes, Alan. 1987b. "The Psychoanalytic Study of the Grimms' Tales with Special Reference to 'The Maiden without Hands' (AT 706)." *Germanic Review* 62 (2): 50–65.

Dundes, Alan. 1991. "Bruno Bettelheim's Uses of Enchantment and Abuses of Scholarship." *Journal of American Folklore* 104 (411): 74–83.

Dundes, Alan. 2005. "Folkloristics in the Twenty-First Century" (AFS Invited Presidential Plenary Address, 2004). *Journal of American Folklore* 118 (470): 385–408.

Dupey, Ana María. 1988. "Tres abordajes a la diversidad cultural: Cultura popular, elitelore y folklore." *Revista de Investigaciones Folclóricas* 3:35–42.

Dussel, Enrique D. (1992) 1995. *The Invention of the Americas: Eclipse of "the Other" and the Myth of Modernity*. Translated by Michael D. Barber. New York: Continuum.

Dussel, Enrique. 1998. "Beyond Eurocentrism: The World-System and the Limits of Modernity." In *The Cultures of Globalization*, edited by Fredric Jameson and Masao Miyoshi. Durham, NC: Duke University Press.

Ellis, John M. 1983. *One Fairy Story Too Many: The Brothers Grimm and Their Tales*. Chicago: University of Chicago Press.

Ellner, Steve, ed. 2014. *Latin America's Radical Left: Challenges and Complexities of Political Power in the Twenty-First Century*. Lantham, MD: Rowman and Littlefield.

Emmerich, Wolfgang. 1971. *Zur Kritik der Volkstumsideologie*. Frankfurt: Suhrkamp.

Epstein, Steven. 1996. *Impure Science: AIDS, Activism, and the Politics of Knowledge*. Berkeley: University of California Press.

Epstein, Steven. 2007. *Inclusion: The Politics of Difference in Medical Research*. Chicago: University of Chicago Press.

Escalante G., Bernarda, and Librado Moraleda. 1992. *Narraciones warao: Origen, cultura, historia*. Caracas: Instituto Caribe de Antropología y Sociología, Fundación La Salle.

Esterly, David. 2012. *The Lost Carving: A Journey to the Heart of Making*. New York: Viking.

Fabian, Johannes. 2000. *Out of Our Minds: Reason and Madness in the Exploration of Central Africa*. Berkeley: University of California Press.

Fanon, Frantz. (1961) 1963. *The Wretched of the Earth*. Translated by Constance Farrington. New York: Grove.

Fanon, Frantz. (1952) 1967. *Black Skin, White Masks*. Translated by Charles Lam Markmann. New York: Grove.

Farmer, Paul. 1992. *AIDS and Accusation: Haiti and the Geography of Blame*. Berkeley: University of California Press.

Farmer, Paul. 2003. *Pathologies of Power: Health, Human Rights, and the New War on the Poor*. Berkeley: University of California Press.

Feintuch, Burt, ed. 1988. *The Conservation of Culture: Folklorists and the Public Sector.* Lexington: University Press of Kentucky.

Feld, Stephen. (1982) 2012. *Sound and Sentiment: Birds, Weeping, Poetics, and Song in Kaluli Expression.* 3rd ed. Durham, NC: Duke University Press.

Feld, Stephen. 1990. "Wept Thoughts: The Voicing of Kaluli Memories." *Oral Tradition* 5 (2–3): 241–66.

Feld, Stephen. 2000. "Sweet Lullaby for World Music." *Public Culture* 12 (1): 145–71.

Fine, Gary Alan. 2008. "The Sweep of Knowledge: The Politics of Grand and Local Theory in Folkloristics." *Journal of Folklore Research* 45 (1): 11–18.

Fine, Gary Alan, and Patricia A. Turner. 2001. *Whispers on the Color Line: Rumor and Race in America.* Berkeley: University of California Press.

Fischman, Fernando, and Javier Pelacoff. 2015. "Reading Memoria Activa's Discourse: Demands for Justice and Identity Symbols." In *Landscapes of Memory and Impunity: The Aftermath of the AMIA Bombing in Jewish Argentina,* edited by Annette H. Levine and Natasha Zaretsky, 44–58. Leiden: Brill.

Flores, Richard. 1995. *Los Pastores: History and Performance in the Mexican Shepherds' Play of South Texas.* Washington, DC: Smithsonian Institution Press.

Flueckiger, Joyce Burkhalter. 2006. *In Amma's Healing Room: Gender and Vernacular Islam in South India.* Bloomington: Indiana University Press.

Foster, George M., and Barbara Gallatin Anderson. 1978. *Medical Anthropology.* New York: Wiley.

Foster, Michael Dylan, and Jeffrey A. Tolbert, eds. 2015. *The Folkloresque: Reframing Folklore in a Popular Culture World.* Logan: Utah State University Press.

Frank, Russell. 2011 *Newslore: Contemporary Folklore on the Internet.* Jackson: University Press of Mississippi.

Frazer, James George. (1922) 1950. *The Golden Bough: A Study in Magic and Religion.* New York: Macmillan.

Freud, Sigmund. (1900) 1965. *The Interpretation of Dreams.* Translated by James Strachey. New York: Avon.

Freud, Sigmund. (1905) 2002. *The Joke and Its Relation to the Unconscious.* Translated by Joyce Crick. London: Penguin.

Freud, Sigmund. (1915) 1946. "Trauer und Melancholie." In *Werke aus den Jahren 1913–1917,* vol. 10 of *Gesammelte Werke,* edited by Anna Freud, 427–46. Frankfurt: S. Fischer Verlag.

Freud, Sigmund. (1916) 1957. "On Transience." In *The Standard Edition of the Complete Psychological Works of Sigmund Freud,* translated and edited by James Strachey, 14:305–7. London: Hogarth.

Freud, Sigmund. (1917) 1957. "Mourning and Melancholia." In *The Standard Edition of the Complete Psychological Works of Sigmund Freud,* translated and edited by James Strachey, 14:243–58. London: Hogarth.

Freud, Sigmund. 1960. *The Psychopathology of Everyday Life.* Translated by Alan Tyson. Edited by James Strachey. New York: Norton.

Garcia, Angela. 2010. *The Pastoral Clinic: Addiction and Dispossession along the Rio Grande.* Berkeley: University of California Press.

García, Jesús Chucho. 1992. *Afroamericano soy.* Caracas: Ediciones del Taller de Información y Documentacion de la Cultura Afrovenezolana.

García Canclini, Néstor. (1990) 1995. *Hybrid Cultures: Strategies for Entering and Leaving Modernity.* Translated by Christopher L. Chiappari and Silvia L. López. Minneapolis: University of Minnesota Press.

García Canclini, Néstor. 1995. *Consumidores y ciudadanos: Conflictos multiculturales de la globalización.* México, D.F.: Grijalbo.

Gershon, Ilana. 2010. *The Breakup 2.0: Disconnecting over New Media*. Ithaca, NY: Cornell University Press.

Gibson, James J. 1997. "The Theory of Affordances." In *Perceiving, Acting, and Knowing*, edited by Robert Shaw and John Bransford, 67–82. Hillsdale, NJ: Lawrence Erlbaum.

Gieryn, Thomas F. 1983. "Boundary-Work and the Demarcation of Science from Non-science: Strains and Interests in Professional Ideologies of Scientists." *American Sociological Review* 48 (6): 781–95.

Gilroy, Paul. 1993. *The Black Atlantic: Modernity and Double Consciousness*. Cambridge, MA: Harvard University Press.

Gingrich, Andre. 1998. "Frontier Myths of Orientalism: The Muslim World in Public and Popular Cultures of Central Europe." In *Mediterranean Ethnological Summer School*, vol. 2, edited by Bojan Baskar and Borut Brumen, 99–127. Ljubljana, Slovenia: Inštitut za Multikulturne Raziskave.

Goffman, Erving. 1961. *Asylums: Essays on the Social Situation of Mental Patients and Other Inmates*. Garden City, NY: Anchor.

Goffman, Erving. 1981. "Response Cries." In *Forms of Talk*, 78–123. Philadelphia: University of Pennsylvania Press.

Goldberg, David Theo. 1993. *Racist Culture: Philosophy and the Politics of Meaning*. Oxford: Blackwell.

Goldstein, Diane. 2001. "Competing Logics and the Construction of Risk." In *Healing Logics: Culture and Medicine in Modern Health Belief Systems*, edited by Erika Brady, 129–40. Logan: Utah State University Press.

Goldstein, Diane E. 2004. *Once upon a Virus: AIDS Legends and Vernacular Risk Perception*. Logan: Utah State University Press.

Goldstein, Diane E., and Amy Shuman, eds. 2016. *The Stigmatized Vernacular: Where Reflexivity Meets Untellability*. Bloomington: Indiana University Press.

Goldstein, Ruth. 2019. "Ethnobotanies of Refusal: Methodologies in Respecting Plant(ed)-Human Resistance." *Anthropology Today* 35 (2): 18–22.

González-Martin, Rachel V. 2017. "A Latinx Folklorist's Love Letter to American Folkloristics: Academic Disenchantment and Ambivalent Disciplinary Futures." *Chiricú* 2 (1): 19–39.

Goodman, Jane E. 2002. "Stealing Our Heritage? Women's Folksongs, Copyright Law, and the Public Domain in Algeria." *Africa Today* 49 (1): 84–97.

Goodman, Jane E. 2005. *Berber Culture on the World Stage: From Village to Video*. Bloomington: Indiana University Press.

Gordon, Avery. 1997. *Ghostly Matters: Haunting and the Sociological Imagination*. Minneapolis: University of Minnesota Press.

Gramsci, Antonio. 1971. *Selections from the Prison Notebooks of Antonio Gramsci*. Edited and translated by Quintin Hoare and Geoffrey Nowell Smith. New York: International.

Grider, Sylvia. 1981. "The Media Narraform: Symbiosis of Mass Media and Oral Tradition." *Arv* 37:125–31.

Grimm, Jacob, and Wilhelm Grimm. (1812/1819) 1987. Prefaces to the First and Second Editions of the *Nursery and Household Tales*. In *The Hard Facts of the Grimms' Fairy Tales*, edited by Maria Tatar, 203–22. Princeton, NJ: Princeton University Press.

Grimm, Jacob, and Wilhelm Grimm. (1816) 1981. Foreword to *The German Legends of the Brothers Grimm*, vol. 1, translated and edited by Donald Ward, 1–11. Philadelphia: Institute for the Study of Human Issues.

Groth, Stefan. 2012. *Negotiating Tradition: The Pragmatics of International Deliberation on Cultural Property*. Göttingen: Universitätsverlag Göttingen.

Gudynas, Eduardo. 2012. "Estado compensador y nuevos extractivismos: Las ambivalencias del progresismo sudamericano." *Nueva sociedad* 237:128–46.

Guha, Ranajit. 1982. "On Some Aspects of the Historiography of Colonial India." In *Subaltern Studies I: Writings on South Asian History and Society*, edited by Ranajit Guha, 1–8. Delhi: Oxford University Press.

Gupta, Akhi. 2012. *Red Tape: Bureaucracy, Structural Violence, and Poverty in India*. Durham, NC: Duke University Press.

Guss, David. 2000. *The Festive State: Race, Ethnicity, and Nationalism as Cultural Performance*. Berkeley: University of California Press.

Gutiérrez, Ramón A. 1991. *When Jesus Came, the Corn Mothers Went Away: Marriage, Sexuality, and Power in New Mexico, 1500–1846*. Stanford, CA: Stanford University Press.

Hafstein, Valdimar. 2004. "The Politics of Origin: Collective Creation Revisited." *Journal of American Folklore* 117 (465): 300–315.

Hafstein, Valdimar. 2018a. "Intangible Heritage as a Festival; or, Folklorization Revisited." *Journal of American Folklore* 131 (520): 127–49.

Hafstein, Valdimar. 2018b. *Making Intangible Heritage: El Condor Pasa and Other Stories from UNESCO*. Bloomington: Indiana University Press.

Hagerty, Alexa S. 2011. "Composing and Decomposing the Dead: Politics and Ethics in the American Funeral Home Movement." MA thesis, University of California, Berkeley.

Hall, Stuart. 1980. "Encoding/Decoding." In *Culture, Media, Language: Working Papers in Cultural Studies 1972–79*, edited by Stuart Hall et al., 128–38. London: Hutchinson.

Hallin, Daniel C. 1986. *The Uncensored War: The Media and Vietnam*. New York: Oxford University Press.

Hand, Wayland D. 1961. Introduction to *Popular Beliefs and Superstitions from North Carolina: The Frank C. Brown Collection of North Carolina Folklore*, 6:xix–xlvii. Durham, NC: Duke University Press.

Hand, Wayland D. 1976. Introduction to *American Folk Medicine: A Symposium*, edited by Wayland D. Hand. Berkeley: University of California Press.

Hand, Wayland D. 1980. *Magical Medicine: The Folkloric Component of Medicine in the Folk Belief, Custom, and Ritual of the Peoples of Europe and America*. Berkeley: University of California Press.

Handler, Richard, and Jocelyn Linnekin. 1984. "Tradition, Genuine or Spurious." *Journal of American Folklore* 97 (385): 273–90.

Hanks, William F. 1996. *Language and Communicative Practices*. Boulder, CO: Westview.

Hanks, William F. 2010. *Converting Words: Maya in the Age of the Cross*. Berkeley: University of California Press.

Haraway, Donna J. 1996. *Modest_Witness@ Second_Millennium.FemaleMan_Meets_ OncoMouseTM: Feminism and Technoscience*. New York: Routledge.

Haraway, Donna J. 2008. *When Species Meet*. Minneapolis: University of Minnesota Press.

Haring, Lee. 2008a. "America's Antitheoretical Folkloristics." *Journal of Folklore Research* 45 (1): 1–9.

Haring, Lee, ed. 2008b. "Grand Theory in Folkloristics." Special issue, *Journal of Folklore Research* 45 (1).

Harries, Karsten. 1983. *The Bavarian Rococo Church: Between Faith and Aestheticism*. New Haven, CT: Yale University Press.

Hartigan, John, Jr. 2017. *Care of the Species: Races of Corn and the Science of Plant Biodiversity*. Minneapolis: University of Minnesota Press.

Harvey, David. 1989. *The Condition of Postmodernity: An Enquiry into the Origins of Culture Change*. Oxford: Blackwell.

Hasan-Rokem, Galit. 2014. "Bodies Performing in Ruins: The Lamenting Mother in Ancient Hebrew Texts." In *Lament in Jewish Thought: Philosophical, Theological,*

     and Literary Perspectives, edited by Ilit Ferber and Paula Schwebel, 33–63. Berlin: De Gruyter.
Hayden, Cori. 2003. *When Nature Goes Public: The Making and Unmaking of Bioprospecting in Mexico*. Princeton, NJ: Princeton University Press.
Heinen, H. Dieter. 1988. "Los Warao." In *Los aborigenes de Venezuela*, vol. 3, edited by Walter Coppens, 585–689. Caracas: Funcación La Salle de Ciencias Naturales, Instituto Caribe de Antropología y Sociología and Monte Avila Editores.
Heinen, Dieter, and Rafael Gassón. 2006. "El verdadero delta indígena: Elementos para una ecología histórica del Delta del Orinoco." *Copérnico* 3 (5): 61–66.
Heller, Monica, and Bonnie McElhinny. 2017. *Language, Capitalism, and Colonialism: Toward a Critical History*. North York, Ontario: University of Toronto Press.
Hepp, Andreas. (2011) 2013. *Cultures of Mediatization*. Translated by Keith Tribe. Cambridge: Polity.
Herder, Johann Gottfried. (1774) 2002. *Philosophical Writings*. Translated and edited by Michael N. Forster. Cambridge: Cambridge University Press.
Herder, Johann Gottfried. (1782–1783) 1833. *The Spirit of Hebrew Poetry*. 2 vols. Translated by James Marsh. Burlington, VT: Edward Smith.
Herder, Johann Gottfried. (1772) 1966. "Essay on the Origin of Language." In *On the Origin of Language: Jean Jacques Rousseau, Essay on the Origin of Languages and Johann Gottfried Herder, Essay on the Origin of Language*, translated by John H. Moran and Alexander Gode. Chicago: University of Chicago Press.
Herder, Johann Gottfried. (1877–1913) 1967. *Sämmtliche Werke*. Vol. 5. Edited by Bernhard Suphan. Hildesheim, Germany: Georg Olms Verlagsbuchhandlung.
Herrera-Sobek, María. 1990. *The Mexican Corrido: A Feminist Analysis*. Bloomington: Indiana University Press.
Herzfeld, Michael. 1982. *Ours Once More: Folklore, Ideology, and the Making of Modern Greece*. Austin: University of Texas Press.
Hill, Jane H. 1995. "The Voices of Don Gabriel: Responsibility and Self in a Modern Mexicano Narrative." In *The Dialogic Emergence of Culture*, edited by Dennis Tedlock and Bruce Mannheim, 97–147. Urbana: University of Illinois Press.
Hill, Jane H. 2008. *The Everyday Language of White Racism*. Chichester, UK: Wiley-Blackwell.
Hindery, Derrick. 2013. *From Enron to Evo: Pipeline Politics, Global Environmentalism, and Indigenous Rights in Bolivia*. Tucson: University of Arizona Press.
Hirschkind, Charles. 2006. *The Ethical Soundscape: Cassette Sermons and Islamic Counterpublics*. New York: Columbia University Press.
Hjarvard, Stig. 2013. *The Mediatization of Culture and Society*. London: Routledge.
Hobsbawm, Eric. 1983. Introduction to *The Invention of Tradition*, edited by Eric Hobsbawm and Terence Ranger, 1–14. Cambridge: Cambridge University Press.
Holbek, Bengt. 1987. *Interpretation of Fairy Tales: Danish Folklore in a European Perspective*. Helsinki: Suomalainen Tiedeakatemia.
Homer. 1963. *The Odyssey*. Translated by Robert Fitzgerald. New York: Anchor.
Howard, Robert Glenn. 2008. "Electronic Hybridity: The Persistent Processes of the Vernacular Web." *Journal of American Folklore* 121 (480): 192–218.
Howard, Robert Glenn. 2011. *Digital Jesus: The Making of a New Christian Fundamentalist Community on the Internet*. New York: New York University Press.
Howard, Robert Glenn. 2012. "How Counterculture Helped Put the 'Vernacular' in Vernacular Webs." In *Folk Culture in the Digital Age: The Emergent Dynamics of Human Interaction*, edited by Trevor Blank, 25–45. Logan: Utah State University Press.
Hufford, David J. 1982. *The Terror That Comes in the Night: An Experience-Centered Study of Supernatural Assault Traditions*. Philadelphia: University of Pennsylvania Press.

Hufford, David J. 1988. "Contemporary Folk Medicine." In *Other Healers: Unorthodox Medicine in America*, edited by Norman Gevitz, 228–64. Baltimore, MD: Johns Hopkins University Press.

Hufford, David J. 1997. "Medicine, Folk." In *Folklore: An Encyclopedia of Beliefs, Customs, Tales, Music, and Art*, edited by Thomas A. Green, 2:544–53. Santa Barbara, CA: ABC-CLIO.

Hufford, Mary. 2004. "Knowing Ginseng: The Social Life of an Appalachian Root." *Cahier de litterature orale* 53–54:265–92.

Hull, Matthew S. 2012. *Government of Paper: The Materiality of Bureaucracy in Urban Pakistan*. Berkeley: University of California Press.

Hurston, Zora Neale. (1935) 1978. *Mules and Men*. Bloomington: Indiana University Press.

Hymes, Dell. 1971. "The Contribution of Folklore to Sociolinguistic Research." *Journal of American Folklore* 84 (331): 42–50.

Hymes, Dell. 1974. *Foundations in Sociolinguistics: An Ethnographic Approach*. Philadelphia: University of Pennsylvania Press.

Hymes, Dell. 1975. "Folklore's Nature and the Sun's Myth." *Journal of American Folklore* 88 (350): 346–69.

Hymes, Dell. 1981. *"In Vain I tried to Tell You": Essays in Native America Ethnopoetics*. Philadelphia: University of Pennsylvania Press.

Hymes, Dell. 1992. "Helen Sekaquaptewa's 'Coyote and the Birds': Rhetorical Analysis of a Hopi Coyote Story." *Anthropological Linguistics* 34 (1–4): 45–72.

Hymes, Dell. 1996. *Ethnography, Linguistics, Narrative Inequality: Toward an Understanding of Voice*. London: Taylor and Francis.

Instituto Nacional de Estadística. 2003. *XII Censo de población y vivienda: Población y pueblos indígenas: Anexo estadístico*. Caracas: Ministerio de Planificación y Desarrollo, Instituto Nacional de Estadística, República Bolivariana de Venezuela.

Irvine, Judith T. 2001. "The Family Romance of Colonial Linguistics: Gender and Family in Nineteenth-Century Representations of African Languages." In *Languages and Publics: The Making of Authority*, edited by Susan Gal and Kathryn A. Woolard, 13–29. Manchester: St. Jerome.

Jaimes, M. Annette, and George A. Noriega. 1988. "History in the Making: How Academia Manufactures the 'Truth' about Native American Traditions." *Bloomsbury Review* 4 (5): 24–26.

Jakobson, Roman. 1960. "Closing Statement: Linguistics and Poetics." In *Style in Language*, edited by Thomas A. Sebeok, 350–77. Cambridge: MIT Press.

Jameson, Fredric. 1981. *The Political Unconscious: Narrative as a Socially Symbolic Act*. Ithaca, NY: Cornell University Press.

Jameson, Fredric. 1991. *Postmodernism, or, the Cultural Logic of Late Capitalism*. Durham, N.C.: Duke University Press.

Jenni, Oskar G., and Bonnie B. O'Connor. 2005. "Children's Sleep: An Interplay between Culture and Biology." *Pediatrics* 115 (1): 204–16.

Jones, Michael Owen, and Patrick A. Polk, with Ysamur Flores-Peña and Roberta J. Evanchuk. 2001. "Invisible Hospitals: Botánicas in Ethnic Health Care." In *Healing Logics: Culture and Medicine in Modern Health Belief Systems*, edited by Erika Brady, 39–87. Logan: Utah State University Press.

Kamenetsky, Christa. 1992. *The Brothers Grimm and Their Critics: Folktales and the Quest for Meaning*. Athens: Ohio University Press.

Kapchan, Deborah. 2007. *Traveling Spirit Masters: Moroccan Gnawa Trance and Music in the Global Marketplace*. Middletown, CT: Wesleyan University Press.

Keane, Webb. 2007. *Christian Moderns: Freedom and Fetish in the Mission Encounter*. Berkeley: University of California Press.

Kirshenblatt-Gimblett, Barbara. 1996. "Topic-Drift: Negotiating the Gap between the Field and Our Name." *Journal of Folklore Research* 33: 245–54.

Kirshenblatt-Gimblett, Barbara. 1998a. *Destination Culture: Tourism, Museums, and Heritage.* Berkeley: University of California Press.

Kirshenblatt-Gimblett, Barbara. 1998b. "Folklore's Crisis." *Journal of American Folklore* 111 (441): 281–327.

Kirshenblatt-Gimblett, Barbara. 2006. "World Heritage and Cultural Economics." In *Museum Frictions: Public Cultures/Global Transformations*, edited by Ivan Karp et al., 161–202. Durham, NC: Duke University Press.

Kitta, Andrea. 2012. *Vaccinations and Public Concern in History: Legend, Rumor, and Risk Perception.* New York: Routledge.

Klein, Melanie. (1940) 1948. "Mourning and Its Relation to Manic Depressive States." In *Contributions to Psycho-Analysis, 1921–1945*, 311–38. London: Hogarth.

Kleinman, Arthur. 1980. *Patients and Healers in the Context of Culture: An Exploration of the Borderland between Anthropology, Medicine, and Psychiatry.* Berkeley: University of California Press.

Kleinman, Arthur. 1988. *The Illness Narratives: Suffering, Healing, and the Human Condition.* New York: Basic Books.

Knorr-Cetina, Karin. 1999. *Epistemic Cultures: How the Sciences Make Knowledge.* Cambridge, MA: Harvard University Press.

Korom, Frank. 2006. *Village of Painters: Narrative Scrolls from West Bengal.* Santa Fe: Museum of New Mexico Press.

Koselleck, Reinhart. 2004. *Futures Past: On the Semantics of Historical Time.* Translated by Keith Tribe. New York: Columbia University Press.

Koven, Mikel J. 2003. "Folklore Studies and Popular Film and Television: A Necessary Critical Survey." *Journal of American Folklore* 116 (460): 176–95.

Kristeva, Julia. (1974) 1984. *Revolution in Poetic Language.* Translated by Margaret Waller. New York: Columbia University Press.

Kristeva, Julia. (1987) 1989. *Black Sun: Depression and Melancholia.* Translated by Leon S. Roudiez. New York: Columbia University Press.

Krohn, Kaarle. (1926) 1971. *Folklore Methodology.* Translated by Roger L. Welsch. Austin: University of Texas Press.

Kroskrity, Paul V., ed. 2000. *Regimes of Language: Ideologies, Polities, and Identities.* Santa Fe, NM: School of American Research.

Lacan, Jacques. (1966) 1977. *Écrit: A Selection.* Translated by Alan Sheridan. New York: Norton.

Lakoff, Andrew. 2005. *Pharmaceutical Reason: Knowledge and Value in Global Psychiatry.* Cambridge: Cambridge University Press.

Lakoff, Andrew. 2017. *Unprepared: Global Health in a Time of Emergency.* Oakland: University of California Press.

Laplanche, Jean. (1992) 1999. *Essays on Otherness.* London: Routledge.

Latour, Bruno. 1987. *Science in Action: How to Follow Scientists and Engineers through Society.* Cambridge, MA: Harvard University Press.

Latour, Bruno. 1999. "Circulating Reference." In *Pandora's Hope: Essays on the Reality of Science Studies*, 24–79. Cambridge, MA: Harvard University Press.

Lau, Kimberly J. 2000. *New Age Capitalism: Making Money East of Eden.* Philadelphia: University of Pennsylvania Press.

Lavandero Pérez, Julio. 1991. *Ajotejana I: Mitos.* Caracas: Ediciones Paulinas.

Lee, Ben, and Edward LiPuma. 2003. "Culture of Circulation: The Imaginations of Modernity." *Public Culture* 14 (1): 191–213.

Lee, Jon. 2014. *An Epidemic of Rumors: How Stories Shape Our Perception of Disease.* Logan: Utah State Unversity Press.
Lefebvre, Henri. (1974) 1991. *The Production of Space.* Translated by Donald Nicholson-Smith. Oxford: Blackwell.
Levine, Lawrence W. 1977. *Black Culture and Black Consciousness: Afro-American Folk Thought from Slavery to Freedom.* Oxford: Oxford University Press.
Limón, José E. 1992. *Mexican Ballads, Chicano Poems: History and Influence in Mexican-American Social Poetry.* Berkeley: University of California Press.
Limón, José E. 1994. *Dancing with the Devil: Society and Cultural Poetics in Mexican-American South Texas.* Madison: University of Wisconsin Press.
Limón, José E. 2007. "Américo Paredes: Ballad Scholar." *Journal of American Folklore* 120 (475): 3–18.
Limón, José E. 2012. *Américo Paredes: Culture and Critique.* Austin: University of Texas Press.
Limón, José E., and M. Jane Young. 1986. "Frontiers, Settlements, and Development in Folklore Studies, 1972–1985." *Annual Review of Anthropology* 15:437–60.
Lipsitz, George. 2001. *American Studies in a Moment of Danger.* Minneapolis: University of Minnesota Press.
Lixfeld, Hannjost. 1994. *Folklore and Fascism: The Reich Institute for German Volkskunde.* Translated and edited by James R. Dow. Bloomington: Indiana University Press.
Lock, Margaret M. 2002. *Twice Dead: Organ Transplants and the Reinvention of Death.* Berkeley: University of California Press.
Locke, John. (1690) 1959. *An Essay concerning Human Understanding.* 2 vols. New York: Dover.
Locke, John. (1690) 1960. *Two Treatises of Government.* New York: New American Library.
Lopez, German. 2020. "Trump's Expert Urged Caution about a Coronavirus Treatment. Trump Hyped It up Anyway." Vox. March 20, 2020. https://www.vox.com/policy-and-politics/2020/3/20/21188397/coronavirus-trump-press-briefing-covid-19-anthony-fauci.
López Morín, José R. 2006. *The Legacy of Américo Paredes.* College Station: Texas A&M University Press.
Lowe, Celia. 2010. "Viral Clouds: Becoming H5N1 in Indonesia." *Cultural Anthropology* 25 (4): 625–49.
Lundby, Knut. 2009. *Mediatization: Concept, Changes, Consequences.* New York: Peter Lang.
MacPhail, Theresa. 2010. "A Predictable Unpredictability: The 2009 H1N1 Pandemic and the Concept of 'Strategic Uncertainty' within Global Public Health." *Behemoth* 3:57–77.
Madsen, William.1964. *The Mexican-Americans of South Texas.* New York: Holt, Rinehart and Winston.
Maes, Mailis, Kristin Kremer, Dick van Soolingen, Howard Takiff, and Jacobus H. de Waard. 2008. "24-Locus of MIRU-VNTR Genotyping Is Useful Tool to Study the Molecular Epidemiology of Tuberculosis among Warao Amerindians in Venezuela." *Tuberculosis* 88 (5): 490–94. https://www.ncbi.nlm.nih.gov/pubmed/18514577.
Magliocco, Sabina. 2018. "Beyond the Rainbow Bridge: Vernacular Ontologies of Animal Afterlives." *Journal of Folklore Research* 55 (2): 39–67.
Malinowski, Bronislaw. 1935. *Coral Gardens and Their Magic: A Study of the Methods of Tilling the Soil and of Agricultural Rites in the Trobriand Islands.* New York: American.
Malinowski, Bronislaw. 1948. *Myth, Science and Religion and Other Essays.* Garden City, NY: Doubleday.

Marcus, George E., and Michael M. J. Fischer. 1986. *Anthropology as Cultural Critique: An Experimental Moment in the Human Sciences*. Chicago: University of Chicago Press.

Marder, Michael. 2013. *Plant-Thinking: A Philosophy of Vegetal Life*. New York: Columbia University Press.

Marder, Michael. 2014. *The Philosopher's Plant: An Intellectual Herbarium*. New York: Columbia University Press.

Martín Barbero, Jesús. (1987) 2003. *De los medios a las mediaciones: Comunicación, cultura y hegemonía*. Mexico City: G. Gili.

Marx, Karl. (1852) 1935. *The Eighteenth Brumaire of Louis Bonaparte*. New York: International Publishers.

Marx, Karl. (1867) 1967. "The Fetishism of Commodities." In *Capital: A Critique of Political Economy*, 1:71–83. New York: International.

McBratney, Michael Frank. 2006. "Tales of Colonel Temple: Critical Folkloristics and Colonial Modernity." MA thesis, Folklore Graduate Program, University of California, Berkeley.

McDowell, John H. 2000. *Poetry and Violence: The Ballad Tradition of Mexico's Costa Chica*. Urbana: University of Illinois Press.

McDowell, John H. 2010. "Rethinking Folklorization in Ecuador: Multivocality in the Expressive Contact Zone." *Western Folklore* 69 (2): 181–210.

Mechling, Jay. 1989. "'Banana Cannon' and Other Folk Traditions between Humans and Nonhuman Animals." *Western Folklore* 48:312–23.

Mechling, Jay. 2001. *On My Honor: Boy Scouts and the Making of American Youth*. Chicago: University of Chicago Press.

Mendoza-Denton, Norma. 2008. *Homegirls: Language and Cultural Practice among Latina Youth Gangs*. Malden, MA: Blackwell.

Menéndez, Eduardo L. 1981. *Poder, estraticación y salud: Analysis de las condiciones sociales y económicas de la enfermedad en Yucatán*. Mexico City: La Casa Chata.

Menéndez, Eduardo L. 2005. "Intencionalidad, experiencia y función: La articulación de los saberes médicos." *Revista de antropología social* 14:33–69.

Menéndez, Eduardo L. 2009. *De sujetos, saberes y estructuras: Introducción al enfoque relacional en el estudio de la salud colectiva*. Buenos Aires: Lugar Editorial.

Menéndez, Eduardo L., and Renée B. Di Pardo.1996. *De algunos alcoholismos y algunos saberes: Atención primaria y proceso de alcoholización*. México: CIESAS.

Menéndez, Eduardo L., and Renée B. Di Pardo. 2009. *Miedos, riesgos e inseguridades: Los medios, los profesionales y los intelectuales en la construcción social de la salúd como catástrofe*. Mexico City: CIESAS.

Mignolo, Walter D. 2000. *Local Histories/Global Designs: Coloniality, Subaltern Knowledges, and Border Thinking*. Princeton, NJ: Princeton University Press.

Miller, Kiri. 2008. "Grove Street Grimm: Grand Theft Auto and Digital Folklore." *Journal of American Folklore* 121 (481): 255–85.

Miller, Theresa L. 2019. *Plant Kin: A Multispecies Ethnography in Indigenous Brazil*. Austin: University of Texas Press.

Mills, Margaret A. 1993. "Feminist Theory and the Study of Folklore: A Twenty-Year Trajectory toward Theory." *Western Folklore* 52 (2–4): 173–92.

Mills, Margaret A. 2008. What('s) Theory? *Journal of Folklore Research* 45 (1): 19–28.

Mills, Margaret A., Peter J. Claus, and Sarah Diamond, eds. 2003. *South Asian Folklore: An Encyclopedia*. New York: Routledge.

Mitchell, Timothy. 2002. *Rule of Experts: Egypt, Techno-Politics, Modernity*. Berkeley: University of California Press.

Montoya, Michael J. 2011. *Making the Mexican Diabetic: Race, Science, and the Genetics of Inequality*. Berkeley: University of California Press.

Mould, Tom. 2011. "Traditionalization." In *Folklore: An Encyclopedia of Beliefs, Customs, Tales, Music, and Art*, vol. 1, edited by Charlie T. McCormick and Kim Kennedy White, 1202–5. Santa Barbara, CA: ABC-CLIO.

Muñoz Martínez, Monica. 2018. *The Injustice Never Leaves You: Anti-Mexican Violence in Texas*. Cambridge, MA: Harvard University Press.

Murphy, Keith M. 2015. *Swedish Design: An Ethnography*. Ithaca, NY: Cornell University Press.

Myers, Fred R. 2002. *Painting Culture: The Making of an Aboriginal High Art*. Durham, NC: Duke University Press.

Myers, Natasha. 2015. "Conversations on Plant Sensing: Notes from the Field." *NatureCulture* 3:35–66.

Myers, Natasha. 2016. "Photosynthesis." *Cultural Anthropology*, January 21, 2016. https://culanth.org/fieldsights/photosynthesis.

Nader, Laura. 1972. "Up the Anthropologist: Perspectives Gained from Studying Up." In *Reinventing Anthropology*, edited by Dell H. Hymes, 284–311. New York: Pantheon.

Naithani, Sadhana. 2001. "An Axis Jump: British Colonialism in the Oral Folk Narratives of Nineteenth Century India." *Folklore* 112:183–88.

Naithani, Sadhana. 2002. "To Tell a Tale Untold: Two Folklorists in Colonial India." *Journal of Folklore Research* 39 (2–3): 201–16.

Naithani, Sadhana. 2006. *In Quest of Indian Folktales: Pandit Ram Gharib Chaube and William Crooke*. Bloomington: Indiana University Press.

Naithani, Sadhana. 2010. *The Story-time of the British Empire: Colonial and Postcolonial Folkloristics*. Jackson: University Press of Mississippi.

Narayan, Kirin, with Urmila Devi Sood. 1997. *Mondays on the Dark Night of the Moon: Himalayan Foothill Folktales*. New York: Oxford University Press.

Nas, Peter J. M. 2002. "Masterpieces of Oral and Intangible Culture: Reflections on the UNESCO World Heritage List." *Current Anthropology* 43 (1): 139–48.

Nasio, Juan-David. 2004. *The Book of Love and Pain: Thinking at the Limit with Freud and Lacan*. Translated by David Pettigrew and François Raffoul. Albany: State University of New York Press.

Neeson, J. M. 1993. *Commoners: Common Right, Enclosure and Social Change in England, 1700–1820*. Cambridge: Cambridge University Press.

Nenola-Kallio, Aili. 1982. *Studies in Ingrian Laments*. Helsinki: Academia Scientiarum Fennica.

Nichter, Mark, ed. 1992. *Anthropological Approaches to the Study of Ethnomedicine*. Montreux, Switzerland: Gordon and Breach.

Nichter, Mark. 2008. *Global Health: Why Cultural Perceptions, Social Representations, and Biopolitics Matter*. Tucson: University of Arizona Press.

Nichter, Mark, and Vinay Kamat. 1998. "Pharmacies, Self Medication, and Pharmaceutical Marketing in Bombay India." *Social Science and Medicine* 47 (6): 779–94.

Noyes, Dorothy. 2008. "Humble Theory." *Journal of Folklore Research* 45 (1): 37–43.

Noyes, Dorothy. 2016. *Humble Theory: Folklore's Grasp on Social Life*. Bloomington: Indiana University Press.

Nuckolls, Janis B. 1999. "The Case for Sound Symbolism." *Annual Review of Anthropology* 28:225–52.

Obeng, Samuel, and Beverly J. Stoeltje. 2002. "Women's Voices in Akan Juridical Discourse." *Africa Today* 49 (1): 21–41.

Ochoa Gautier, Ana María. 1996. "Plotting Musical Territories: Three Studies in Processes of Recontextualization of Musical Folklore in the Andean Region of Colombia." PhD diss., Indiana University.

Ochoa Gautier, Ana María. 2003. *Entre los deseos y los derechos: Un ensayo crítico sobre políticas culturales*. Bogota: Instituto Colombiano de Antropología e Historia.

Ochoa Gautier, Ana María. 2006. "Sonic Transculturation, Epistemologies of Purification and the Aural Public Sphere in Latin America." *Social Identities* 12 (6): 803–25.

Ochoa Gautier, Ana María. 2014. *Aurality: Listening and Knowledge in Nineteenth-Century Colombia*. Durham, NC: Duke University Press.

Ochs, Elinor, Ruth C. Smith, and Carolyn E. Taylor. 1996. "Detective Stories at Dinnertime: Problem Solving through Co-Narration." In *Disorderly Dialogues: Narrative, Conflict, and Inequality*, edited by Charles L. Briggs, 95–113. Oxford: Oxford University Press.

O'Connor, Bonnie B. 1995. *Healing Traditions: Alternative Medicine and the Health Professions*. Philadelphia: University of Pennsylvania Press.

O'Connor, Bonnie B., and David J. Hufford. 2001. "Understanding Folk Medicine." In *Healing Logics: Culture and Medicine in Modern Health Belief Systems*, edited by Erika Brady, 13–35. Logan: Utah State University Press.

Ó Giolláin, Diarmuid. 2000. *Locating Irish Folklore: Tradition, Modernity, Identity*. Cork: Cork University Press.

Olsen, Dale A. 1996. *Music of the Warao of Venezuela: Song People of the Rain Forest*. Gainesville: University Press of Florida.

Omi, Michael, and Howard Winant. 1994. *Racial Formation in the United States: From the 1960s to the 1990s*. New York: Routledge.

O'Neill, Sean Patrick. 2013. "Translating Oral Literature in Indigenous Societies: Ethnic Aesthetic Performances in Multicultural and Multilingual Settings." *Journal of Folklore Research* 50 (1–3): 217–50.

Ong, Aihwa, and Stephen J. Collier, eds. 2005. *Global Assemblages: Technology, Politics, and Ethics as Anthropological Problems*. Malden, MA: Blackwell.

Oring, Elliott. 1981. *Israeli Humor: The Content and Structure of the Chizbat of the Palmah*. Albany: SUNY Press.

Oring, Elliott. 1984. *The Jokes of Sigmund Freud: A Study in Humor and Jewish Identity*. Philadelphia: University of Pennsylvania Press.

Oring, Elliott. 1992. *Jokes and Their Relations*. Lexington: University Press of Kentucky.

Oring, Elliott. 1998. Review of Alan Dundes, *From Game to War and Other Psychoanalytic Essays on Folklore*. *Western Folklore* 57:63–64.

Oring, Elliott. 2012. *Just Folklore: Analysis, Interpretation, Critique*. Los Angeles: Cantilever.

Oring, Elliott. 2015. "What Freud Actually Said about Jokes." Paper presented at the American Folklore Society Annual Meeting, Longbeach, CA.

Ortiz, Renato. 1985. *Cultura brasileira e identidade nacional*. São Paulo: Editora Brasilense.

Ortiz, Renato. 1992. *Românticos e folcloristas: Cultura popular*. São Paulo: Olho d'Agua.

Ortner, Sherry B. 1995. "Resistance and the Problem of Ethnographic Refusal." *Comparative Studies in Society and History* 37 (1): 173–93.

Ortner, Sherry B. 2003. *New Jersey Dreaming: Capital, Culture, and the Class of '58*. Durham, NC: Duke University Press.

Osborn, Henry A. 1962. "Warao Phonology and Morphology." PhD diss., Indiana University.

Pandolfo, Stefania. 2018. *The Knot of the Soul: Madness, Psychoanalysis, Islam*. Chicago: University of Chicago Press.

Paredes, Américo. 1958. *With His Pistol in His Hand: A Border Ballad and Its Hero*. Austin: University of Texas Press.

Paredes, Américo. 1974. "José Mosqueda and the Folklorization of Actual Events." *Aztlan* 4:1–29.

Paredes, Américo. 1993. *Folklore and Culture on the Texas-Mexican Border*. Edited by Richard Bauman. Austin: Center for Mexican American Studies, University of Texas at Austin.

Paredes, Américo, and Richard Bauman, eds. (1971) 1972. *Toward New Perspectives in Folklore*. Austin: University of Texas Press and the American Folklore Society.
Peirce, Charles S. (1940) 1955. "Logic as Semiotic: The Theory of Signs." In *Philosophical Writings of Peirce*, edited by Justus Buchler, 98–119. New York: Dover.
Pennycook, Alastair. 2018. *Posthumanist Applied Linguistics*. London: Routledge.
Petryna, Adriana. 2002. *Life Exposed: Biological Citizens After Chernobyl*. Princeton, NJ: Princeton University Press.
Petryna, Adriana. 2009. *When Experiments Travel: Clinical Trials and the Global Search for Human Subjects*. Princeton, NJ: Princeton University Press.
Petryna, Adriana, Andrew Lakoff, and Arthur Kleinman, eds. 2006. *Global Pharmaceuticals: Ethics, Markets, Practices*. Durham, NC: Duke University Press.
Peuckert, Will-Erich. 1948. "Zur Situation der Volkskunde: Die Nachbarn." *Jahrbuch für vergleichende Volkskunde* 1:130–35.
Pigg, Stacy Leigh. 2001. "Languages of Sex and AIDS in Nepal: Notes on the Social Production of Commensurability." *Cultural Anthropology* 16 (4): 481–541.
Poovey, Mary. 1998. *A History of the Modern Fact: Problems of Knowledge in the Sciences of Wealth and Society*. Chicago: University of Chicago Press.
Postero, Nancy. 2017. *The Indigenous State: Race, Politics, and Performance in Plurinational Bolivia*. Oakland: University of California Press.
Povinelli, Elizabeth A. 2016. *Geontologies: A Requiem to Late Liberalism*. Durham, NC: Duke University Press.
Prasad, Leela. 2007. *Poetics of Conduct: Oral Narrative and Moral Being in a South Indian Town*. New York: Columbia University Press.
Preston, Richard. 1994. *The Hot Zone*. New York: Random House.
Quijano, Aníbal. 2000. "Coloniality of Power, Eurocentrism, and Latin America." *Nepantla*, 1 (3): 533–80.
Rabinow, Paul. 1996. *Making PCR: A Story of Biotechnology*. Chicago: University of Chicago Press.
Rabinow, Paul. 2003. *Anthropos Today: Reflections on Modern Equipment*. Princeton, NJ: Princeton University Press.
Rabinow, Paul. 2008. *Marking Time: On the Anthropology of the Contemporary*. Princeton, NJ: Princeton University Press.
Raheja, Gloria Goodwin. 1996. "Caste, Colonialism and the Speech of the Colonized: Entextualization and Disciplinary Control in India." *American Ethnologist* 23 (3): 494–513.
Ralph, Laurence. 2014. *Renegade Dreams: Living through Injury in Gangland Chicago*. Chicago: University of Chicago Press.
Rapp, Rayna, Deborah Heath, and Karen-Sue Taussig. 2001. "Genealogical Dis-ease: Where Hereditary Abnormality, Biomedical Explanation, and Family Responsibility Meet." In *Relative Matters: New Directions in the Study of Kinship*, edited by Sarah Franklin and Susan MacKinnon, 384–412. Durham, NC: Duke University Press.
Rev. 2020. "Donald Trump and Coronavirus Task Force News Conference Transcript: March 15." Rev Transcript, published March 15, 2020. Accessed March 21, 2020. https://www.rev.com/blog/transcripts/donald-trump-andcoronavirus-task-force-news-conference-transcript-march-15.
Riles, Annelise. 2004. "Real Time: Unwinding Technocratic and Anthropological Knowledge." *American Ethnologist* 31 (3): 392–405.
Riles, Annelise, ed. 2006. *Documents: Artifacts of Modern Knowledge*. Ann Arbor: University of Michigan Press.
Risling Baldy, Cutcha. 2015. "Coyote Is Not a Metaphor: On Decolonizing, (Re)claiming and (Re)naming Coyote." *Decolonization: Indigeneity, Education and Society* 4 (1): 1–20.

Rival, Laura M. 2016. *Huaorani Transformations in Twenty-First-Century Ecuador: Treks into the Future of Time*. Tucson: University of Arizona Press.

Robb, John Donald. 1980. *Hispanic Folk Music of New Mexico and the Southwest: A Self-Portrait of a People*. Norman: University of Oklahoma Press.

Roberts, John W. 1989. *From Trickster to Badman: The Black Folk Hero in Slavery and Freedom*. Philadelphia: University of Pennsylvania Press.

Roberts, John W. 1999. "'Hidden Right Out in the Open': The Field of Folklore and the Problem of Invisibility." *Journal of American Folklore* 112 (444): 119–39.

Roberts, John W. 2008. "Grand Theory, Nationalism, and American Folklore." *Journal of Folklore Research* 45 (1): 45–54.

Rodríguez, Juan Luís. 2008. "The Translation of Poverty and the Poverty of Translation in the Orinoco Delta." *Ethnohistory* 55 (3): 417–38.

Róheim. Géza. 1992. *Fire in the Dragon and Other Psychoanalytic Essays on Folklore*. Edited by Alan Dundes. Princeton, NJ: Princeton University Press.

Romano-V., Octavio I. 1968. "The Anthropology and Sociology of Mexican-Americans: The Distortion of Mexican-American History." *El Grito* 2 (1): 13–26.

Rosa, Jonathan. 2019. *Looking Like a Language, Sounding Like a Race: Raciolinguistic Ideologies and the Learning of Latinidad*. New York: Oxford University Press.

Rosaldo, Renato. 1985. "Chicano Studies, 1970–1984." *Annual Review of Anthropology* 14:405–27.

Rosaldo, Renato. 1989. *Culture and Truth: The Remaking of Social Analysis*. Boston: Beacon.

Rosaldo, Renato. 1991. "Fables of the Fallen Guy." In *Criticism in the Borderlands: Studies in Chicano Literature, Culture, and Ideology*, edited by Héctor Calderón and José David Saldívar, 84–97. Durham, NC: Duke University Press.

Rosaldo, Renato. 2014. *The Day of Shelly's Death: The Poetry and Ethnography of Grief*. Durham, N.C.: Duke University Press.

Rosenberg, Charles E. 1992. *Explaining Epidemics and Other Studies in the History of Medicine*. Cambridge: Cambridge University Press.

Rubel, Arthur J. 1966. *Across the Tracks: Mexican-Americans in a Texas City*. Austin: University of Texas Press.

Russo, Peggy A. 1992. "Uncle Walt's Uncle Remus: Disney's Distortion of Harris's Hero." *Southern Literary Journal* 25 (1): 19–32.

Said, Edward. 1978. *Orientalism*. New York: Pantheon Books.

Salas, Yolanda. 1987. *Bolívar y la historia en la conciencia popular*. Caracas: Instituto de Altos Estudios de América, Universidad Simón Bolívar.

Salas, Yolanda. 2003. "En nombre del pueblo: Nación, patrimonio, identidad y cigarro." In *Políticas de identidades y diferencias sociales en tiempos de globalización*, edited by Daniel Mato, 147–72. Caracas: FACES.

Saldívar, Ramón. 2006. *The Borderlands of Culture: Américo Paredes and the Transnational Imaginary*. Durham, NC: Duke University Press.

Samuels, David W. 2013. "Ethnopoetics and Ideologies of Poetic Truth." *Journal of Folklore Research* 50 (1–3): 251–83.

Sanders, Charles. 1932. *The Collected Papers of Charles Sanders Peirce*. Vol. 2: *Elements of Logic*, edited by Charles Hartshorne and Paul Weiss. Cambridge: Cambridge University Press.

Santner, Eric L. 1990. *Stranded Objects: Mourning, Memory, and Film in Postwar Germany*. Ithaca, NY: Cornell University Press.

Sapir, Edward. 1949. *Selected Writings of Edward Sapir in Language, Culture and Personality*. Edited by David G. Mandelbaum. Berkeley: University of California Press.

Sassen, Saskia. 2006. *Territory, Authority, Rights: From Medieval to Global Assemblages*. Princeton, NJ: Princeton University Press.

Saussure, Ferdinand de. (1916) 1959. *A Course in General Linguistics*. Tanslated by Wade Baskin. New York: McGraw-Hill.

Sawin, Patricia. 2002. "Performance at the Nexus of Gender, Power, and Desire: Reconsidering Bauman's Verbal Art from the Perspective of Gendered Subjectivity as Performance." *Journal of American Folklore* 115 (455): 28–61.

Sawyer, Suzana, and Edmund Terence Gomez, eds. 2012. *The Politics of Resource Extraction: Indigenous Peoples, Multinational Corporations, and the State*. New York: Palgrave Macmillan.

Schechner, Richard. 1985. *Between Theater and Anthropology*. Philadelphia: University of Pennsylvania Press.

Scheper-Hughes, Nancy. 1996. "Theft of Life: Globalization of Organ Stealing Rumors." *Anthropology Today* 12 (3): 3–11.

Scheper-Hughes, Nancy, and Margaret M. Lock. 1987. "The Mindful Body: A Prolegomenon to Future Work in Medical Anthropology." *Medical Anthropology Quarterly* 1 (1): 6–41.

Scher, Philip W. 2002. "Copyright Heritage: Preservation, Carnival and the State in Trinidad." *Anthropological Quarterly* 75 (3): 453–84.

Scher, Philip W. 2016. "*Landship*, Citizenship, Entrepreneurship and the Ship of State in Barbados: Developing a Heritage Consciousness in a Postcolonial State." *Western Folklore* 75 (3–4): 313–51.

Scherzinger, Martin Rudoy. 1999. "Music, Spirit Possession and the Copyright Law: Cross-Cultural Comparisons and Strategic Speculations." *Yearbook for Traditional Music* 31:102–25.

Schieffelin, Bambi B., Kathryn A. Woolard, and Paul V. Kroskrity, eds. 1998. *Language Ideologies: Practice and Theory*. Oxford: Oxford University Press.

Schmiesing, Ann. 2014. *Disability, Deformity, and Disease in the Grimms' Fairy Tales*. Detroit: Wayne State University Press.

Schulthies, Becky. 2019. "Partitioning, Phytocommunicability and Plant Pieties." *Anthropology Today* 35 (2): 8–12.

Scott, James C. 1985. *Weapons of the Weak: Everyday Forms of Peasant Resistance*. New Haven, CT: Yale University Press.

Sekaquaptewa, Helen. 1978. *Iisaw: Hopi Coyote Stories*. Produced by Larry Evers. Video, 17:47. Words and Place: Native Literature from the American Southwest 4. http://parentseyes.arizona.edu/wordsandplace/sekaquaptewa.html.

Sekoff, Jed. 1999. "The Undead: Necromancy and the Inner World." In *The Dead Mother: The Work of André Green*, edited by Gregorio Kohon, 109–27. London: Routledge.

Seremetakis, C. Nadia. 1991. *The Last Word: Women, Death, and Divination in Inner Mani*. Chicago: University of Chicago Press.

Servicio de Apoyo Local, A. C. (SOCSAL). 1998. Registro sociodemográfico Warao de Punta Pescador. Photocopy. Caracas: SOCSAL.

Shapin, Steven. 1994. *A Social History of Truth: Civility and Science in Seventeenth-Century England*. Chicago: University of Chicago Press.

Shaul, David Leedom. 2002. *Hopi Traditional Literature*. Albuquerque: University of New Mexico Press.

Sherzer, Joel, 1983. *Kuna Ways of Speaking: An Ethnographic Perspective*. Austin: University of Texas Press.

Shuman, Amy. 1986. *Storytelling Rights: The Uses of Oral and Written Texts by Urban Adolescents*. Cambridge: Cambridge University Press.

Shuman, Amy. 1993. "Dismantling Local Culture." *Western Folklore* 52 (2–4): 345–64.

Shuman, Amy. 2016. "Culturally Available Narratives in Parents' Stories about Disability." In *The Routledge International Handbook on Narrative and Life History*, edited by

Ivor Goodson, Ari Antikainen, Pat Sikes, and Molly Andrews, 237–48. London: Routledge.

Silverman, Carol. 2012. *Romani Routes: Cultural Politics and Balkan Music in Diaspora*. New York: Oxford University Press.

Silverstein, Michael. 1976. "Shifters, Linguistic Categories, and Cultural Description." In *Meaning in Anthropology*, edited by Keith Basso and Henry Selby, 11–55. Albuquerque: University of New Mexico Press.

Silverstein, Michael. 1993. "Metapragmatic Discourse and Metapragmatic Function." In *Reflexive Language: Reported Speech and Metapragmatics*, edited by John A. Lucy, 33–58. Cambridge: Cambridge University Press.

Singer, Merrill, and Hans Baer, eds. 1995. *Critical Medical Anthropology*. Amityville, NY: Baywood.

Smith, Kalim H. 2005. "Language Ideology and Hegemony in the Kumeyaay Nation: Returning the Linguistic Gaze." MA thesis, University of California, San Diego.

Smith, Kalim H. 2007. "Performing Indigenous Language Ideologies: The Legend of Nightfire and the Politics of Language and Race in Contemporary Indian Country." Lecture presented at the Center for Race and Gender, University of California, Berkeley, October 4.

Smith, Linda Tuhiwai. 1999. *Decolonizing Methodologies: Research and Indigenous Peoples*. London: Zed.

Soja, Edward. 1989. *Postmodern Geographies: The Reassertion of Space in Critical Social Theory*. London: Verso.

Spitulnik, Debra. 2002. "Mobile Machines and Fluid Audiences: Rethinking Reception through Zambian Radio Culture." In *Media Worlds: Anthropology on New Terrain*, edited by Faye D. Ginsburg, Lila Abu-Lughod, and Brian Larkin, 337–54. Berkeley: University of California Press.

Spivak, Gayatri Chakravorty. 1988. "Can the Subaltern Speak?" In *Marxism and the Interpretation of Culture*, edited by Cary Nelson and Lawrence Grossberg, 271–313. Urbana: University of Illinois Press.

Sprat, Thomas. (1667) 1958. *History of the Royal Society*, edited by Jackson I. Cope and Harold Whitmore Jones. St. Louis, MO: Washington University Studies.

Stagl, Justin. 1995. *A History of Curiosity: The Theory of Travel, 1550–1800*. Chur, Switzerland: Harwood.

Star, Susan Leigh, and James R. Griesemer. 1989. "Institutional Ecology, 'Translations' and Boundary Objects: Amateurs and Professionals in Berkeley's Museum of Vertebrate Zoology, 1907–39." *Social Studies of Science* 19 (3): 387–420.

Stebbins, Kenyon Ranier. 2001. "Going Like Gangbusters: Transnational Tobacco Companies 'Making a Killing' in South America." *Medical Anthropology Quarterly* 15 (2): 147–70.

Stein, Mary Beth. 1987. "Coming to Terms with the Past: The Depiction of 'Volkskunde' in the Third Reich since 1945." *Journal of Folklore Research* 24 (2): 157–85.

Stengers, Isabelle. 2005. "The Cosmopolitical Proposal." In *Making Things Public: Atmospheres of Democracy*, edited by Bruno Latour and Peter Weibel, 994–1003. Cambridge, MA: MIT Press.

Stewart, Kathleen. 2008. "Weak Theory in an Unfinished World." *Journal of Folklore Research* 45 (1): 71–82.

Stewart, Kathleen. 2012. "Precarity's Forms." *Cultural Anthropology* 27 (3): 518–25.

Stewart, Susan. 1991. *Crimes of Writing: Problems in the Containment of Representation*. New York: Oxford University Press.

Stocking, George W., Jr. 1968. *Race, Culture, and Evolution: Essays in the History of Anthropology*. New York: Free Press.

Stoeltje, Beverly J. 1988. "Gender Representations in Performance: The Cowgirl and the Hostess." *Journal of Folklore Research* 25:219–41.
Stoler, Ann Laura. 1995. *Race and the Education of Desire: Foucault's History of Sexuality and the Colonial Order of Things*. Durham, NC: Duke University Press.
Stone, Kay. 1975. "Things Walt Disney Never Told Us." *Journal of American Folklore* 88 (347): 42–50.
Strathern, Marilyn. 2000. "Afterword: Accountability . . . and Ethnography." In *Audit Cultures: Anthropological Studies in Accountability, Ethics and the Academy*, edited by Marilyn Strathern, 279–304. London: Routledge.
Strömbäck, Jesper. 2008. "Four Phases of Mediatization: An Analysis of the Mediatization of Politics." *International Journal of Press/Politics* 13 (3): 228–46.
Tangherlini, Timothy R. 1999. "Remapping Koreatown: Folklore, Narrative, and the Los Angeles Riots." *Western Folklore* 58 (2): 149–73.
Tatar, Maria. 1987. *The Hard Facts of the Grimms' Fairy Tales*. Princeton, NJ: Princeton University Press.
Tatar, Maria. 1992. *Off with Their Heads! Fairy Tales and the Culture of Childhood*. Princeton, NJ: Princeton University Press.
Taylor, Anne-Christine. 2001. "Wives, Pets, and Affines: Marriage among the Jivaro." In *Beyond the Visible and the Material: The Amerindianization of Society in the Work of Peter Pivière*, edited by Laura Rival and Neil Whitehead, 45–56. Oxford: Oxford University Press.
Taylor, Diana. 2003. *The Archive and the Repertoire: Performing Cultural Memory in the Americas*. Durham, NC: Duke University Press,
Tedlock, Dennis. 1983. *The Spoken Word and the Work of Interpretation*. Philadelphia: University of Pennsylvania Press.
Teuton, Christopher B., with Hastings Shade, Sammy Still, Sequoyah Guess, and Woody Hansen. 2012. *Cherokee Stories of the Turtle Island Liars' Club*. Chapel Hill: University of North Carolina Press.
Thompson, E. P. 1963. *The Making of the English Working Class*. London: V. Gollancz.
Thompson, Tok. 2010. "The Ape that Captured Time: Folklore, Narrative, and the Human-Animal Divide." *Western Folklore* 69:395–420.
Thompson, Tok. 2018. "Folklore beyond the Human: Toward a Trans-Special Understanding of Culture, Communication, and Aesthetics." *Journal of Folklore Research* 55:69–91.
Trask, Haunani-Kay. 1991. "Natives and Anthropologists: The Colonial Struggle." *Contemporary Pacific* 3 (1): 159–77.
Treichler, Paula A. 1999. *How to Have Theory in an Epidemic: Cultural Chronicles of AIDS*. Durham, NC: Duke University Press.
Trouillot, Michel-Rolph. 1991. "Anthropology and the Savage Slot: The Poetics and Politics of Otherness." In *Recapturing Anthropology: Working in the Present*, edited by Richard G. Fox, 17–44. Santa Fe, NM: School of American Research.
Tsing, Anna. 2005. *Friction: An Ethnography of Global Connection*. Princeton, NJ: Princeton University Press.
Tsing, Anna. 2015. *The Mushroom at the End of the World: On the Possibility of Life in Capitalist Ruins*. Princeton, NJ: Princeton University Press.
Tucker, Elizabeth. 1992. "Text, Lies and Videotape: Can Oral Tales Survive?" *Children's Folklore Review* 15 (1): 25–32.
Tylor, Edward B. (1871) 1889. *Primitive Culture: Researches into the Development of Mythology, Philosophy, Religion, Language, Art and Custom*. New York: Henry Holt.
Unwerth, Matthew von. 2005. *Freud's Requiem: Mourning, Memory, and the Invisible History of a Summer Walk*. New York: Riverhead.

Urban, Greg. 1988. "Ritual Wailing in Amerindian Brazil." *American Anthropologist* 90 (2): 385–400.

Urban, Greg. 2001. *Metaculture: How Culture Moves through the World.* Minneapolis: University of Minnesota Press.

Urciuoli, Bonnie. 1996. *Exposing Prejudice: Puerto Rican Experiences of Language, Race, and Class.* Boulder, CO: Westview.

Urry, John. 2007. *Mobilities.* Cambridge: Polity.

Vaz da Silva, Francisco. 2002. *Metamorphosis: The Dynamics of Symbolism in European Fairy Tales.* New York: Peter Lang.

Velasco, Alejandro. 2015. *Barrio Rising: Urban Popular Politics and the Making of Modern Venezuela.* Oakland: University of California Press.

Velásquez, Teresa A. 2018. "Tracing the Political Life of Kimsacocha: Conflicts over Water and Mining in Ecuador's Southern Andes." *Latin American Perspectives* 45 (5): 154–69.

Vilhena, Luis Rodolfo. 1997. *Projeto e missão: O movimento folclórico brasileiro 1947–1964.* Rio de Janeiro: Funarte.

Villalba, Julian A., Yushi Liu, Mauyuri K. Alvarez, Luisana Calderon, Merari Canache, Gaudymar Cardenas, Berenice Del Nogal, Howard E. Takiff, and Jacobus H. De Waard. 2013. "Low Child Survival Index in a Multi-dimensionally Poor Amerindian Population in Venezuela." *PLoS ONE* 8 (12): e85638.

Viveiros de Castro, Eduardo. 2004. "Exchanging Perspectives: The Transformation of Objects into Subjects in Amerindian Ontologies." *Common Knowledge* 10 (3): 463–84.

Vološinov, V. N. (1929) 1973. *Marxism and the Philosophy of Language.* Translated by Ladislav Matejka and I. R. Titunik. New York: Seminar Press.

Waitzkin, Howard. 1991. *The Politics of Medical Encounters: How Patients and Doctors Deal with Social Problems.* New Haven, CT: Yale University Press.

Wald, Priscilla. 2008. *Contagious: Cultures, Carriers, and the Outbreak Narrative.* Durham, NC: Duke University Press.

Warner, Michael. 2002. *Publics and Counterpublics.* New York: Zone.

Watts, Michael J. 2005. "Righteous Oil? Human Rights, the Oil Complex, and Corporate Social Responsibility." *Annual Review of Environment and Resources* 30:373–407.

Weffer Cifuentes, Laura. 2008. "En los últimos 2 meses han fallecido 16 waraos por enfermedad desconocida." *El Nacional*, August 7.

Weidman, Amanda J. 2006. *Singing the Classical, Voicing the Modern: The Postcolonial Politics of Music in South India.* Durham, NC: Duke University Press.

White, Hayden. 1978. *Tropics of Discourse: Essays in Cultural Criticism.* Baltimore, MD: Johns Hopkins University Press.

White, Luise. 2000. *Speaking with Vampires: Rumor and History in Colonial Africa.* Berkeley: University of California Press.

Wiget, Andrew. 1987. "Telling the Tale: A Performance Analysis of a Hopi Coyote Story." In *Recovering the Word: Essays on Native American Literature*, edited by Brian Swann and Arnold Krupat, 297–336. Berkeley: University of California Press.

Wilbert, Johannes. 1975. *Warao Basketry: Form and Function.* Los Angeles: Museum of Cultural History, University of California. Los Angeles.

Wilbert, Johannes. 1976. "To Become a Maker of Canoes: An Essay in Warao Enculturation." In *Enculturation in Latin America: An Anthology*, edited by Johannes Wilbert, 303–58. Los Angeles: UCLA Latin American Center Publications.

Wilbert, Johannes. 1980. "Genesis and Demography of a Warao Subtribe: The Winikina." In *Demographic and Biological Studies of the Warao Indians*, edited by Johannes Wilbert and Miguel Layrisse, 13–47. Los Angeles: UCLA Latin American Center Publications.

Wilbert, Johannes. 1987. *Tobacco and Shamanism in South America.* New Haven, CT: Yale University Press.

Wilbert, Johannes. 1996. *Mindful of Famine: Religious Climatology of the Warao Indians.* Cambridge, MA: Harvard University Center for the Study of World Religions.

Wilbert, Werner. 1996. *Fitoterapia Warao: Una teoría pnéumica de la salud, la enfermedad y la terapia.* Caracas: La Salle de Ciencias Naturales, Instituto Caribe de Antropología y Sociología.

Wilbert, Werner. 2001. "Warao Spiritual Ecology." In *Indigenous Traditions and Ecology: The Interbeing of Cosmology and Community*, edited by John A. Grim, 377–410. Cambridge, MA: Center for the Study of World Religions, Harvard Divinity School.

Wilbert, Werner, and Cecilia Ayala Lafée Wilbert. 2011. "Fitoterapia warao: Fundamentos teóricos." In *Perspectivas en salud indígena: Cosmovisón, enfermedad y políticas públicas*, edited by Germán Freire, 307–24. Quito: Ediciones Abya Yala.

Wilce, James M. 1998. *Eloquence in Trouble: The Poetics and Politics of Complaint in Rural Bangladesh.* New York: Oxford University Press.

Williams, Raymond. 1973. *The Country and the City.* New York: Oxford University Press.

Williams, Raymond. 1977. *Marxism and Literature.* Oxford: Oxford University Press.

Williams, Raymond. 2003. *Television: Technology and Cultural Form.* Edited by Ederyn Williams. London: Routledge.

Wilson, William A. 1976. *Folklore and Nationalism in Modern Finland.* Bloomington: Indiana University Press.

Wittgenstein, Ludwig. (1953) 1972. *Philosophical Investigations.* Translated by G.E.M. Anscombe. Oxford: Basil Blackwell.

Wojcik, Daniel. 2009. "Spirits, Apparitions, and Traditions of Supernatural Photography." *Visual Resources: An International Journal of Documentation* 25 (1–2): 109–36.

Wolf, Eric R. 1982. *Europe and the People without History.* Berkeley: University of California Press.

Yoder, Don. 1972. "Folk Medicine." In *Folklore and Folklife: An Introduction*, edited by Richard M. Dorson, 191–215. Chicago: University of Chicago Press.

Young, Katharine, ed. 1993. *Bodylore.* Knoxville: University of Tennessee Press.

Young, Katharine. 1997. *Presence in the Flesh: The Body in Medicine.* Cambridge, MA: Harvard University Press.

Zentella, Ana Celia. 1997. *Growing Up Bilingual: Puerto Rican Children in New York.* Malden, MA: Blackwell.

Zipes, Jack David. 1979. *Breaking the Magic Spell: Radical Theories of Folk and Fairy Tales.* Austin: University of Texas Press.

Zola, Irving Kenneth. 1972. "Medicine as an Institution of Social Control." *Sociological Review* 20:487–504.

Index

A

Aarne-Thompson: *The Types of the Folktale*, 91
acoustics. *See* lamentation; materiality; poetics
aesthetics: entextualization and, 146; and form, 26–27, 60, 61, 85, 220; and Freud, 137–139, 145; and media, 216
affect: dreams and jokes, 142–143, 145; early years, 12, 16; and entextualization, 148–152, 155, 157; and folklore, 89, 106, 113, 131; mediatized, 249–253, 255–260; in mourning, 172–178, 181, 188; traditionalization and, 214, 220, 226, 230
affordances: defined, 24; and form, 226–227, 230, 259
African American folklore, 59, 116. *See also* Hurston, Zora Neale; Levine, Lawrence; Roberts, John W.
AIDS. *See* HIV/AIDS epidemic
alabados (hymns), 15. *See also* La Cofradía del Nuestro Padre Jesús Nazareno
alabanza (hymn of praise), 22
alfalfa, 7–10
Altheide, David, 219, 221
American Indian Movement, 82
Americanist tradition in linguistics, 55–60, 69, 73
Angosto-Ferrández, Luís, 268, 284. *See also* progressive extractivism
anticolonial, 38, 63, 112, 114, 157, 266–268. *See also* Indigenous University of Venezuela; Moraleda, Librado
anti-immigrant, 66, 240–243
anti-racist approaches, 38, 63, 130, 224, 249, 267
anti-Semitism, 120–123, 140–141, 289
anti-vaccine movements, 202, 258, 260–261. *See also* biomedicine, rejection of
Anzaldúa, Gloria, 27
Appadurai, Arjun: on globalization, 67; incarceration by culture, 49, 83, 184, 224–225; and representation in South Asia, 117, social life of objects, 23, 207

Aragón, José Rafael, 20; New Mexico, 20. *See also* wood-carving
Arbery, Ahmaud, 288
aspen, 4, 21–24, 43
assemblages: and erasure, 182–183; global, 209; and mediatization, 220–221; multispecies, 276, 278; as project, 129
Aubrey, John: place in folkloristics, 27, 55, 91–92, 100, 106–108, 130, 193, 210; and media, 215; and traditionality/coloniality, 108–110, 121–122; view of communicability, 88–89, 91–92. *See also* Dorson, Richard; traditionality
audience: design, 148; and epidemic narratives, 212, 236, 243, 247, 249, 252, 254–258; and performance, 12, 87, 139–140, 144, 145, 148, 149, 158, 214, 220. *See also* performance; reception
Austin, J. L., 27, 36, 67
authenticity and folkloristics, 93, 127, 210. *See also* Bendix, Regina
autoatención (medical labor performed by non-professionals), 203–204. *See also* Menéndez, Eduardo L.
avian influenza, 237, 247, 253
Ayala Lafée, Cecilia, 278, 285n5. *See also* phytotherapy; play

B

Bacchilega, Cristina, 128
bacteria, 4, 37–38, 165, 241. *See also* cholera
Bakhtin, M.M.: chronotope, 227, 241; and heteroglossia, 61, 109, 142; and genre, 76, 142. *See also* epidemic chronotope; performance
"Ballad of Gregorio Cortez," 80–83, 86–87, 288. *See also* Paredes, Américo
Barlow, Kathleen, 273
Bateson, Gregory, 4, 73, 146
bats, 4, 41, 49n14, 182, 264, 282. *See also* rabies; transmission; viruses
Bauman, Richard: and entextualization, 74, 146–147, 157; and Paredes, 82, 85, 126–127,

193; performance-centered approach, 12, 27, 36, 58, 61, 66, 126, 142, 144–145, 149, 247, 252; technology and folklore, 92, 126, 129–130, 217; and traditionalization, 213, 222–223, 226, 258–259; and vernacular philology, 27, 62–63, 74, 96, 129

Bausinger, Hermann: critique of folklore and National Socialism, 120–121; on folklore and technology, 58, 92, 126, 129–130, 217; and traditionalization, 213, 222–224; folklore and spatialization, 230

bees, 9–10
Beltrán, Héctor, 231
Bendix, Regina, 93, 127, 210, 222
Benjamin, Walter, 24, 72, 131, 205
Bettelheim, Bruno, 151
Bhabha, Homi, 114, 116
Biehl, João, 201
Bigott Foundation, 220, 226. *See also* folkloric nationalism; commodification
bilingualism, 38–40, 81
biomedicine: inequalities and, 202, 206–207, 288; and knowledge/practice, 203–204, 208, 249–250, 253, 255, 261; relation to "folk" medicine, 31, 84, 195–201, 210–211, 260; rejection of, 202, 258, 260–261
Blache, Martha, 123
Black Atlantic, 103, 112. *See also* Gilroy, Paul
Blackwell, Thomas, 121
Blank, Trevor, 216
Boas, Franz, 66, 69, 88, 132n8
bodylore, 207. *See also* embodiment; Young, Katherine
Boellstorff, Tom, 216–217
Bolívar, Símon, 123
Bolivarian socialist revolution, 32, 47, 181, 188, 264, 266–268, 284
border thinking, 27, 82, 113–114, 118. *See also* Anzaldúa, Gloria; Mignolo, Walter
borders. *See* boundary crossing; boundary-work
boundary crossing, 58–62, 65n4, 225. *See also* Bauman, Richard; Hymes, Dell
boundary objects, 69–70, 76–77n2, 210, 249. *See also* Griesemer, James R.; Star, Susan Leigh
boundary-work, 128, 137–138, 210; defined, 45; and disciplinarity, 54–57, 60–64, 64–65n2, 90, 92, 95, 104, 110, 125, 210; Paredes' rejection of, 80–81, 222–223; and reification of "media," 215–219, 227, 236–239, 257. *See also* disciplinarity; Dorson, Richard; Gieryn, Thomas

Bourdieu, Pierre, 73, 212n2, 227–228
Bourke, John Gregory, 127
Bowker, Geoffrey C., 182–183, 203, 209
Boyd, E., 20, 25
Brentano, Clemens, 230
Briggs's Principles for Unlearning, 44
British American Tobacco, 220
British colonialism, 102, 108–119, 121, 127, 132n9, 224
Bronner, Simon, 54, 106, 136, 234n1
Brown, Michael, 26
Brunvand, Jan, 126, 259
Burke, Kenneth, 27
Butler, Judith, 162, 185

C

Camden, William, 103, 105–106
Canguilhem, Georges, 145
canoe, 31–33, 271–274, 276–278, 282–283, 285
cante fable, 30, 75–76. *See also* mixed genre
Carr, Gerald L., 67–68, 71–75
carving. *See* wood carving
capitalism: coloniality of folklore and, 110, 122; and extractivism, 264, 284; and traditionality, 82, 91, 100, 107, 110–111, 229; and retraditionalization, 224
cartographies, communicable, 87–88, 98, 249, 279. *See also* communicability
Casas, Bartolomé de las, 104, 110
Castells, Manuel, 124, 219
Catholicism: conversion and indigeneity, 30–31, 103–104, 110; New Mexican context, 14–26. *See also* wood carving
CBS Evening News, 229–239, 251
Center for Land Grant Studies, 26
Certeau, Michel de, 212
Chakrabarty, Dipesh, 101–102, 107, 116, 131n2, 225
Chaube, Pandit Ram Gharib, 113, 118–119. *See also* Naithani, Sadhana
Chávez, Alex, 61–62. *See also huapango arribeño*
Chávez Frías, Hugo (Venezuelan President), 32, 166, 180–183, 186, 188, 267–268, 284
Cheng, Anne, 162, 186
cholera, 37–38, 40, 43, 165, 182, 197, 202, 207, 270, 287–288
circulation, 71, 87, 93, 202
Clarke, Adele, 200
classification: epistemic, 55, 59–60, 188, 202; and indigeneity, 30, 182, 267, 285; and traditionality, 70, 91

Clifford, James, 23, 26, 67, 81, 83, 86, 105–106, 114, 124, 200, 224, 267
Cocchiara, Giuseppe, 110
La Cofradía del Nuestro Padre Jesús Nazareno (The Confraternity of Our Father Jesus the Nazarene), 15
Cohen, Lawrence, 199
Cold War, 55, 57, 131
collecting, colonial, 102, 112–114, 117, 132n6, 224
colonial relativity, 70–71
colonial: anti-, 38, 63, 112, 114, 157, 266–268; British, 102, 108–119, 121, 127, 132n9, 224; and capitalism, 110, 122; collection, 102, 112–114, 117, 132n6, 224; de-, 63, 101–104, 266, 284–285; and ritual, 101–103; and traditionality, 108–110, 115–123; violence, 71, 73, 80, 103–104, 107, 110–111, 119, 123, 131, 160n10, 186–188, 224–225, 289. *See also* postcolonial
coloniality of folkloristics, 100–131
commodification: and folklore, 92, 215–216, 223, 227, 229–230; of language, 66–67, 72; of nature, 268, 284; research on, 93, 117, 199, 207, 209
communicability, 78–99, 105, 208, 249, 288. *See also* circulation; COVID-19; phytocommunicability
communicable models, 87–90, 93–94, 96–98, 208–209
communicative technologies: and boundary-work, 57, 126, 216; and epidemics, 261
community-driven research, 31, 40–42, 60–61; 74, 165–168, 175–178, 181–189, 272–274, 283–284. *See also* rabies; *Stories in the Time of Cholera*
condensation, 142–143, 156–157. *See also* dreams; entextualization; Freud, Sigmund
contagion narratives, 239–262
Córdova, NM, 14–29, 152–153, 157. *See also* wood carving
Coronil, Fernando, 122, 267
corrido (ballad), 80, 83, 85–88, 288. *See also* "Ballad of Gregorio Cortez"; Paredes, Américo
Couldry, Nick, 214, 219. *See also* mediatization
countryside, and construction of "folklore," 88, 91, 100–101, 106–111, 132n5, 193, 228–230
Couric, Katie, 239–242, 246–247, 248, 251. *See also* journalism

COVID-19 pandemic: 38, 47, 202, 205, 236–237, 245, 248, 250, 255, 287–288, 290
Crapanzano, Vincent, 163, 174
critical border studies. *See* border thinking
critical epidemiology, 197, 200, 211, 287
critical geography: approach to spatiality, 200, 205; and folkloristic analysis, 212n2–3. *See also* Lefebvre, Henri; Tangherlini, Timothy
Crooke, William, 111–113, 118–119, 132n7. *See also* Chaube, Pandit Ram Gharib; Naithani, Sadhana
cultures of circulation, 71

D

Das, Veena, 116, 117, 142, 187, 202, 204, 207, 210
Daunarani (Mother of the Forest), 34, 271–273, 276, 278, 281. *See also* myth; phytotherapy
Daxelmüller, Christoph, 120
décima (ten-line stanza of poetry), 85
decolonial: 63, 266; and phyto-socialism, 284–285; studies, 101–104
decontextualization, 27, 146
Dégh, Linda, 28, 215
deherotu (performer of myths), 34, 35, 153, 157, 271–273, 276, 283, 286n1; and gender, 36
de la Cadena, Marisol, 283, 285n2
Deleuze, Gilles, 94, 128–129, 221, 227
Delta Amacuro, 3, 30–42, 48–49n13, 158–159, 161, 164–190, 207, 267, 288
Derrida, Jacques, 4, 67, 94, 140, 265
design, architectural, 267–270, 274–276
Desmodus rotundus. *See* bats
Devy, Ganesh N., 128
diabetes, 199, 259
diagnosis: and categories, 67, 182–183, 203, 208–209; and phyotherapy, 278–279; as process, 36, 158, 161, 164, 166–167, 177–178, 188, 198, 273, 281–282
differential identity, 82, 126. *See also* Bauman, Richard
Dirks, Nicholas, 112, 116
disability studies, 124, 145, 206, 209, 221, 224, 289
disciplinarity, 53–64, 64–65n2, 90–92, 95, 104, 110, 125, 210
discourse-centered approach, 28
disease, and communicability, 208, 235–262, 288; in Delta Amacuro, 42, 47, 48n9, 48–49n13, 49n14, 161, 164, 166, 178, 182,

183, 197, 208, 212, 264–286; and folkloristics of health, 195–197, 201–204, 206, 208–212; and medical anthropology, 125, 198–200, 206, 209
Disney(fication), 215–216, 230–231
displacement, psychic, 143
ditches, 8–9, 11–12
DNA: of performance, 238, 261; scientific claims around, 238
Dobie, Frank, 94
documents, anthropology of, 74–75
Dorson, Richard: "fakelore" and boundary-work, 55–56, 58, 61, 83, 215, 222; genealogy of folkloristics, 27, 53, 91–92, 94, 100, 104–108, 110–112, 114–115, 119, 130, 131n1–2, 193–194
double consciousness, 84, 118. *See also* Du Bois, W.E.B.
Dow, James, 64–65n2, 120–121
dreams: and healing, 36, 109, 208, 283; in Freud, 136–137, 141–143, 145–147, 163; in *moyotu* ritual, 273
Du Bois, W.E.B., 84, 118, 186–187
dugout canoe. *See* canoe
dump rake, 7–9, 293
Dundes, Alan: boundary-work, 57, 64–65n2; on "folk," 80, 126; and psychoanalysis, 45–46, 57, 135–137, 144, 151, 156, 157, 159n1; on technology and folklore, 92, 126, 216, 219; on theory and folklore, 53–54, 57
Dussel, Enrique, 101–104. *See also* decolonial studies

E

elders: as mentors, 5–25, 28–29, 152–153; and processes of circulation, 19–20, 72–73, 75–76. *See also plática de los viejitos de antes*
embodiment: acoustics of, 173; and condensation, 156–157; folkloristics of health and, 207, 265; mediatization and, 216–217, 223, 252, 255; and mobility, 67, 107, 182; and performance, 75–76, 135, 149
Emmerich, Wolfgang, 120–121
Enlightenment, 58, 62, 89, 100, 121
entextualization, 27, 74, 90, 92, 107, 125, 127, 146–151, 154–155, 157–159, 226, 254
epidemic: cholera, 37–38, 40, 43, 165, 182, 197, 202, 207, 270, 287–288; rabies, 5, 41–43, 47, 49n14, 164–188, 274, 266, 273–274, 279–285. *See also* pandemics
epidemic chronotope, 241–242, 248
epidemic narratives. *See* contagion narratives

epidemiology. *See* critical epidemiology
Epstein, Steve, 200
Esterly, David, 24
ethics: extractivism and, 275, 284; and narrative, 76; 117; and politics of circulation, 40, 70–71, 73. *See also* colonial relativity; ethnographic refusal; progressive extractivism
ethnographic authority, 23, 82–85, 124–125, 186–187; Paredes' critique of, 83–85. *See also* community-driven research
ethnographic refusal, 21–24, 69–70, 73–74, 152–153. *See also* O'Neill, Sean Patrick; Ortner, Sherry
ethnography, future directions, 259, 265; interviewing and, 21–24, 83, 186; and mobility, 186; and polyphony, 81
ethnography of speaking, 27, 54, 58, 140, 201. *See also* Bauman, Richard; Hymes, Dell
ethnomedicine, 194, 198–199, 204. *See also* folk medicine
ethnopoetics, 45, 66–77
Eurocentrism: critique of Marder, 265–266, and folkloristics, 45, 78, 91, 105, 114–115, 131, 131n1
Evers, Larry, 75
expertise, 67, 72, 112, 200, 208, 243–247, 250–258
extractivism. *See* progressive extractivism

F

Fabian, Johannes, 112
failure, as stimulus for knowledge production, 21–24, 42–44
"fakelore," 55–56, 83, 92, 97, 215, 222. *See also* boundary-work; Dorson, Richard
Fanon, Frantz, 118, 155, 157–158, 179, 186–187
Farmer, Paul, 202, 260
Feaster, Patrick, 92, 126
feminism. *See* gender: feminist critiques
Fernández, María, 37, 43. *See also* lamentation; mourning
festival, 109, 127, 223, 271; *nahanamu*, 32–35
fidelity ideology. *See* intertextual transparency, ideology of
film: Disney and folklore, 215–216, 230; and narrative of I'isaw, 75–76; and newscast genre, 251–252; and traditionalization, 226
Fine, Gary Alan, 57–58
Fischman, Fernando, 123
Flores, Richard, 93
Floyd, George, 288–290

Flueckiger, Joyce Burkhalter, 117, 119
"the folk": as construction, 101; invocations of, 54–55, 80, 83, 87–88, 90–91, 97, 137, 195
Folk-Lore Society, 106, 111–112
folk medicine, 193–199, 203–204, 208, 235. *See also* folkloristics of health; Hand, Wayland; Hufford, David; O'Connor, Bonnie; Yoder, Don
folk music, 6, 14, 17–18, 61–62, 127. *See also huapango arribeño*; Ochoa Gautier, Ana María; Robb, John Donald
folklore cosmopolitanisms, 90. *See also* Grimm, Jacob and Wilhelm
"folkloresque," 223
folkloric nationalism, 100–101, 112, 120–123, 212n1, 220
"folklorismus," 222
folkloristics: coloniality of, 100–131; and disciplinarity, 54–57, 60–64, 64–65n2, 90, 92, 95, 104, 110, 125, 210; and Eurocentricism, 45, 78, 91, 105, 114–115, 131, 131n1; and mediatization, 213–263; Paredes's challenge to, 45, 59–60, 78–99, 115, 117, 124–127, 131, 149, 158, 194, 221–223
folkloristics of health: 46–47, 193–212; and "swine flu" narrative, 235–262
folklorization, 83, 123, 222–223, 232. *See also* McDowell, John; Paredes, Américo
form: and intertextuality, 164, 226, 258–259; and mediatization, 226–227, 229–230, 236, 251, 258–259
Foster, Michael Dylan. *See* "folkloresque"
fragments, narrative, 142–143, 146, 149–150, 229. *See also* Das, Veena; dreams; Freud, Sigmund
Frazer, James, 113
Freud, Sigmund: and aesthetics, 137–139, 145; and anti-Semitism, 140–141; on dreams, 136–137, 141–143, 145–147, 163; and fragments, 142–143, 146; and gender, 139–140; *The Joke and Its Relation to the Unconscious*, 136–143, 145–147, 163; and sexuality, 136, 138–143; "On Transience," 172, 178–179. *See also* "Mourning and Melancholia"
fruit trees, 10, 13, 18, 281

G

Garcia, Angela, 162
García, Jesús Chucho, 123
García Canclini, Néstor, 93, 122–123, 127, 212n1
Garner, Eric, 288

gender: and canoes, 271–273; feminist critiques, 81–82, 94–95, 149, 203, 230; ethnopoetics and, 69, 74; and Freud, 139–140; and healing, 36, 283; intersubjectivity and, 298; and plants, 272–273, 277–279, 283; and positionality, 25, 27, 116–117, 124, 135, 147, 149, 155, 157, 206, 224
genealogies, folkloristic, 54–63, 78–79, 88, 94–95, 100–102, 104–115, 130, 131n1, 132n10, 193; of modernity, 102–104, 107–108; multi-genealogical approach, 128–131
genre: in circulation, 87, 181; and entextualization, 147, 150–152; epistolary, 158–159; fairytale, 229; Freud's examination of, 138, 140, 142; and Indian folklore, 113, 118–119; oral, 31, 217, 231; and mediatization, 47, 231, 251, 258–259; mixed, 74, 76; Paredes' experiment with, 81, 83, 85–86; and performance, 60–61, 153; and traditionalization, 226–227
gentrification, 6–7, 9–10, 152. *See also* land appropriation; whiteness
genocide, 120–122, 225, 288
geography. *See* critical geography; historical-geographic approach
German: language and Freud, 139, 163, 168; folkloristics, 64–65n2, 101, 120–122, 217; nation-state construction, 100–101, 120–122, 139
Gibson, James, 24, 226. *See also* affordances
Gieryn, Thomas, 45, 54–55, 92. *See also* boundary-work
Gilpin, Laura, 17, 24
Gilroy, Paul, 103, 112. *See also* Black Atlantic
Gingrich, Andre, 122
Goffman, Erving, 140, 147–148, 172–175. *See also* response cries
Goldstein, Diane, 197, 260, 261, 295
Gómez, Herminia, 38–40, 43
Gómez, Norbelys, 40–42, 158, 164–166, 181, 183–184, 273. *See also* nurses
Gómez, Tirso, 40–42, 164, 166, 181, 184–185, 273. *See also* healing
González-Martin, Rachel, 130
Goodman, Jane, 209
Gordon, Avery, 81
gossip: in circulation, 83, 87; in fieldwork, 25, 35, 40, 61, 271; health-related, 202; and mobility, 68. *See also* Shuman, Amy
Gramsci, Antonio, 9. *See also* resistance
Grant, Oscar, 288
Grider, Sylvia, 216

grief. *See* mourning
Griego, (Mrs.) Emma, 13–14, 37
Griego, Peter Jr., 13
Griesemer, James R., 69–70, 76–77n2, 210. *See also* boundary objects
Grimm, Jacob and Wilhelm, 87, 90, 100–101, 105, 129, 137, 214, 216, 223, 228–233, 235–236
Groth, Stefan, 209
Guattari, Félix, 94, 128–129, 221, 227
Gudynas, Eduardo, 263, 267. *See also* progressive extractivism
Guss, David, 220

H

H1N1 ("swine flu"), 47, 236–263
Haburi (myth of), 272–273, 276. See *also* canoe; Daunarani; *moyotu*; myth
Hafstein, Valdimar, 209, 233
Hallin, Daniel C., 80, 236–237, 243, 250, 252–253, 261, 262n1. *See also* journalism; mediatization
Hand, Wayland, 195. *See also* folk medicine
Haraway, Donna, 203, 238
Haring, Lee, 53–54, 71
Hasan-Rokem, Galit, 152
Hayden, Cori, 199
Hayden, White, 105, 206
healing: Bay Area, 231; scholarship and, 47, 125, 201, 204–205, 208, 211, 261; and Warao practices, 31, 35, 37, 41, 165, 187, 212, 277–278, 281–282. *See also* phytotherapy
hebu ("spirit" or "pathogen"), 32, 36, 164. See also *wisidatu*
Hepp, Andreas, 214, 219. *See also* mediatization
Herder, Johann Gottfried, 89–90, 100, 110, 118, 121–122, 230
heritage research, 96, 98, 127, 194, 209, 223–224, 227, 232–233
Herzfeld, Michael, 101
Hirschkind, Charles, 175, 232
historical-geographic approach, 91
HIV/AIDS epidemic, 197, 200, 260. *See also* Epstein, Steven; Goldstein, Diane
Hjarvard, Stig, 214, 219
hoa (particular class of "spirits" or "pathogen"), 36
hoarotu (healer skilled in extracting *hoa*), 35–36, 270. *See also* dreams; healing
Hobsbawm, Eric, 97, 221
horsebeans, 29, 152. *See also* proverbs
horses, 7–10, 28, 83, 229
hotarao (non-indigenous persons), 33–34, 48n12, 157, 285n1
Howard, Robert Glenn, 126, 216, 232
huapango arribeño (competitive musical performance), 61–62. *See also* Chávez, Alex
Hufford, David, 195–198, 211. *See also* folk medicine
Hunt, George, 132n8
Hurston, Zora Neale, 82
Hymes, Dell: and circulation, 70–71; dialogue, 75; ethnography of speaking, 27, 58; interdisciplinary and, 65n4, 66, 201; myth, 160n8, 160n10; performance, 27, 36, 58, 66, 75; poetics, 70–72; on texts, 61; and traditionalization, 213, 222–224
hyper-cathexis, 162, 164, 188; definition of, 13. *See also* Freud, Sigmund; mourning

I

iconicity, 76n1, 141, 151–155, 158, 173, 185. *See also* Peirce, Charles S.; photography
ideological labor, 227
ideology: of circulation, 67–68, 71; constructed nature, 40, 96, 234; debates over pro-Indigenous, 269; language, 73; of media, 47, 214, 219–221, 224–234, 236, 242, 251, 258–259; medical, 205–209; of mobility, 209; modernity as, 107; and phytocommunicability, 265–266; domination and, 81, 102, 120–122; scientific, 57
ideology of metapragmatic transparency, 229
I'isaw (Hopi narrative), 75–76, 153–155. *See also* Sekaquaptewa, Helen
Immigration and Customs Enforcement (ICE), 240–241
immobility: of cultural forms, 45, 67–70, 73, 182, 205, 210, 290
imperialism, 70, 80, 94, 102–104, 288. *See also* coloniality; violence
indexicality, 67, 68, 71–74, 76n1, 141, 151, 158, 242, 277. *See also* Peirce, Charles S.
India, 101, 109, 111–120, 125, 127–128, 131, 132
indigenous socialism, 32, 266–269. *See also* Indigenous University of Venezuela; Moraleda, Librado; Muaina
Indigenous University of Venezuela, 167–168, 181, 267. *See also* Moraleda, Librado
infanticide, 38–40
internalization, subjective, 147–155, 157–158, 162, 170–171, 175, 289. *See also*

hyper-cathexis; Klein, Melanie; mourning; Nasio, Juan-David
intertextual transparency, ideology of, 69, 71, 90, 229
interviewing: journalistic, 242–245; and media research, 237, 252; and the politics of knowledge, 21–24, 30, 186–187, 202
invention of tradition, 97–98, 221. *See also* Hobsbawm, Eric
Ireland, folklore of, 110, 112, 127, 132n5. *See also* Ó Giolláin, Diarmuid
iterability, 37, 67, 140, 171, 176. *See also* Derrida, Jacques; mourning; performance

J
Jakobson, Roman, 27, 139, 142, 144–146, 159n3, 234n2. *See also* performance; poetics
jokes: circulation and performance, 19, 25, 93, 216; Freud's study of, 136–143, 145–146, 163; indexicality and, 151; Paredes' analysis of, 80–84
Journal of American Folklore, 58, 132n15–16
journalism: critical engagement with, 42, 166, 181–185, 287–288; and epidemics, 47, 205–206; 211, 228, 236–237, 239–262, 287–288; and folklore, 127, 233, 259–260; temporality of, 236, 241–242, 248, 251–252. *See also* epidemic chronotope

K
Kamat, Vinay, 204, 207, 210
Kapchan, Deborah, 209
Kariña people, 30
Keane, Webb, 70, 91, 207, 265. *See also* missionaries; poetics
KHM (Kinder- und Hausmärchen), 228–231. *See also* Grimm, Jacob and Wilhelm
Kirshenblatt-Gimblett, Barbara, 57, 96, 127, 209, 223, 227. *See also* metaculture
Kitta, Andrea, 198
Klein, Melanie, 46, 147–148, 150, 170–171, 188
Kleinman, Arthur, 198, 206
knowledge production: and biomedicine, 203–204, 208, 249–250, 253, 255, 261; early lessons, 22–24, 43; and ethnography, 125, 187–188; and mediatization, 215–219, 227, 236–239, 257; as political project, 41–42, 180–181; and reification, 55–60, 68, 72, 86, 90–92, 97–98, 119, 123, 124–131, 157–158, 200, 206–207, 210–211, 223; stakes of, 40
Korom, Frank J., 117

Kristeva, Julia, 46, 148–149, 162, 172–174. *See also* semiotic process
Kroeber, Alfred, 69
Krohn, Kaarle, 91
Kumeyaay (language and nation), 73, 231. *See also* Smith, Kalim
Kwamuhu (town in Delta Amacuro State, Venezuela), 37, 44, 48–49n13. *See also* lamentation; tuberculosis

L
labor, 25, 29, 39, 64, 72, 203–204, 224, 233, 267, 279. *See also* autoatención
Lacan, Jacques, 46, 57, 147–148, 157, 171–172, 175
Lakoff, Andrew, 74, 237, 254
lamentation: acoustics of, 161–162, 171, 173–174, 181, 187–188; collective aspect of, 175; in Delta Amacuro, 5, 37, 41, 43, 46, 161, 164, 168–170, 175–178, 183, 184, 274; and entextualization, 60, 150, 158–159; poetics of, 171, 181, 187–188
land, appropriation of, 6–7, 9–10, 25–27, 29–30, 34–35, 42–43, 70–71, 80, 104, 110, 224, 268. *See also* gentrification; labor; violence
language ideologies, 68, 73, 108, 125. *See also* intertextual transparency, ideologies of
language revitalization, 68, 71–72
Laplanche, Jean, 46, 162, 171–172
Latour, Bruno, 55, 85, 182, 199, 202–203, 209
Lau, Kimberly, 197
Lee, Jon, 85, 251, 256
Lefebvre, Henri, 124, 200, 205, 212n2. *See also* critical geography
legends: and health, 197, 202, 256; in journalism, 259–260; New Mexican, 12, 19, 22, 25, 60, 224; Paredes' analysis of, 83–86, 88, 93, 127–128, 288; and psychoanalysis, 136, 142
Levine, Lawrence, 116
Limón, José, 60, 78, 81–82, 93, 127–128, 159n1
linguistic anthropology, 3, 30, 45, 56, 58, 65n4, 66–68, 75, 125, 201, 212n2, 234
Lipset, David, 273
LiPuma, Edward, 71, 85
literacy, as binary with orality or illiteracy, 75, 80, 90, 92, 100–101, 104, 106–107, 196, 215, 229
Lixfeld, Hannjost, 120
Lock, Margaret, 199
Locke, John, 71, 100, 108, 157, 193
López, George, 14, 17, 19, 23

López, José Dolores, 14, 18, 21, 25
López, Silvianita, 14, 19, 23, 28–29, 60, 152–153. *See also* proverbs
López Morín, José, 81
Lowe, Celia, 237
Lowth, Robert, 121
Luhmann, Niklas, 237
Lundby, Knut, 214, 219. *See also* mediatization

M

Macotera, Florencia, 43, 164–166, 175–177, 181. *See also* lamentation; mourning
MacPhail, Theresa, 250, 253. *See also* H1N1
Madsen, William, 84, 94
Maduro, Nicolás (Venezuelan President), 188
magical nominalism, 125
malaria, 31, 37, 202
Malinowski, Bronislaw, 27
Mantini-Briggs, Clara, 37–42, 158, 164–167, 178, 181, 183–184, 197, 272–273, 280–281
Marder, Michael, 47, 264–266, 275, 278, 282–283. *See also* ontologies; plant-human relations
Mariusa (region of Delta Amacuro State, Venezuela), 32–38, 270–273
Martín Barbero, Jesús, 123, 127, 214, 216, 218, 234. *See also* mediatization
Marx, Karl, 72, 115–116, 188
materiality, 23, 74, 207; acoustic, 170–171; and embodiment, 207, 223–224, 234; and language, 141; phytocommunicability and, 264, 278, and semiotics, 148–151, 157; and text, 72–73, 91
McBratney, Michael, 112, 132n6
McDowell, John, 86, 222–223
Mechling, Jay, 126, 159n2
media: anthropology, 66; reification of, 213–219, 227, 236–239, 257
mediation, 218. *See also* Martín Barbero, Jesús
mediatization, 47, 213–234, 235–262
medical anthropology, 125, 197–206, 209–211, 236, 257–260
Meek, Barbra, 67–68, 71, 73–75
memory: and folkloristics, 79, 123, 131, 238; psychic, 143, 179
Menéndez, Eduardo L., 197, 200, 203–204, 205, 207–208, 210, 257, 278. *See also* autoatención; folkloristics of health; medical anthropology, relationality
mentorship: dialogics of, 4, 42–44, 46, 155–156, 158–159; impact of, 13, 22–23, 43, 45, 157, 290–291

metacommunication, 4, 148, 229. *See also* Bateson, Gregory
metaculture: of modernity, 68, 70; and heritage, 96, 223, 227, 233. *See also* Kirshenblatt-Gimblett, Barbara; Urban, Greg
metapragmatics, 68, 72, 86, 229. *See also* ideology of metapragmatic transparency
Mexico, border with US, 25–26, 29, 42–43, 80–82, 99n3, 239–243, 251, 255–257
Mignolo, Walter, 102–104, 108, 113, 118
military and folkloristics, 127
Miller, Theresa, 278
Mills, Margaret, 54, 59, 61, 63, 117–118
missionaries: and folklore, 102–103, 110–111, 113, 119, 224; and language, 70–71, 73; and Warao, 30–31, 48n7–8. *See also* colonial relativity
Mitchell, Timothy, 72
mixed genre, 74, 76, 142. *See also* Bakhtin, M.M.
mobility: and embodiment, 67, 107, 182; and ethnography, 186; and immobility, 45, 67–70, 73, 182, 205, 210, 290; and modeling, 55, 91, 182–183, 199–201, 203, 209, 238, 261; and statistics, 67, 107, 182–183, 209; and technology, 67, 73, 182
models, communicable. *See* communicable models
modernity: co-production with traditionality, 57, 62–63, 78, 80, 82, 88, 100–132, 196, 212n1, 214–215, 220, 227; and socialism, 274
Montoya, Michael, 199. *See also* diabetes
Moraleda, Conrado, 32, 34, 40, 158, 164, 166–167, 181–184, 187, 272
Moraleda, Enrique, 32, 40–42, 158, 164, 166–167, 175–176, 180–181, 184–188, 273–274
Moraleda, Librado, 32, 34, 180–181, 267, 273, 284. *See also* indigenous socialism; Muaina
Moraleda, Teodoro, 31–33, 40
Moraleda, Tomasa, 31–32
Morales, Evo (Bolivian President), 268
mortality, child, 37, 48n9, 166, 279–281
Mould, Tom, 234n1
mourning: acoustics of, 172–178; anthropology as, 186–190; Butler and grievability, 185–186; Du Bois on, 186; and Klein's work, 170–171; and Kristeva, 172–174; and Laplanche, 171–172; and Nasio, 171; and Rosado, 172. *See also* Freud, Sigmund; lamentation

"Mourning and Melancholia," 161–164, 178, 180, 186, 188
Movimiento al Socialismo, 32, 267
moyotu (builder of canoes), 273–274, 276, 282–283. *See also* canoe; wood carving
Muaina (town in Delta Amacuro State, Venezuela), 32, 43, 164–190, 267–286. *See also* epidemics; indigenous socialism; Moraleda, Librado
multigenealogical approach, 79, 102, 124–132
multispecies relations, 5–14, 24, 76, 154–155, 188, 237, 290. *See also* plant-human relations
Muñoz Martínez, Monica, 288
Murako (town in Delta Amacuro State, Venezuela), 37, 48–49n13. *See also* tuberculosis
Murphy, Keith, 268. *See also* design
museums: and folkloristics, 4, 96, 127, 194, 207, 224; and wood carving, 14, 20, 23, 27
Myers, Fred, 26
Myers, Natasha, 278, 281. *See also* plant-human relations; sensorium
mysterious epidemic. *See* rabies
myth: of Daunarani and Haburi, 34, 271–273, 276; and folkloristics, 103, 136; of the *hotarao* (non-indigenous peoples), 34, 157, 285n1; and performance, 150, 153–155; of the Sun, 36, 153; Warao, 31, 34–37, 153, 271–274, 276–277, 283, 285. *See also deherotu*; Rivera, Santiago

N

Nabasanuka (town in Delta Amacuro State, Venezuela), 31, 36, 40
Nader, Laura, 125, 204–205
nahanamu (annual festival), 32–25. *See also* Mariusa; *wisidatu*
Naithani, Sadhana, 45, 101
namubaka (disparaging term for non-indigenous person), 270
Narayan, Kirin, 117
narrative. *See* communicability; fragments; storytelling; transmission
Nas, Peter, 209
Nasio, Juan-David, 147, 171, 174, 185, 289. *See also* Lacan, Jacques; unconscious: ivy analogy
National Socialism, 120–122
nationalism, 64n1, 89, 100, 112, 120–123, 130–131, 212n1, 220. *See also* folkloristic nationalism
Native American: and folkloristics, 116; marginalization in scholarship, 78, 95, 289;
narrative, 75–76, 153–155; politics of language, 73–74, 231
naturalism, as perspective, 24, 107, 264–265, 275, 282. *See also* Viveiros de Castro, Eduardo
Navajo language, 29
New Mexico, 5–30, 42, 60, 138, 224. *See also* Córdova, NM; mentorship; unlearning; wood carving
Nichter, Mark, 199, 204, 207, 210. *See also* ethnomedicine; global health
nonhuman, 4, 47, 147–149, 155, 187, 200, 212, 226, 229, 248, 264, 267, 283, 293. *See also* alfalfa; aspen; bacteria; bats; canoes; ditches; dump rake; *hebu*; horses; ontologies; palm trees; viruses
Noyes, Dorothy, 57, 61, 63, 234n1
nurses, 38, 40–43, 165, 206, 269, 278–279, 281

O

O'Connor, Bonnie, 195–198, 211
Ó Giolláin, Diarmuid, 101, 127, 132n5. *See also* Irish folklore
O'Neill, Sean Patrick, 67–69
Ochoa Gautier, Ana María, 127
Old Man Hawkins, 10–13, 18, 22, 24, 47, 156
Ong, Aihwa, 67, 209
ontologies: of disease, 36, 75–76; associated with modernity, 215; mythic, 75–76, 272–273; nonhuman, 4, 6; and plants, 47, 263–265, 275, 281, 284. *See also* multispecies relations
oral histories, 27, 83, 85, 119, 121
orality. *See* literacy
Orientalism, 103, 110, 121–122
origin stories: and caste, 119; of folkloristics, 55, 105, 128; and journalism, 242, 251, 255–256; Latin American folklore and, 122; as models of circulation, 69; and traditionality, 227, 230; Warao, 272–273, 285n1
Oring, Elliott: on Dorson, 131n1; folklore and psychoanalysis, 136, 138, 141; on journalism and folklore, 259–60
Ortiz, Renato, 122–123, 127
Ortner, Sherry, 70, 125
Osborn, Henry A., 48, 190. *See also* missionaries; Warao language
outbreak narratives. *See* contagion narratives
Outbreak, 251–252. *See also* contagion narratives; film

P

palm trees, 4, 30–33, 267, 269–272, 278
pandemics: COVID-19, 38, 47, 202, 205, 236–237, 245, 248, 250, 255, 287–288; H1N1, 47, 236–263; as X-raying society, 38, 202
Pandolfo, Stefania, 187
Paredes, Américo: challenge to folkloristics, 45, 59–60, 78–99, 115, 117, 124–127, 131, 149, 158, 194, 221–223; and communicable models, 79–81, 83–94; critiques of, 81–82; 94; on ethnographic authority and whiteness, 81–84; on racialized state violence, 80–83, 94, 98, 288. *See also* "Ballad of Gregorio Cortez"
patriarchy, and folklore, 82, 88–89, 93, 122–123, 230–231. *See also* Herder, Johann Gottfried
Peirce, Charles S., 141, 151, 173, 185. *See also* iconicity; indexicality
performance: -centered approach, 12, 27, 28, 36, 46, 54, 58, 61, 66, 116, 135, 137, 144–145, 149, 247, 252; and audience, 12, 87, 139–140, 144, 145, 148, 149, 158; poetics of, 135–160, 208, 236–238, 241, 260–262, 288; and preparedness, 236–237, 241, 254–255, 257–258, 260; and scale, 152–153, 155; and science, 238–239, 251–252, 261; and social media, 260, 288–290. *See also* Bauman, Richard; Hymes, Dell
performativity: of circulation, 71, 76; and language, 27, 36, 67. *See also* Austin, J. L.; Derrida, Jacques
Peuckert, Will-Erich, 120
pharmaceuticals, 74, 199, 201, 204–205, 207
philology, 121. *See also* vernacular philology
photography: in fieldwork, 24–25, 41, 167; and iconicity, 151, 185; and witnessing, 41, 181–186, 232, 238
phytocommunicability, 266, 271, 273, 276–285
phyto-design, 275–276
phytotherapy, 36, 47, 278–283, 285n5. *See also yarokotarotu*
Pizarro, Indalesio, 166, 180–181, 267, 270, 273–274, 276. *See also* phyto-design
Pizarro, Mamerto, 164–169, 171, 173, 175–181, 183, 186–190, 267, 268, 270–271, 273–274, 279, 281. *See also* lamentation; rabies
plant-human relations, 29, 47, 264–285. *See also* ontologies; phytotherapy
plática de los viejitos de antes (talk of the elders of bygone days), 19, 224

play: and epistemology, 64, 81, 84; jokes, 140–141; in memory, 9, 11–13, 168; and phytotherapy, 278
poetics: and acoustics, 170–172, 187, 188, 246, 258; and folkloristics, 54, 57, 70–71, 80, 82, 104; of mourning, 13–14, 37, 45–46, 164, 171–174; and performance, 135–160, 208, 236–238, 241, 260–262, 288; and psychoanalysis, 135–159, 164. *See also* ethnopoetics; lamentation
Poovey, Mary, 58
postcolonial: folkloristics, 116; studies, 70–71, 101–104, 107–108, 112–120, 224–225
Postero, Nancy, 269
practice: as framework for folkloristics of health, 205–209, 211, 212n2; analytics and mediatization, 227–228. *See also* Bourdieu, Pierre
Prague School, 234n2
Prasad, Leela, 117
preparedness, and performance, 236–237, 241, 254–255, 257–258, 260
progressive extractivism, 264–285. *See also* Gudynas, Eduardo
proverbs, 6, 19, 25, 28–29, 60, 90, 121, 142, 150, 152–153, 217, 229, 235
psychoanalysis: folkloristics and, 45–46, 57, 135–138, 141–142, 144, 151, 156, 157, 159n1; and mourning, 5, 43, 46, 161–164, 167–168, 170–174, 188; and semiosis, 37, 142–143, 148–149. *See also* Freud, Sigmund; performance; poetics
public folklore, 63, 93, 123, 211, 234
public health, 37–42, 47, 167, 196–202, 207–208, 211–212, 228, 237, 241, 247, 249–255, 258–262, 287. *See also* pandemics

Q

Quijano, Aníbal, 101–103, 108

R

rabies, 5, 41–43, 47, 49n14, 164–188, 266, 273–274, 279–285. *See also* bats; diagnosis; epidemic; Muaina
Rabinow, Paul, 200, 237
race and ethnic studies, 59, 61, 84, 156, 234
racialization, 5, 29, 38–40, 78, 80, 93, 103–104, 107, 110–111, 119–123, 131, 141, 157–158, 160n10, 179–181, 207, 230, 261, 288–290
racism: and aesthetics, 26; and indigeneity, 30, 38–40, 78, 95, 182, 267, 285, 289; and linguistic anthropology, 66, 69–73; and

Paredes' legacy in folklore, 78–79; and positionality, 27–29; psychic toll, 155, 179, 181, 186; and universality, 95, 158, 230. *See also* anti-racist approaches; Du Bois, W.E.B.; Fanon, Frantz

Raheja, Gloria, 113, 116

reality-testing, 14, 162–164, 169–170, 179–181, 188–189. *See also* Freud, Sigmund

reception: and communicability, 87, 96–97; critique of media, 215–216, 219, 226; and health, 67–68, 207–208, 252, 255–258; racialized, 95, 110, 114, 203. *See also* communicability

recontextualization, 12, 27, 84, 143, 147, 254

recording technologies: and folklore, 28, 92, 98, 126, 217, 225, 231; role in ethnography, 21–22, 24, 28, 37, 60, 70, 76, 165

reification: and folkloristics, 55–60, 68, 72, 86, 90–92, 97–98, 119, 123, 124–131, 157–158, 200, 206–207, 210–211, 223; and "media," 213–219, 227, 236–239, 257

relationality, perspective, 195–198, 203–208, 211, 279. *See also* Menéndez, Eduardo

remediation, 129–130, 228

reported speech, 86–87, 148. *See also* entextualization; Vološinov, V.N.

repression, psychic, 138–140. *See also* jokes; Oring, Elliott; sexuality

resistance, 68, 265; and ethnographic writing, 4–5, 43–44, 46; and folkloristics debates, 46, 120, 126; Gramscian, 9; political, 29, 83, 94, 104, 112, 224

response cries, 147–148, 172–175. *See also* Goffman, Erving

revolution. *See* Bolivarian socialist revolution

Risling Baldy, Cutcha, 75, 116, 153

ritual: and Catholicism, 14–15, 37; and coloniality, 101–103; Venezuelan context, 31–37, 176, 275–276, 283. *See also* healing; lamentation

Rival, Laura, 277–278

Rivas, Anita, 43, 183–184

Rivera, María, 36, 40, 60. *See also* phytotherapy

Rivera, Santiago, 33–36, 60, 153, 157, 271

Robb, John Donald, 14–17

Roberts, John W., 59–60, 116, 124, 130

Róheim, Géza, 151

Romantic Nationalism: and folklore, 80, 89, 100, 120

Rosaldo, Renato, 81, 172

Royal Society, 108, 131n4, 193. *See also* Aubrey, John; Locke, John

Rubel, Arthur J., 84, 94

Russian Formalism, 142, 234n2

S

Said, Edward, 116

saints, 18–23, 25–26. *See also* Catholicism; woodcarving

Salas, Yolanda, 123, 220

Saldívar, Ramón, 82, 94, 99n3

salud colectiva. *See* public health

Samuels, David W., 68, 70–71, 73

Santner, Eric, 174

Santuario de Chimayó, 14, 16, 23

Sapir, Edward, 69, 229

SARS (Severe Acute Respiratory Syndrome): 2003 epidemic, 238, 247, 253, 259. *See also* COVID-19

Sassen, Saskia, 67, 209

Saussure, Ferdinand de, 140, 151

Sawin, Patricia, 135, 149

scale: and circulation, 72, 84, 86, 93, 209; clinical space, 201, 206, 209; folkloristics and, 103–104, 127; mourning practices, 181–182; and performance, 152–153, 155; and theory, 59

Schechner, Richard, 252

Scheper-Hughes, Nancy, 199

Scher, Philip, 209, 227, 233

Scherzinger, Martin, 209

Schmiesing, Ann, 230–231

science: and boundary-work, 45, 54–57, 60–64, 64–65n2, 90, 92, 95, 104, 110, 125, 210, 238–239, 247, 255, 260–261; and erasure, 28; health hierarchies and, 195–196, 199, 202, 206–209, 211, 288; and hegemony, 27, 73, 84, 100–101, 107–108, 124–125, 130–131, 211, 238; modeling and mobility, 55, 91, 182–183, 199–201, 203, 209, 238, 261; as performance, 238–239, 251–252, 261; reification and, 91, 257

science and technology studies (STS), 23–24, 45, 47, 54, 68, 194, 200, 236–237

Scott, James, 116

Sekaquaptewa, Emory, 76

Sekaquaptewa, Helen, 75–76, 153–155. *See also* I'isaw

semiotic process, 148–149, 173–174. *See* Kristeva, Julia

Señor Olguín, 7–10, 13, 18, 22, 42, 48

sensorium, 5–14, 175, 226, 232, 269–270, 276–285

Serematakis, Nadia, 175

sexuality: in myth, 153, 270–273; patriarchal, 82, 88–89, 230–231; positionality and, 81, 124, 149, 155–156, 206, 209, 221, 224, 289; in psychoanalysis, 136, 138–143; racialized, 155
shadchen (marriage broker), 136, 144
shamanism, 35, 207, 231
Shaul, David, 75
Sherzer, Joel, 28
Shuman, Amy, 53, 87, 204
Silverstein, Michael, 72, 86
Simmel, Georg, 221
slow scholarship, 24, 48n3. *See also* Stengers, Isabelle
Smith, Kalim, 73
Smith, Linda Tuhiwai, 70
Snow, Robert, 219, 221
slavery, 112, 289
social death, 38–40, 186–188
social media: and circulation, 129, 205, 216; folk medicine and, 196, 205; and performance, 260, 288–290; and research, 205, 237, 241, 255–256, 258
socialism. *See* Bolivarian socialist revolution; indigenous socialism
Soja, Edward, 124
space: and epistemology, 59, 107, 215, 269–270, 275–276, 283; and indexicality, 76n1; and mediatization, 215, 230, 238–239; and power, 40, 103, 106–107, 112, 205–206, 273–276, 283, 290
Spanish language: and indigenous languages, 34, 39, 180–181; media, 26, 83; New Mexican, 6–7, 10, 16, 18, 20, 60, 224; and power, 152
Spivak, Gayatri, 116
Star, Susan Leigh, 69–70, 76–77n2, 182–183, 203, 209–210. *See also* boundary objects
statistics: mobility of, 67, 182–183, 209; role in narrativizing epidemics, 259, 288. *See also* Bowker, Geoffrey; Star, Susan Leigh
state, constructions of, 199–200, 218, 247
Stengers, Isabelle, 48
Stewart, Jon, 256–257, 260
Stewart, Kathleen, 188
Stewart, Susan, 217
stigma: and disability, 145, 209; and health, 55, 137–138, 255, 259; racialized, 38–40, 157–158, 179–181
Stoeltje, Beverly, 28
structural violence. *See* violence
Stories in the Time of Cholera, 38–40, 42, 165

storytelling, 5–14, 20, 24, 39–40, 69, 72–73, 88, 109, 121, 156, 159n4, 173, 194, 202–203, 215, 257. *See also* circulation
Strömbäck, Jesper, 219
"swine flu" pandemic. *See* H1N1

T

Tangherlini, Timothy, 212n3
taro (*Colocasio esculenta*), 30
Tatar, Maria, 151, 229–230
Taylor, Anne-Christine, 276
Taylor, Breonna, 288
Taylor, Diana, 238, 261
technology: bio-, 199, 201; and folklore, 57–58, 80, 92, 100–101, 106–107, 126, 129–130, 217; as form of determinism, 215–216, 219. *See also* Bausinger, Hermann; Benjamin, Walter; science and technology studies
Tedlock, Dennis, 159n4
Temple, Richard Carnac, 111–112, 132n6–7
temporality: and indexicality, 76n1, 152; of mourning, 162–163, 168–169, 171–172; and narrative, 40, 69, 72, 75; and pandemic, 235–236, 238, 248, 252; as relates to plants, 277; and traditionalization, 223–226, 230–231
Teuton, Christopher, 116
Texas Rangers, 80, 87, 94, 98. *See also* Paredes, Américo; violence, colonial and racialized
text. *See* intertextual transparency, ideology of
theory, 1, 17–18, 45, 116, 121; in folkloristics, 53–64; postcolonial, 115, 117; psychoanalytic, 45–46, 135–159, 161–164, 170–172, 173–174, 178–179, 185–186, 188–189, 289–290; vernacular, 11, 22–24, 43, 61, 62–63, 84–85
Tolbert, Jeffrey. *See* "folkloresque"
Torres, Manuel, 35–36, 40, 153. *See also* dreams; healing; *hoarotu*
Torres, Odilia, 279–281, 286n6
Torres Rivas, Elbia, 41–42, 168, 179–180, 183–186, 280
tourism, 14, 19–20, 26, 96, 127–128, 194, 222, 225, 231. *See also* Bendix, Regina; Kirshenblatt-Gimblett, Barbara; traditionalization; UNESCO
traditionality/coloniality, 101, 115–123
traditionalization: and critique of "media," 213–234; and news production, 235–262; temporality of, 194
translation, 68–69, 71, 73, 77n2, 117, 118, 230, 285n2; as journalistic practice, 249, 262n3; of "Mourning and Melancholia," 161–163,

189n1; and racism, 38–40. *See also* de la Cadena, Marisol; Risling Baldy, Cutcha

transmission: in medical context, 42, 178, 196–197, 203, 239, 250, 281; of stories, 41, 58, 72, 85–93, 126, 141, 180, 215–216, 224, 226, 229. *See also* circulation; temporality

Treichler, Paula, 259

Trinidad, 34, 233

Trouillot, Michel-Rolph, 95

Trump, Donald (American President), 250, 262, 288, 290

Tsing, Anna, 59, 67, 68, 74, 96, 281–282, 298

tuberculosis, 31, 37, 48–49n13, 202

Tylor, Edward B., 113

U

unconscious: ivy analogy, 171; as problematic binary, 137–143; Paredes' critique, 83, 88. *See also* communicability; Freud, Sigmund; jokes; Nasio, Juan-David

UNESCO (United Nations Educational, Scientific and Cultural Organization): ethnography of, 233; and traditionalization, 225; and intangible heritage regulation, 98, 209, 232

universality: and psychoanalysis, 136, 140, 157–158, 163, 187; intervention in folklore and health, 201; and mediatization, 219; and racialization, 95, 230; religious traditions in India, 119; subaltern critiques of, 102, 116; theory and, 58–59

unlearning: as project, 4–5, 22–23, 27, 44–48, 290–291; and Paredes' legacy, 79, 96. *See also* Briggs's Principles for Unlearning

Unwerth, Matthew von, 178–179. *See also* Freud, Sigmund

Urban, Greg, 68, 70

Urry, John, 67, 73, 182

V

vaccines, 202, 207, 238–241, 247–248, 258

vampire bats. *See* bats

Vaz da Silva, Francisco, 151

Venezuela: anthropology of, 48n8, 123, 272–273, 277–279, 281, 285n5; author's work in, 3, 10, 29–43, 46, 47, 60, 74, 138, 161, 164–171, 175–188, 197, 207–208, 264–286; and British American Tobacco, 220, 226; as petro-state, 268–269. *See also* Bolivarian socialist revolution; Delta Amacuro

vernacular philology, 27, 74, 129. *See also* Bauman, Richard

vernacularity: and circulation, 96; and critical epidemiology, 287; critique of cultural forms, 101, 117, 127–128; and the internet, 126, 216; relation to theory, 54, 62–64, 208, 261; romanticization of, 204

Vibrio cholerae. *See* cholera

violence: colonial, 71, 73, 80, 103–104, 107, 110–111, 119, 123, 131, 160n10, 186–188, 224–225, 289; extractivist, 283–284; institutional, 123; racialized, 5, 78, 80, 93, 103–104, 107, 110–111, 119, 121, 123, 131, 141, 160n10, 261, 288–290; sexual, 39–40, 89, 139–140, 153, 289; structural, 40, 42, 122, 127, 186–188, 261, 288–290; symbolic, 73, 141, 169, 180–183, 272–273, 276

viruses, 4, 187, 236–242, 246–262, 282, 288–290

Viveiros de Castro, Eduardo, 24, 265–266, 276, 283. *See also* ontologies

Voices of Modernity, 53, 57, 59, 63, 64n1, 80, 88, 93, 100, 107–108, 130–131, 132n8, 137, 193–194, 215, 229, 265

Volkskunde, 120–122

Vološinov, V.N., 148

W

Waitzkin, Howard, 206

Wald, Priscilla, 251, 259. *See also* contagion narratives

walking, as folklore collection technique, 106–107; and mobility, 182. *See also* Aubrey, John

Warao: collaboration with, 74, 165–168, 175–178, 181–189; as ethnic classification, 30, 182, 267; language, 30–31, 33–34, 38–39, 48n7, 60, 267, 271; and missionaries, 30–31, 48n7–8; mortality rates amongst, 31, 48n9, 48–49n13; relationship to plants and healing, 278–285; social movement, 32, 180–181, 266; textual production, 267

"Warao Radio" (word of mouth transmission in Delta Amacuro), 41, 180

Weidman, Amanda, 92

Weigle, Marta, 21, 25

White, Hayden, 105–106, 206

White, Luise, 132n9, 202

whiteness, 6–7, 18, 23, 57, 59, 78, 84, 89, 94–95, 102–103, 107, 122, 128, 130, 131n1, 155, 230. *See also* González-Martin, Rachel; politics of knowledge

Wiget, Andrew, 75, 153, 160n9

Wilbert, Johannes, 48n8–9, 273

Wilbert, Werner, 278–279, 281, 285n5. *See also* phytotherapy
Williams, Brian, 247, 251, 260
Williams, Raymond, 28, 132n5, 206–207, 219, 226–227, 230
Wilson, William, 101
WIPO (World Intellectual Property Organization), 98, 209
wisidatu (healer skilled in extracting *hebu*), 273, 276–277, 281–283
Wittgenstein, Ludwig: on boundary-work, 53, 64; and language games, 17–18, 20, 36, 43
Wojcik, Daniel, 232

Wolf, Eric, 104
Wood, Robert, 121
wood carving, 14–24. *See also*; Córdova, NM; saints

Y

yarokotarotu (phytotherapist), 278–280, 283
Yoder, Don, 196
Young, Katharine, 159, 206

Z

Zapata, Paulino, 38
Zipes, Jack, 216, 229

www.ingramcontent.com/pod-product-compliance
Lightning Source LLC
Chambersburg PA
CBHW070906030426
42336CB00014BA/2310